Human Insulin

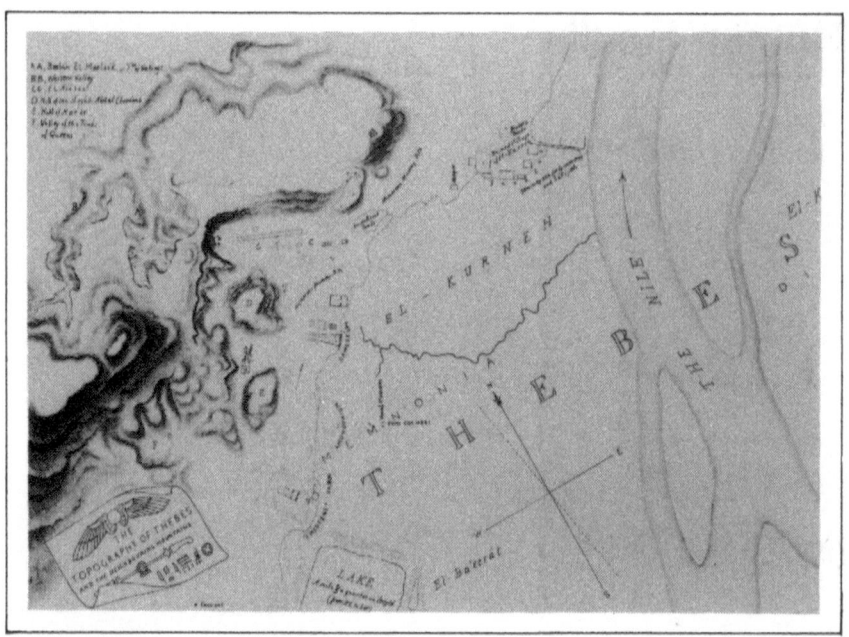

Topography of Thebes and the neighbouring mountains by Edward Lane (ca. 1826–1827)

Human Insulin
Clinical Pharmacological Studies in Normal Man

D. R. Owens, M.D.

Department of Medicine
University of Wales College of Medicine
Cardiff, Wales

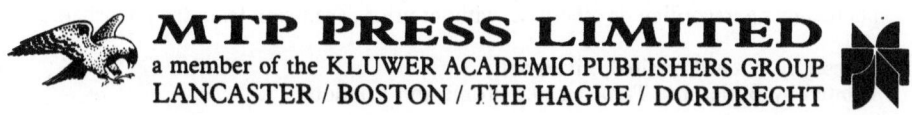

MTP PRESS LIMITED
a member of the KLUWER ACADEMIC PUBLISHERS GROUP
LANCASTER / BOSTON / THE HAGUE / DORDRECHT

To
Jennifer
Rachel and Rebecca

Published in the UK and Europe by
MTP Press Limited
Falcon House
Lancaster, England

British Library Cataloguing in Publication Data

Owens, D.R.
 Human insulin : clinical pharmacological studies
 in normal man.
 1. Diabetes—Chemotherapy 2. Insulin—
 Therapeutic use
 I. Title
 616.4′62061   RC661.I6

 ISBN-13:978-94-010-8347-8   e-ISBN-13:978-94-009-4161-8
 DOI:10.1007/978-94-009-4161-8

Published in the USA by
MTP Press
A division of Kluwer Boston Inc
190 Old Derby Street
Hingham, MA 02043, USA

Library of Congress Cataloging in Publication Data

Owens, D. R.
 Human insulin.

 Bibliography: p.
 Includes index.
 1. Insulin—Physiological effect. I. Title.
 [DNLM: 1. Insulin—administration & dosage.
 WK 820 097h]
 QP572.I5O94   1986   615′.365   86–2848
 ISBN-13:978-94-010-8347-8

Typeset by Witwell Limited, Liverpool
Printed by Butler and Tanner Ltd., Frome and London

Contents

4   Clinical–pharmacological studies

Preface

Since insulin became available for the treatment of diabetes in 1922 a number of major advances have been made, which include the modification of insulin to vary its timing of action, its purification, and latterly, the production of human insulin. Human insulin in quantities sufficiently large for therapy has been made available by two techniques developed in parallel during the late 1970s. These involve either (i) formulation in *E. coli* bacteria suitably encoded by DNA recombinant methods of the A- and B-chains of human insulin followed by a chain combination reaction ('biosynthetic' human insulin) or (ii) enzymatic conversion (transpeptidation) of porcine insulin brought to react with a threonine ester by porcine trypsin in a mixture of water and organic solvents, yielding human insulin ('semi-synthetic' human insulin).

This book includes the first clinical–pharmacological studies of each of the highly purified 'semi-synthetic' human insulin preparations: Actrapid® HM; Monotard® HM; Protaphane® HM; Actraphane® HM; and Ultratard® HM (Novo Industri A/S, Copenhagen). The preliminary studies established their safety and efficacy relative to their porcine and bovine counterparts emphasising the relevance of species and formulation on the pharmacokinetics and biological responses to insulin.

Additional investigations with human insulin demonstrated the influence of insulin concentration, site of administration, the addition of aprotinin to insulin and the mixing of 'short-' and 'intermediate-acting' formulations on insulin 'bioavailability'. Examination of the 'within' and 'between' subject day-to-day variation in absorption and the effect of subcutaneous insulin also demonstrates the dominating influence of insulin responsiveness.

The 'human bio-assay' studies in normal man have provided material for Health Authorities in order to make the 'semi-synthetic' human insulins available for clinical use. The findings from the single-dose studies cannot, however, be extrapolated to diabetic patients, as attempts to characterise the timing of action of insulin preparations in normal subjects have limited clinical relevance.

In the author's opinion the studies indicate the importance of species and pharmaceutical formulation on the 'bioavailability' and hypoglycaemic 'potency' of insulin. Awareness of the considerable influence of many different factors on the absorption and response to insulin provides a basis for improving the quality of 'conventional' insulin treatment. Alterations in the formulation, purity and species of insulin, and the adoption of different regimens, have been designed to improve the quality of insulin treatment. The ultimate constraint in insulin treatment, however, lies with the patient. The contribution of human insulin in the evolution of insulin treatment remains to be established.

1
Introduction

1.1 HISTORICAL INTRODUCTION TO DIABETES AND ITS TREATMENT

1.1.1 The clinical syndrome of diabetes mellitus

A papyrus discovered in one of the tombs of the nobles (scribes, artists and artisans) at El Assassif, Thebes, Egypt in 1862 (Frontispiece), later acquired by the German Egyptologist, Georg M. Ebers (1837–1898), and therefore called the 'Ebers Papyrus' (Leake, 1952), possibly represents the first known medical text describing diabetes and its treatment (Figure 1.1). The 'Ebers Papyrus', a teaching text, was written about 1500 BC during the 18th Dynasty (the brilliant period of Egyptian culture) when ancient Thebes rose to its political and religious zenith, marking the beginning of the New Kingdom, 1567–1080 BC (18th to 20th Dynasties).

Inscribed on the document was a prescription for the treatment of 'over-abundant urine', consisting of 'bones, wheat grains, fresh grits, green lead earth and water', with the instructions to 'let stand moist, strain and take for four days'.

Sweetness in urine was first recorded in India by Susruta around 400 BC (Ayur Vedic/Sanskrit scriptures), who referred to '*madhumeha*' (honey urine) and noted that the urine in cases of '*ikshumeha*' (sugar urine) was assailed by flies (Frank, 1957). The clinical description resembles diabetes mellitus with its treatment reliant upon elaborate diets, herbal and mineral agents and exercise (Barach, 1949; Sathe, 1969).

Apollonius of Memphis and Demetrius of Apamea are reputed to be the first to use the name 'diabetes' during the 3rd century BC. Aurelius Cornelius Celsus (1st century AD) described in De Medicina (Translated by W. G. Spence, 1960), a condition characterised by polyuria requiring treatment by restricting dietary intake. The term 'diabetes' ($\delta\iota\alpha\beta\alpha\acute{\iota}\nu\omega$) was introduced into medical nomenclature by Aretaeus of Cappadocia (ca. AD 30–90). The name originates from the Greek verb 'diabaino', which means 'go through', and 'diabetes' – 'the thing the fluid runs through, i.e. a syphon' (Hirsch, 1883; Reed, 1954; Henschen, 1969). Aretaeus described diabetes in his book on the *Therapeutics of Chronic Disease* (translated by Adams, 1856; Figure 1.2).

Galen (AD 129–199), the Greek philosopher and physician, also described a

1

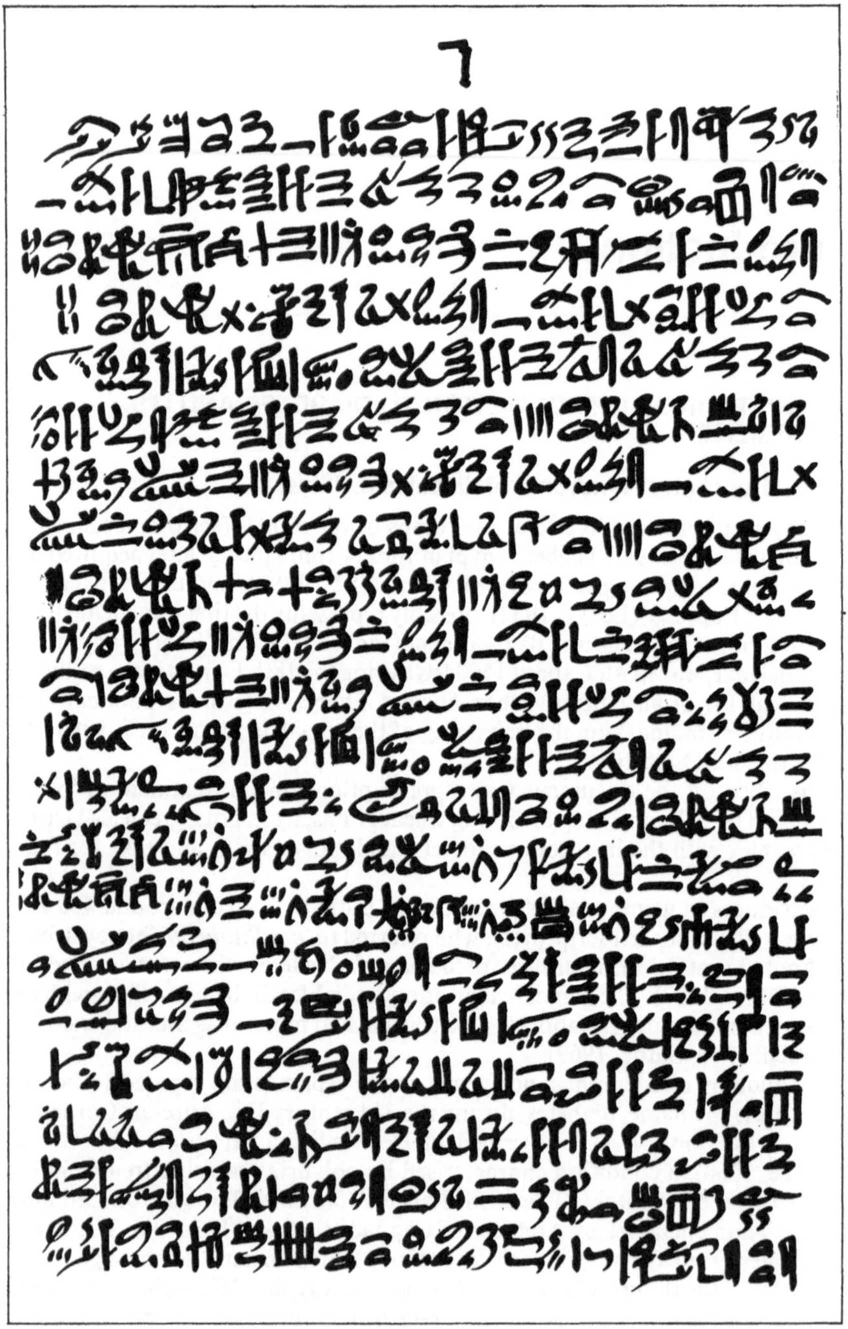

Figure 1.1 A page from Ebers Papyrus (ca. 1500 BC)

"Diabetes is a wonderful affection, not very frequent among men, being a melting down of the flesh and limbs into urine. The patients never stop making water, but the flow is incessant, as if the opening of aqueducts. Life is short, disgusting and painful; thirst unquenchable; excessive drinking, which, however, is disproportionate to the large quantity of urine for more urine is passed, and one cannot stop them either from drinking nor making water. Or if for a time they abstain from drinking, their mouth becomes parched and their body dry; the viscera seems as if scorched up; they are affected with nausea, restlessness and a burning thirst; and at no distant term they expire."

Figure 1.2 Description of diabetes: Aretaeus of Cappadocia

disease likely to be diabetes, referring to it as 'diarrhoea of the urine' – a cause of the thirst experienced with the disease due to weakness of the kidneys (King, 1964). Also, during the following centuries reference to conditions that could be diabetes was made by several authors: Tchang-Thoug-King, the Chinese Hippocrates, ca. AD 200; Aetios of Amida, ca. AD 600.

In the 7th century AD, detailed descriptions of the symptoms of diabetes mellitus and its complications appeared in the Chinese medical literature. The sweet taste of diabetic urine was documented by Zhen Quan and Zhen Liyan of Sui and T'ang Dynasties in a book called *Effective Recipes of the Past and Present 572 AD* (Jiang, 1982; Figure 1.3). Obesity was also recognised as an important aetiological factor, with diet and exercise the prime forms of treatment (Miyasita, 1980).

The next account of diabetes appeared from the Persian physicians Rhazes (AD 860–932) and Avicenna (AD 980–1037), who in his medical encyclopaedia *Canon* noted that diabetics suffered great thirst, exhaustion, loss of sexual function, furunculosis, phthisis and gangrene (Papaspyros, 1964; Medvei, 1982).

During the 16th century the Swiss physician and alchemist Philippus Aureolus Theophrastus Bombastus of Hohenheim (1493–1541), 'Paracelsus', pronounced that diabetes was a general disease caused by an alteration of the blood composition, and advised the testing of the urine, but failed to taste the evaporated urine, mistaking its appearance for saltpetre. The lipaemia of diabetes mellitus was later described by the Belgian physician, Johannes Baptista van Helmont (1577–1644) (Garrison, 1929).

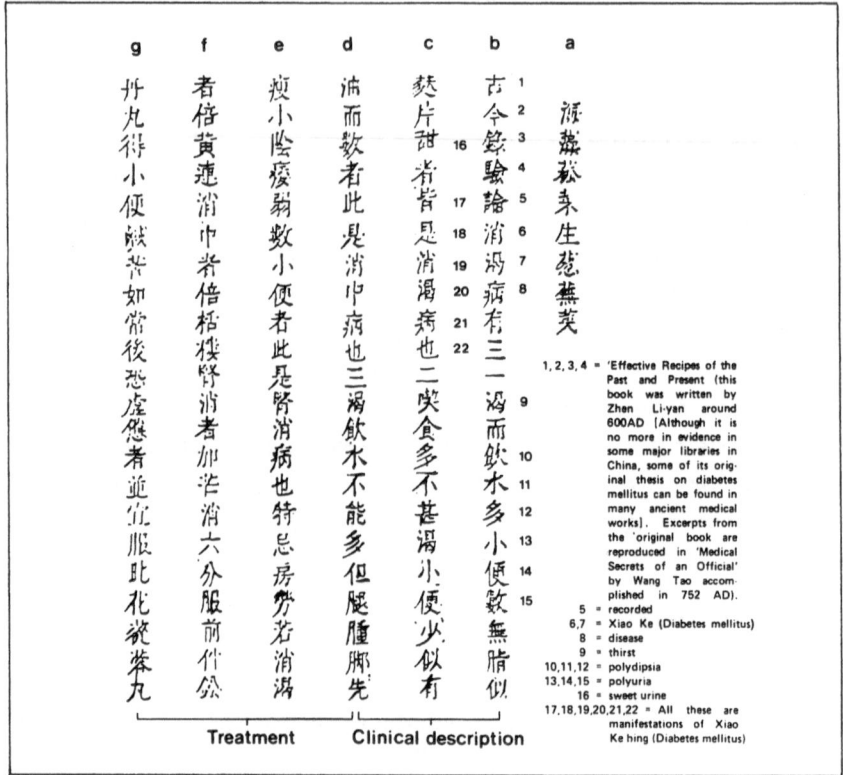

Figure 1.3 Record of the sweetness of diabetic urine: Zhen Liyan

The modern history of diabetes began when Thomas Willis (1621–1675) re-described the presence of glycosuria in certain cases of diabetes ('the pissing evil') in *Pharmaceutice Rationalis* (Willis, 1674) and concluded that this must be preceded by the appearance of sweetness in the blood. It was not until 1774 that Matthew Dobson (1745–1784) demonstrated that the sweetness of urine and serum was due to the presence of sugar (Dobson, 1776), which was later shown to be glucose (Chevreul, 1815). Interestingly, Johann Conrad à Brunner (1653–1727) observed that removing the pancreas from dogs produced the characteristic signs of diabetes (Brunner, 1682), although he failed to make the connection since his experimental animals rapidly recovered due to incomplete removal of the pancreas.

It was not until von Mering (1849–1908) and Minkowski (1858–1931) carried out a complete surgical removal of the pancreas of a dog in 1889 that the ensuing polyuria was associated with the secretion of large quantities of sugar (von Mering and Minkowski, 1890; Naunyn, 1898, 1903). However, during the preceding hundred years a number of notable observations and discoveries were made: Cawley (1788) suggested the relationship between chronic pancreatitis and diabetes; Rollo (1797) and Bouchardat (1875) re-emphasised the importance of dietary management, while Trommer (1841), von Fehling (1848) and Bouchardat (1875), contributed to the demonstration of glucose in the urine. Classical clinical descriptions included that of diabetic coma by Prout (1785–1850) and Küssmaul (1874) and xanthoma diabeticum by Addison and Gull in 1851 (Rolleston, 1936; Barach, 1949). In 1849, Claude Bernard (1813–1878), discovered the glycogenic function of the liver (Bernard, 1849, 1857, 1877), and demonstrated glycosuria following the puncturing of the floor of the fourth ventricle of the brain 'piqûre diabétique'. In 1870 he also observed that his dogs remained well despite blocking the pancreatic exocrine ducts.

Soon after the observations of von Mering and Minkowski, Laguesse (1861–1927) suggested that the absence of 'islets' of cells described earlier in 1869 by Langerhans (1849–1888) could be responsible for diabetes (Laguesse, 1893), but it was only in 1901 that Opie (1873–1971) demonstrated the association between degeneration of the 'islets of Langerhans' and diabetes (Opie, 1901). During this period, several workers confirmed the earlier observation of the preservation of the islet cells following obstruction of the pancreatic ducts and atrophy of the exocrine pancreas (Arnozan and Vaillard, 1884; Schultze, 1900; Ssobolew, 1902; MacCullum, 1909; Kirkbride, 1912; Kamimura, 1917; Barron, 1920). In 1912, Massaglia clearly demonstrated that destruction of the islets of Langerhans did result in glycosuria (IDF Special Committee, 1971). These findings naturally initiated the search for the factor capable of controlling the metabolism of carbohydrates, and the name 'insulin' was proposed for this hypothetical hormone (De Meyer, 1909; Sharpey-Schäfer, 1916).

1.1.2 The discovery of insulin

An extensive search, which was to involve many investigators, began during the last decade of the 19th century to isolate the active factor produced by the islets of Langerhans (Table 1.1).

Table 1.1 Attempts at insulin extraction

Capparelli	1892	Sjöquist	1908
Comby	1892	Lépine	1909
Battistini	1893	Pratt	1910
White	1893	Knowlton and Starling	1911
Vanni	1895	Scott	1911
Hougounena and Doyou	1897	Massaglia and Zannini	1912
Blumenthal	1898	Murlin and Kramer	1913
Hédon	1898	Clark	1916
Zuelzer	1903–1914	Kleiner and Meltzer	1919
Gley	1905	Paulesco	1916
De Witt	1906		1920–1921
Rennie and Fraser	1907	Banting and Best	1921–1922

Early unsuccessful endeavours to extract the hormone involved using water, saline, ethanol and glycerol as extractives. Attempts were made in 1912 by

Massaglia and Zannini, as well as Scott, to obtain the hypothetical hormone, using techniques involving pancreatic duct ligation, which were also unsuccessful, although De Witt's extract in 1906 undoubtedly had glycolytic properties (De Witt, 1906; Scott, 1912; IDF Special Committee, 1971).

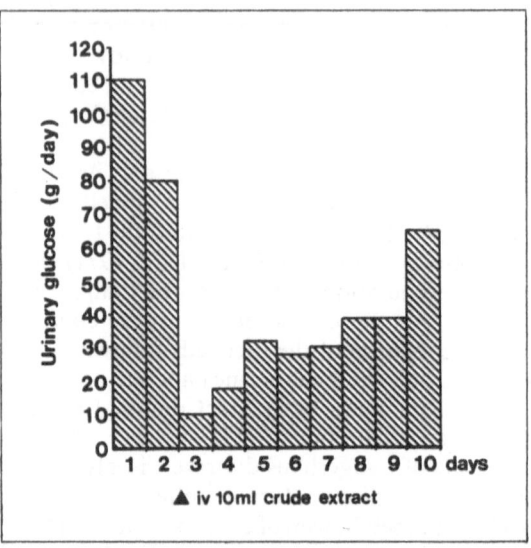

Figure 1.4 Effect of an early pancreatic extract on the glycosuria of a diabetic male patient aged 65 years (adapted from Zuelzer, 1908)

In 1908 Georg Ludwig Zuelzer (1870–1949) achieved a favourable response to his pancreatic extract on glycosuria (and ketonuria) in diabetics (Zuelzer, 1908; Figure 1.4). Severe side effects, such as convulsions, which were attributed to impurities (in the absence of blood sugar measurements) were observed following the administration of his extract. By 1914 Zuelzer's extract had been purified by Reuter, and was shown to be capable of producing marked convulsive episodes in his dogs. This was again believed to be a direct toxic effect, heralding the termination of his research which came so near to isolating insulin. Soon afterwards in 1916, Paulesco (1869–1931) observed that an intravenous injection of an aqueous solution of pancreatic extract in a diabetic dog was followed by rapid and short-lived symptomatic relief. In 1920 his studies clearly demonstrated that his pancreatic extract 'Pancreine' was capable of lowering blood sugar, ketones, urea and urine volume in both normal and depancreatised dogs (Paulesco 1921a–d; 1923a, b). Paulesco presented his extensive findings to the Roumanian Society of Biology between 21st April and 23rd June 1921. These were later published during June 1921 (Paulesco, 1921d), with the expressed intention of extending the studies to man (Paulesco, 1924).

Independently, Banting (1891–1941), an orthopaedic surgeon, and Best (1899–1978), newly graduated as a physiologist/biochemist, began working together on 16th May 1921 under Professor Macleod in the Department of Physiology at the University of Toronto. Banting was prompted into trying to isolate the internal secretion of the pancreas by the publication of Barron (1920), which stated that obstruction of the pancreatic duct leads to atrophy of the exocrine pancreas, the islets remaining intact.

Extracts of degenerated pancreas injected intravenously into a depancreatectomised dog on 30th July 1921 appeared promising by the lowering of blood sugar. Further studies followed during which Banting and Best also observed the symptoms and signs of severe hypoglycaemia in response to an overdose of the pancreatic extract, which they called 'Isletin'. In this phase of their investigations over 75 doses of extract were administered to ten different diabetic animals. Banting and Best first presented their results to the Physiology Journal Club of the University of Toronto on 14th November 1921, being a prelude to their first publication in February of the following year (Banting and Best, 1922a).

With the exhaustion of pancreatic tissue from dogs in which the pancreatic ducts had been ligated 7–10 weeks previously, active extracts were then obtained from intact glands. In order to be sure that trypsin activity was avoided, Banting and Best used foetal calf pancreas (Banting and Best 1922b; Banting, 1929; Best, 1956, 1962). Further developments included the extraction of ox pancreas which yielded adequate amounts of insulin provided that the whole gland was placed in acid aqueous alcohol without delay (Banting et al., 1922a). In the light of these results Macleod (1922) expressed the possibility of administering the pancreatic extract to treat diabetic patients. On the afternoon of 11th January 1922, Banting and Best's extract – prepared from whole beef pancreas by acid ethanol extraction, vacuum evaporated, washed with toluene and appearing thick and brown – was administered by Dr. Ed Jeffrey to a young patient, Leonard Thompson, under the care of Dr. Walter Campbell at the Toronto Hospital (Banting et al, 1922b; Best, 1956). A moderate fall in blood sugar was observed following subcutaneous administration of 7.5 ml of Banting and Best's serum into each buttock, followed days later by severe local reactions (Burrow et al, 1982; Figure 1.5).

Treatment was resumed on 23rd January with a more purified extract prepared by Collip who had joined the team in December 1921. 'Collip's serum' was given frequently over the first 24 hours, producing a marked fall in blood sugar and glycosuria with the disappearance of ketonuria with clear symptomatic improvement (Collip, 1922, 1923; Figure 1.5).

During February 1922 six other diabetic patients in Dr. Campbell's clinic at Toronto General Hospital were also treated with insulin with marked clinical improvement (Banting et al, 1923). In April 1922 the extract name was accepted as insulin and, after a brief setback, the supply of insulin from Eli Lilly in Indianapolis, USA, was well and truly on its way by May 1922. The story of this epoch-making discovery has been retold a number of times in the literature (Banting, 1926, 1929; Best, 1962, 1972; Wrenshall et al, 1962; Papaspyros, 1964; Colwell, 1968; Macleod, 1978; Poulsen, 1982; Bliss, 1982a,b; Jackson, 1982; Mayer, 1982).

During the summer of 1922 insulin was being produced commercially by the Connaught Laboratories of the University of Toronto and Eli Lilly in Indianapolis, USA. Over the ensuing years many other insulin manufacturers started to produce insulin (Table 1.2), emphasising the overwhelming need for

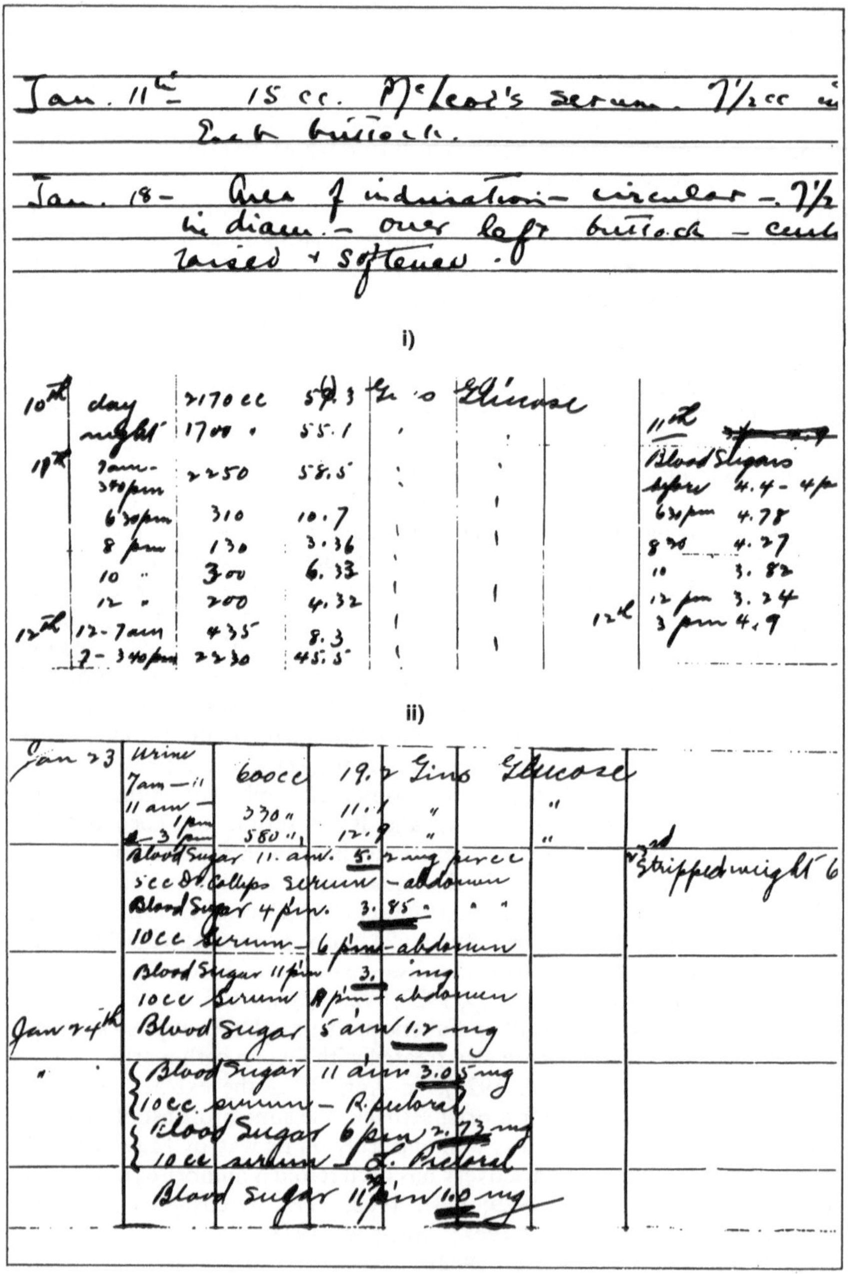

Jan. 11th — 15 cc. McLeod's serum. 7½ cc in each buttock.

Jan. 18 — Area of induration — circular — 7½ in diam. — over left buttock — central raised + softened.

i)

10th day 2170 cc 59.3 Gm's Glucose
night 1700 " 55.1
11th 7am–3.40pm 2250 58.5
6.30pm 310 10.7
8 pm 130 3.36
10 " 300 6.33
12 " 200 4.32
12th 12–7am 435 8.3
7–3.40pm 2230 45.5

11th Blood Sugars
before 4.4 – 4pm
6.30pm 4.78
8.30 4.27
10 3.82
12 pm 3.24
12th 3 pm 4.9

ii)

Jan 23 Urine
7am — 11 600cc 19.2 Gms Glucose
11 am — 1pm 330 " 11.1 " "
— 3 pm 580 " 12.9 " "
Blood Sugar 11. am. 5.2 mg per cc
5cc Dr. Collip's serum — abdomen
Blood Sugar 4 pm. 3.85 " "
10cc serum — 6 pm — abdomen
Blood Sugar 11 pm 3. mg
10cc serum 8 pm — abdomen
Jan 24th Blood sugar 5 am 1.2 mg
" " Blood Sugar 11 am 3.05 mg
10cc. serum — R. pectoral
Blood Sugar 6 pm 2.73 mg
10 cc serum L. Pectoral
Blood sugar 11.30 pm 1.0 mg
2nd Stripped weight 6

Figure 1.5 Hospital record of first patient (Leonard Thompson, aged 14 years) to receive insulin: (i) Macleod's serum, (ii) Dr. Collip's serum, during January 1922 at the Toronto General Hospital, Canada

Table 1.2 Insulin manufacturers

Name	Started production
Connaught Laboratories, Canada	1922
Eli Lilly, USA	1922
Allen and Hanbury	1923
Boots Pure Drug Company, UK	1923
British Drug Houses, UK	1923
Burroughs Wellcome, UK	1923
Commonwealth Serum Laboratories, Australia	1923
Farbwerke Hoechst, FRG	1923
Nordisk Insulinlaboratorium, Denmark	1923
NV Organon, The Netherlands	1923
E.R. Squibb & Sons, USA	1924
Novo Industri A/S, Denmark	1925
Swiss Serum and Vaccine Inst., Switzerland	1938
Hormon-Chemie, Munich, FRG	1945
Weddel Pharmaceuticals, UK	1950s

this life-giving treatment which has since benefited untold millions of diabetics.

1.1.3 Summary

Notable milestones in the history of diabetes mellitus and insulin treatment are listed in Table 1.3. Insulin heralded the end of an era in which the insulin-requiring diabetic was sentenced to a shortened life of suffering, enduring severe starvation, (Naunyn, 1903; Allen, 1913; Joslin, 1916; Allen et al, 1919), intermittent and terminal infections. To all such otherwise doomed patients insulin was a true miracle, and its discovery set in motion developments in treatment for the good of the insulin-requiring diabetic patient.

Table 1.3 Notable milestones in the history of diabetes[1], mellitus[2] and insulin treatment[3]

Ebers Papyrus	1500 BC	H.C. von Fehling	1848
The Ayur Veda of Charak		Claude Bernard	1849
and Susruta	600–400 BC	Paul Langerhans	1869
Demetrius of Apamea	30 BC	A. Kussmaul	1874
Celsus and Aretaeus[1]	30 BC–AD 90	A. Bouchardat	1875
Galen	AD 129–199	J. von Mering and	
Zhen Liyan	AD 572	O. Minkowski	1889
Rhazes	AD 860–932	E. Laguesse	1893
Avicenna	980–1037	C. H. von Noorden	1895
'Paracelsus'–Theophrastus	1493–1541	E. L. Opie	1901
Bombastus von Hohenheim		L. W. Ssobolew	1902
Thomas Willis[2]	1674	J. de Meyer	1909
J. Conrad Brunner	1682	F. M. Allen	1913
Matthew Dobson	1774	E. P. Joslin	1916
John Rollo	1797	N. C. Paulesco[3]	1921
Michel Eugene Chevreul	1815	F. G. Banting and	
		C. H. Best[3]	1921

1.2 THE EVOLUTION OF INSULIN

Introduction

The introduction of insulin heralded the end of the 'Pre-insulin Era', otherwise known as the 'Frustration Era' (Colwell, 1968). The ability of insulin to restore an otherwise doomed patient to life set the scene just over 60 years ago for a non-stop revolution in insulin treatment (Mirouze, 1983). The acceptance of this new therapy posed a series of new questions requiring urgent attention, including the manufacture of insulin to meet clinical demands, the need for several injections each day, and the observation that local reactions such as irritation, swelling and even abscesses occurred at the injection sites.

Banting, Best and Collip's demonstration that the extraction of normal adult ox pancreas with acidified aqueous alcohol could yield insulin in appreciable amounts, provided the whole gland was placed in aqueous ethanol without delay, served as a basis for future developments in the manufacture of insulin (Banting and Best, 1922b; Collip, 1922). Their further success owed much to J. B. Collip (1923) who, by manipulating the technique of fractional precipitation, achieved and demonstrated the isolation of the active principle.

Since insulin became available in its crudest form, parallel advances have occurred in production, purification and the modification of insulin into different pharmaceutical formulations.

1.2.1 Production of insulin

The production of crude insulin is illustrated in Figure 1.6. In summary, the pancreas glands are deep-frozen as soon as possible after extirpation to inhibit bacterial and enzymatic decomposition prior to extraction. Aqueous acid/ethanol is then used for extraction, followed by neutralisation of the extract and evaporation of ethanol, thereby ensuring protection of the insulin against enzymatic breakdown, removal of fatty acid material and concentration of the extract. Insulin and other peptides are next salted out from the non-proteinaceous material. The salt-cake is then dissolved in water and the pH adjusted to 5.0–5.5 (close to the iso-electric point for insulin), resulting in an amorphous precipitate containing 50–60% insulin.

Shortly after the introduction of extracts of animal pancreas glands as unmodified 'short-acting' insulin for the treatment of diabetes mellitus, immunological side effects attracted considerable attention (Williams, 1922; Tuft, 1928), emphasising the need for purification of the insulin. The first step in its purification was based on studies by Abel (1926, 1927 et al), where he described its crystallisation. Subsequently it was demonstrated that zinc ions (Scott, 1934) or certain other metal ions (Schlichtkrull, 1956) had to be added to secure crystallisation. Normally, the amorphous insulin is crystallised at least twice (Figure 1.6), i.e. the first crystallisation step is carried out in an acetone–zinc-containing citrate buffer, followed by a second crystallisation process usually involving the acetate–salt method (Schlichtkrull, 1958).

The general principles for the production of crystalline insulin have

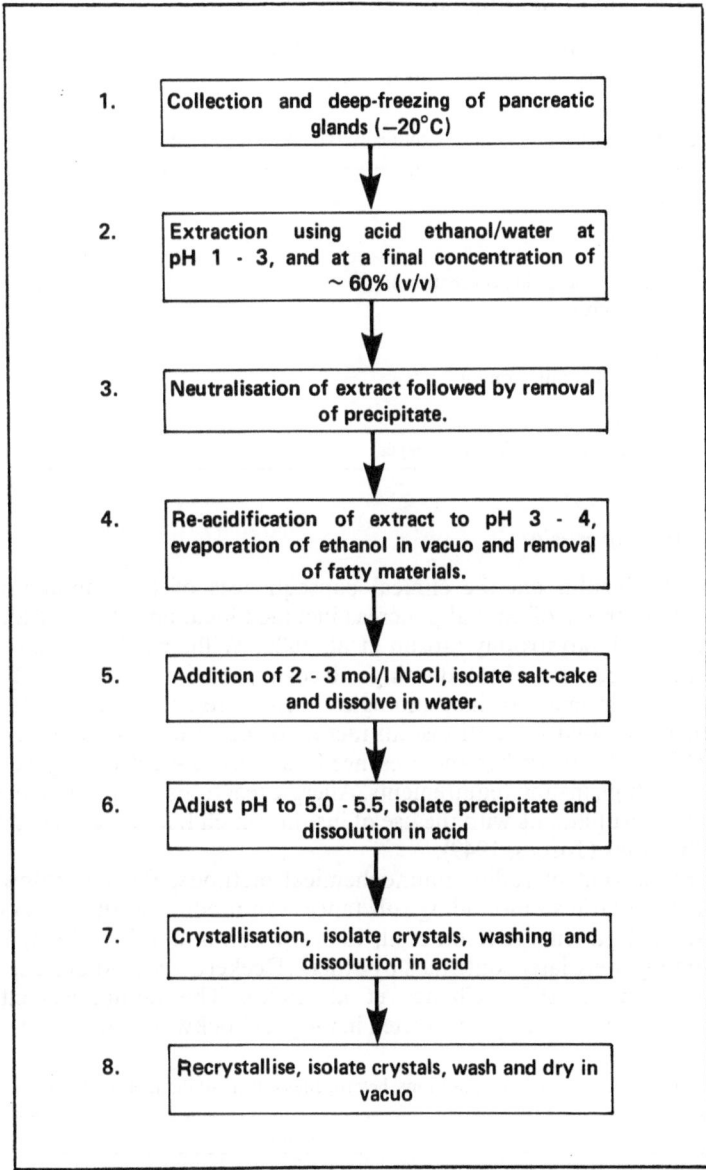

Figure 1.6 Insulin production from pancreatic glands (after Brange et al, 1985)

remained essentially unchanged over the past 40–50 years (Romans et al, 1940; Schlichtkrull et al, 1975).

Insulins purified by recrystallisation were first introduced into clinical practice in the late 1940s.

1.2.2 Purity and immunogenicity of insulin

Various factors may play a part in determining the immunogenicity of individual insulin preparations (Table 1.4).

Table 1.4 Factors known to influence the immunogenicity of insulin

Insulin
  Purity
  Species
  pH
  Solubility and zinc concentration
  Retarding agents

Others
  Mode of administration
  Age
  Infection
  Constitutional variation (Ir genes)

1.2.2.1 Insulin purity

Early in the insulin era the clinical consequences of the immunological reactions to extracts of animal pancreas included local and systemic allergic reactions and lipodystrophy (Joslin et al, 1922; Williams, 1922; Lawrence, 1925; Tuft, 1928; Joslin, 1946). Banting and co-workers in 1938 were the first to report the development of immunological 'insulin resistance' in a patient in whom they localised the anti-insulin factor to the serum globulin fraction. Lowell (1944) also described the presence of an insulin-neutralising factor in patients with high insulin requirements. Allergic reactions disappeared or were reduced in most patients with the use of insulin which had undergone several recrystallisations (Jorpes, 1949).

With the advent of radioimmunochemical methods, Berson, Yalow and co-workers found insulin-binding substances (antibodies) in the serum of all insulin-treated patients (Berson et al, 1956; Berson and Yalow, 1964, 1966). These findings were later confirmed by others (Deckert, 1964; Andersen, 1972, 1973; Root et al, 1972; Chance et al, 1976). The immunogenicity of homologous insulin was demonstrated in the pig (Lockwood and Prout, 1965;

Table 1.5 Impurities in insulin preparations: heterogeneity of crystallised or recrystallised insulin

Authors	Methods
Hafenist and Craig, 1952	Countercurrent distribution
Carpenter, 1958	Partition chromatography
Thomson and O'Donnell, 1960; Cole, 1960	Anion- or cation-exchange chromatography
Mirsky and Kawamura, 1966	Disc electrophoresis
Steiner, 1967; Steiner et al, 1968	Gel filtration

Brunfeldt and Deckert, 1966), cow (Renold et al, 1966) and humans (Deckert et al, 1972) and amorphous insulin was shown to be more immunogenic than recrystalised insulin in rabbits (Brunfeldt and Deckert, 1964), all suggesting that impurities function as adjuvants with regard to insulin antibody formation (Schlichtkrull et al, 1974).

Several authors have described impurities in commercially available insulins (Harfenist and Craig, 1952; Carpenter, 1958; Thompson and O'Donnell, 1960, Cole, 1960; Mirsky and Kawamura, 1966; Steiner, 1967; Steiner et al, 1968; Table 1.5).

Steiner and co-workers (1968) fractionated crystalline insulin into components according to molecular size by gel filtration, i.e. a high molecular weight a-component (mol. wt. $\geqslant$15,000), a b-component (mol. wt. ~ 9,000) and a c-component (mol. wt. <6,000) (Figure 1.7). Using ion-exchange chromatographic techniques, Steiner and co-workers were able to identify the constituents of the b-component as proinsulin, intermediates and a dimer of insulin (Steiner, 1967; Steiner and Oyer, 1967; Steiner et al, 1968). Others have confirmed these findings (Chance et al, 1968; Schmidt and Arens, 1968). The

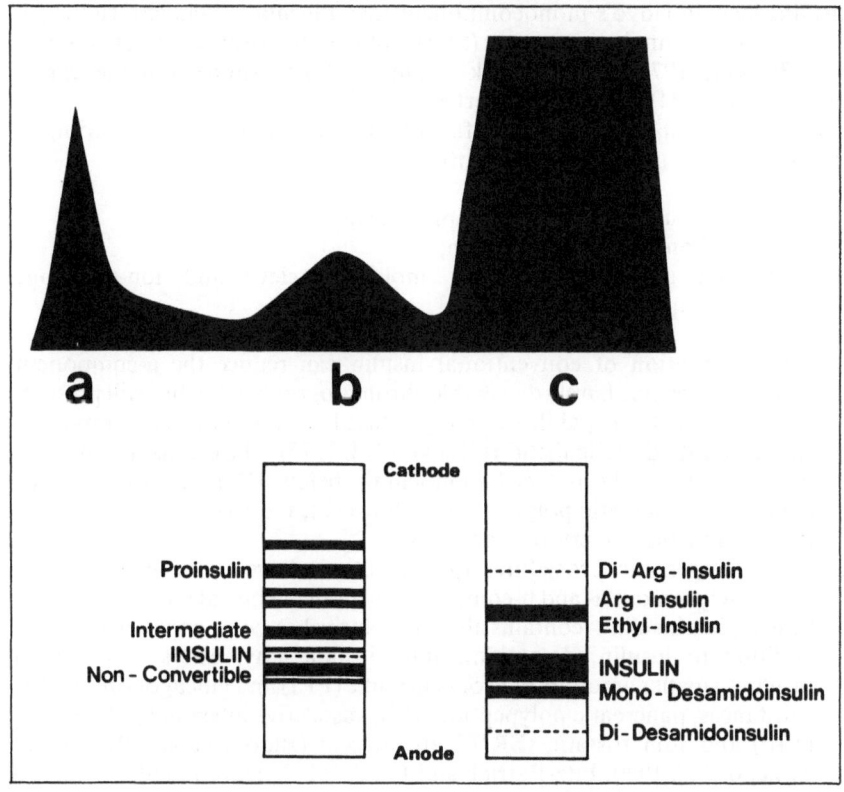

Figure 1.7 Gel filtration of once-crystallised porcine insulin on Bio-gel P-30 and disc electrophoresis of b- and c-component with approximate positions of protein contents

c-component comprised the true Sanger insulin, monodesamidoinsulins, monoarginine and monoethyl insulins (Schlichtkrull et al, 1972, 1974). In the a-component there are a large number of undefined proteins with high molecular weights (Steiner et al, 1968).

It has been demonstrated that impurities in recrystallised insulin preparations were primarily responsible for the formation of circulating insulin antibodies (Schlichtkrull et al, 1970, 1972, 1974; Root et al, 1972). Therefore, based on these findings, it was considered necessary to produce insulins devoid of peptides capable of inducing antibody formation (Schlichtkrull et al, 1974, 1975). A method based on anion-exchange chromatography, developed for the removal of impurities detected by disc electrophoresis and gel filtration, was introduced in 1970 (Jørgensen et al, 1970). With the advent of a proinsulin radioimmunoassay (Yip and Logothetopoulus, 1969; Heding et al, 1974), the once chromatographed insulin was shown to contain up to 500 ppm (ppm = parts per million by weight of dry insulin) proinsulin-like immunoreactivity (PLI). An additional chromatographic step was then introduced to reduce PLI to less than 1 ppm (Schlichtkrull et al, 1974; Jørgensen et al, 1982). Twice-chromatographed insulins include Novo's monocomponent (MC) insulins (Schlichtkrull et al, 1974), Eli Lilly's single component (SC) insulins (Chance et al, 1976; Galloway and Bressler, 1978) and Nordisk Insulin Laboratorium's porcine rarely immunogenic (RI) insulins (Deckert et al, 1974).

Insulins available for clinical use fall into three main categories according to the methods of purification (Schlichtkrull, 1979):

1. crystallised but non-chromatographed insulin;
2. crystallised and gel-filtered insulin;
3. crystallised insulin purified by molecular sieve and ion-exchange chromatography.

1. Recrystallisation of conventional insulin can reduce the a-component content to become barely detectable chromatographically, but still present, as revealed by the capability of recrystallised insulin to form a-component specific antibodies (Schlichtkrull et al, 1974, 1975). The proinsulin content, however, cannot be reduced significantly below 1% (10,000 ppm). The content of pancreatic polypeptide is, however, reduced below 25 ppm in three to five times recrystallised insulins.
2. Chromatographic procedures (gel filtration) have to be employed to completely remove a- and b-component peptides. This category of insulin – 'single-peak insulin' – contains almost exclusively c-component proteins. In addition to insulin, desamidoinsulin, insulin ethyl esters and arginyl insulins, smaller amounts of proinsulin-like (PLI) and glucagon-like (GLI) substances, pancreatic polypeptide (PP), vasoactive intestinal polypeptide (VIP) and somatostatin (SRIF) are present (Bloom et al, 1976, 1978; Mizuno et al, 1980; Fitz-Patrick and Patel, 1981). The content of PLI can vary from 10 to 2000 ppm in this category of insulin preparations.
3. The third category of insulin having undergone an additional step of chromatographic purification, shows essentially one band only when

analysed by disc gel electrophoresis. However, this group of insulins can be further subdivided according to the content of proinsulin-like immunoreactive (PLI) material. Generally, insulins with detectable amounts of proinsulin (PLI $\geqslant$ 1 ppm) also contain detectable amounts of PP and GLI when subjected to sensitive radioimmunoassay (RIA) techniques.

Table 1.6 Purity of monocomponent (MC) insulins characterised by radioimmunological analyses: Bovine and Porcine MC-Insulin (after Bloom et al, 1976)

Proinsulin (PLI)	<1ppm
Glucagon (GLI)	<0.01ppm
Pancreatic polypeptide (PP)	<0.01ppm
Vasoactive intestinal polypeptide (VIP)	<0.01ppm
Somatostatin (SRIF)	<0.01ppm

Some analytical data of pharmaceutical preparations of Monocomponent (MC) insulin are presented in Table 1.6. Therefore, insulin purity should be estimated by a combination of analytical procedures, as different methods yield different compositions of hormonal contaminants (Jørgensen et al, 1982). More recently, high-performance liquid chromatography has been introduced to determine insulin purity and potency (Jørgensen et al, 1982; Kroeff and Chance, 1982; Pingel et al, 1982; Welinder and Andresen, 1982).

1.2.2.2 Clinical implications of the quest for insulin purity

Unwanted immunological side effects of insulin treatment are summarised in Table 1.7. The purification of insulin has progressed since the first step, that of crystallisation (Abel, 1926; Scott, 1934; Scott and Fisher, 1935), to the presently available 'highly purified' insulins (Schlichtkrull, 1974; Chance et al, 1976; Deckert et al, 1974). The effect of purity on the complications of insulin therapy, including insulin allergy, lipodystrophy and insulin antibody formation has been well established, although the clinical relevance of these antibodies is still being debated (Andersen and Egeberg, 1977; Andersen, 1980; Kurtz and Nabarro, 1980; Alberti and Nattrass, 1978; Heding et al, 1980a; Home and Alberti, 1982).

Table 1.7 Side effects (immunological) of insulin treatment

  (i) Allergy
 (ii) Lipoatrophy
(iii) Insulin antibodies
 (iv) Insulin requirements, resistance
  (v) Altered metabolic control
 (vi) Placental transfer of insulin antibodies
(vii) Induced autoimmunity
(viii) Late diabetic complications

(i) Insulin allergy

Allergic reactions either disappeared or were reduced in most patients following the introduction in the late 1940s of recrystallised insulin (Jorpes,

1949; Heiskell et al, 1959). Allergic reactions to the recrystallised insulins also improved with the introduction of highly purified insulins (Andreani et al, 1972; Korp and Levett, 1973; Teuscher, 1975; Bruni et al, 1977). Changeover to highly purified insulins is not, however, always accompanied by improvement (Christy et al, 1977; Leslie, 1977; Reisner et al, 1978). Some authors have noted a higher incidence of local allergic reactions with the modified insulins compared to regular insulin (Paley, 1950). The true incidence of insulin allergy is not known, with local allergic reaction still occurring in approximately 10% of patients, even when treated with some highly purified insulins (Galloway et al, 1982d). Insulin purified to monocomponent specifications does not appear to induce antibodies of the IgE class, irrespective of the insulin species (Falholt, 1982). It is important, however, to establish, in patients with insulin allergy, whether there was previous intermittent insulin treatment, other allergies, the presence of atopy or a family history of atopy, insulin resistance and/or lipoatrophy.

(ii)   Lipodystrophy: lipoatrophy

About one-third of all patients treated with conventional insulins develop lipoatrophy to a greater or lesser degree (Renold et al, 1957; Wright et al, 1979). The prevalence is highest in young female patients (Renold et al, 1957). Transfer of affected patients to highly purified insulins has resulted in the total or partial disappearance of the atrophic areas (Bruni et al, 1977; Teuscher, 1975; Galloway and Bressler, 1978; Wright et al, 1979; Teuscher, 1974; Hulst, 1976; Devlin and Parameswaran, 1975).

Patients with lipoatrophy generally have higher levels of circulating insulin antibodies (Reeves et al, 1980; Witters et al, 1977). Immunofluorescent examination of tissue from the edge of lipoatrophic areas indicates the presence of immunological components such as IgM, C3 and fibrin in the walls of dermal vessels. Such findings are suggestive of local immune complex formation and complement fixation (Reeves, 1980; Reeves et al, 1980), resulting in inflammatory destruction of subcutaneous tissue. The prevalence of lipoatrophy is very low in patients treated solely with highly purified insulins (Deckert et al, 1974; Wright et al, 1979; Galloway et al, 1982d).

(iii)   Insulin antibodies

Switching patients from conventional recrystallised insulin preparations to the highly purified insulins has been accompanied by a fall in insulin antibody titres in most patients (Andreani et al, 1972; Andreani, 1973; Lavaux et al, 1973; Korp and Levett, 1973; Mirouze et al, 1973; Schlichtkrull et al, 1974; Czyzyk et al, 1974; Bruni et al, 1973, 1977; Devlin and Parameswaran, 1975; Yue and Turtle, 1975; Galloway and Bressler, 1978; Asplin et al, 1978; Kurtz et al, 1980).

Patients with lipoatrophy and/or insulin resistance usually have a high insulin-binding capacity (Witters et al, 1977). It has also been demonstrated that most patients on bovine insulin have circulating antibodies to the C-peptide fraction of bovine proinsulin, which fall dramatically following conversion from conventional to purified insulin, underlining the importance of purity of the insulin preparations as a major determinant of insulin immunogenicity (Schlichtkrull et al, 1970, 1974, 1975; Root et al, 1972).

(iv) Insulin dosage requirements

When patients have been converted to highly purified porcine insulin from conventional insulins, this is accompanied by a dosage reduction, especially in those patients requiring a relatively high daily dose (Oakley, 1976; Mustaffa et al, 1977; Asplin et al, 1978). Whilst a dramatic fall in requirements may occur (Evans and Smith, 1976; Logie and Stowers, 1976; Asplin et al, 1978), in the majority of patients a gradual fall is observed (Andreani, 1973; Andreani et al, 1974). It is difficult to make general recommendations regarding dosage reductions when switching patients from conventional to highly purified insulins (Alberti and Nattrass, 1978; Home and Alberti, 1982). The dosage requirements necessary are dependent on the quantitative, and also qualitative, characteristics of the prevailing insulin antibodies (Witters et al, 1977; Kurtz et al, 1978; Reeves, 1980; Walford et al, 1980, 1982).

(v) Altered metabolic control

Several authors have documented either (a) better metabolic control following the introduction of highly purified insulins compared to the earlier conventional insulin preparations (Lavaux et al, 1973; Asplin et al, 1978), (b) no change (Yue and Turtle, 1975; Klaff et al, 1978) or (c) even deterioration (Fankhauser, 1969; Dixon et al, 1975). Asplin et al (1978) observed higher circulating free insulin concentrations in patients following conversion from conventional to highly purified insulins. The use of highly purified porcine insulin in patients on conventional insulins with high antibody levels is associated with a more rapid onset of action (Nosadini et al, 1981). Patients with high antibody titres tend to have more severe late hypoglycaemic attacks (Berson and Yalow, 1960; Munkgaard Rasmussen et al, 1975) and impaired recovery from hypoglycaemia (Bolli et al, 1983). Others have demonstrated considerable influence of insulin-binding antibodies on insulin pharmacokinetics (Bollinger et al, 1964; Kurtz et al, 1977; Roy et al, 1980; Sodoyez and Sodoyez-Goffaux, 1984). Low affinity/high capacity antibodies blunt and delay the free insulin peaks very dramatically (Kurtz et al, 1977; Kruse, 1981).

In addition, it has been inferred that insulin antibodies can depress endogenous insulin secretion (Ludvigsson and Heding, 1976), thereby compromising the achievement of good diabetes control (Yue et al, 1978; Gonen et al, 1979). The negative relationship between high insulin antibodies and low C-peptide levels in juvenile diabetics beyond the remission phase implies an inhibitory effect of the insulin antibodies on endogenous beta cell function (Andersen, 1972; Heding et al, 1980a). Such findings are consistent with the observation that insulin antibodies cause beta cell degranulation. The constant depletion of insulin from the beta cells due to the presence of insulin antibodies with high binding capacities may enhance the process of beta cell destruction. There is a strong clinical impression that the remission phase in newly diagnosed insulin-dependent diabetics occurs more frequently and lasts longer in the absence of detectable insulin antibodies. While this may be a contributory factor, improved primary care must be of paramount importance, as has been demonstrated by Mirouze and co-workers (1978, 1982a). Antibodies may also interact with the insulin receptors (De Pirro et al, 1980). Therefore, antibodies are a disadvantage in the attempt to achieve good metabolic control.

(vi)   Placental transfer of insulin antibodies

It is known that insulin antibodies can cross the placental barrier (Spellacy and Goetz, 1963; Starzynska et al, 1969; Nakagawa et al, 1973) and result in increased foetal beta cell activity (Phelps et al, 1978; Heding et al, 1980b). Neonatal hypoglycaemia also appears more frequently in infants with antibodies to insulin and glucagon (Nakagawa et al, 1973; Villalpando and Drash, 1979; Heding et al, 1980b).

(vii)   Autoimmunity

Conventional insulin-treated patients, in addition to having insulin antibodies, develop antibodies to other contaminant peptides such as PP, PLI, a-component, glucagon, VIP and SRIF (Bloom et al, 1976, 1979; Villalpando and Drash, 1979; Heding et al, 1980a). In contrast, patients treated with highly purified insulin do not have detectable antibodies to these contaminants (Bloom et al, 1979). Consequently transfer from conventional insulins is accompanied by a fall in such antibodies (Heding et al, 1980a; Kurtz et al, 1980). However, the full significance of such a state of induced autoimmunity is not known.

(viii)   Late complications

The formation of insulin antibodies and the development of morphological changes in the kidneys of animals have been demonstrated following immunisation with impure insulin (Mauer et al, 1972; Wehner et al, 1973). Acceleration of severe diabetic complications by high antibody levels in diabetics has also been proposed (Andersen and Egeberg, 1977; Andersen, 1980). The influence of antibodies on the bioavailability of insulin may, directly or indirectly, contribute to the development of severe vascular complications (Nabarro et al, 1979; Stout, 1979).

Other late non-vascular complications may occur due to the induced autoimmunity caused by hormonal contaminants in conventional insulins (Bloom et al, 1979).

1.2.2.3   Other considerations: insulin species, etc.

Unravelling the immune response to insulin is inherently difficult due to the many interrelated variables that cannot be isolated. The factors influencing the immunogenicity of insulin preparations, in addition to purity, include: species

(Berson and Yalow, 1959; Anderson, 1973; Reeves, 1980), pH (Deckert and Grundahl, 1970), zinc concentration (Arquilla et al, 1978), presence of protamine as a retarding agent (Kern and Langer, 1939; Samuel, 1977; Kurtz et al, 1983), mode of administration (Reeves, 1980), age and sex (Andersen, 1972; Åkerblom and Mäkela, 1977), the presence of infection (Czyzyk et al, 1974) and constitutional variation in immune responsiveness (Reeves, 1980; Reeves et al 1984a,b; cf. Table 1.4).

The greater antigenicity of beef and pork insulin in man was first demonstrated by Berson and Yalow (1959). It has also been recognised that patients develop antibodies earlier with bovine than with porcine insulin (Hurn et al, 1969), due to the greater immunogenicity of beef insulin impurities compared to the corresponding pork insulin contaminants (Schlichtkrull et al, 1972). Root et al (1972) also reported that beef a- and b-components were more immunogenic in rabbits than their pork counterparts. Others have confirmed that bovine insulin preparations are more immunogenic than porcine insulin of equal purity in both animals (Neubauer and Schöne, 1978) and man (Chance et al, 1976; Reeves, 1980). Mixed beef/pork insulins are more immunogenic than either insulin alone, possibly due to a greater number of immunogenic carrier determinants (Keck, 1975, 1977).

The A-chain loop of the insulin molecule appears to provide a crucial carrier determinant in the response to haptenic determinants located elsewhere on the molecule (Keck, 1975). Alanine in the B-30 position of the B-chain appears also to influence the immunoreactivity of insulin antibodies and may be an immune determinant (Kumar and Miller, 1970; Kumar, 1979).

In addition, it is known that during storage, transformation products are formed (Schlichtkrull et al, 1975). Deamidation occurs on storage, being greater in acid solution (Jackson et al, 1972) and at high storage temperature (Jørgensen et al, 1982). The deamidation products, however, retain full biological potency (Carpenter, 1966; Chance, 1972) and are of low immunogenicity (Schlichtkrull et al, 1975). Dimerisation and polymerisation products are also formed on storage (Schlichtkrull et al, 1975). The rate of formation of di- and polymerisation products increases dramatically with increasing temperature (Jørgensen et al, 1982). These products have a much reduced potency but are not significantly immunogenic (Schlichtkrull et al, 1975). Bovine insulin, being the more lipophilic, has the greatest tendency to form non-dissociable polymers, which may in part explain the greater antigenicity of bovine insulin preparations (Kurtz and Nabarro, 1980).

1.2.3 Human insulin

Introduction

During the second decade of insulin therapy several clinicians postulated possible theoretical benefits to the diabetic patient of treatment with human compared with animal species insulin (Karr et al, 1931; Lewis, 1937). Lowell (1944) reported the presence of circulating insulin antibodies in a diabetic patient with insulin allergy and insulin resistance, whose serum contained a neutralising factor against beef/pork but not human insulin. Berson, Yalow and co-workers (Berson et al, 1956; Berson and Yalow, 1959), soon after introducing their radioimmunochemical methods for the study of insulin antibodies, observed the marked variations in affinity of such antibodies to different species of insulin. In 1961 Yalow and Berson also demonstrated that porcine and human insulins reacted either identically or differently in their radioimmunoassay depending on the antisera used, confirming that human and porcine insulins have different affinities towards certain antibodies (Yalow and Berson, 1961).

The discovery, using human cadaveric pancreas, that the amino acid sequence of human insulin was different from other mammalian insulins (Nicol and Smith, 1960), stimulated the chemists along several different pathways to produce human insulin.

Human insulin has been prepared by four different methods utilising:

1.2.3.1   Human cadaveric pancreas.
1.2.3.2   Total peptide synthesis from amino acids.
1.2.3.3   Enzymatic conversion of porcine insulin to human insulin.
1.2.3.4   Recombinant DNA technology.

1.2.3.1   Human cadaveric pancreas

Crystalline human insulin was first prepared in the early 1960s from human cadaveric pancreas glands (Nicol and Smith, 1960; Mirsky et al, 1963; Smith, 1964; Kimmel and Pollock, 1967; Brunfeldt et al, 1969; Shapcott and O'Brien, 1970). The relatively small yield allowed the amino acid composition and sequence of human insulin to be determined by Nicol and Smith (1960). They showed that the amino acid sequence A1–A7 and A11–A21 was the same for human and all other mammalian species of insulin (Brown et al, 1955; Ryle et al, 1955; Harris et al, 1956; Ishihara et al, 1958). The only differences found in the A-chain were in the sequence of the three amino acids at positions 8, 9 and 10. For human insulin the sequence is Thr.Ser.Ileu as in the pig, dog and sperm whale, etc. compared to Ala.Ser.Val in bovine insulin (Figure 1.8; Table 1.8). The amino acid sequence of the B-chain showed the presence of threonine as C-terminal amino acid in human insulin, compared to alanine in both porcine and bovine insulins.

During the late 1960s relatively small amounts of human insulin became available and were used as reference material in the insulin radioimmunoassay or in physicochemical identity tests. The first human insulin international

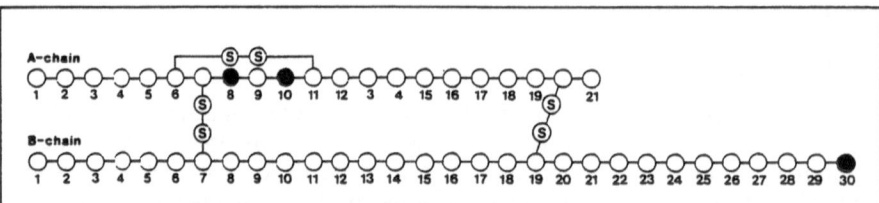

Figure 1.8   Basic structure of insulin: human, bovine and porcine

Table 1.8 Species differences in amino acid sequence of mammalian insulins

	Positions			
	'A' Chain			'B' Chain
	8	9	10	30
Beef	Alanine	Serine	Valine	Alanine
Pork	Threonine	Serine	Isoleucine	Alanine
Human	Threonine	Serine	Isoleucine	Threonine
Other species				
Dog	Threonine	Serine	Isoleucine	Alanine
Sperm whale	Threonine	Serine	Isoleucine	Alanine
Rabbit	Threonine	Serine	Isoleucine	Serine
Sei whale	Alanine	Serine	Threonine	Alanine

reference standard for immuno- and radio-receptor binding assays was established in 1975 by a WHO Expert Committee (WHO Technical Report, 1975). At this time sterile recrystallised neutral, soluble human insulin derived from human pancreatic glands was used clinically in a limited way to carry out skin testing in insulin-allergic patients (Kreines, 1965), pharmacokinetic studies (Akre et al, 1964; Ørskov and Christensen, 1969; Sönksen et al, 1973) and short-term clinical studies (Deckert et al, 1972).

Such material was totally inadequate for therapeutic purposes, thereby prompting scientists during the 1970s to attempt to synthesise human insulin using a variety of different methods (Markussen, 1977).

1.2.3.2 Total peptide synthesis

Meienhofer and co-workers, in 1963, achieved the first full synthesis of sheep insulin (Meienhofer et al, 1963), to be followed soon afterwards by crystalline bovine insulin (Kung et al, 1966). In 1974 Sieber and co-workers successfully completed the total chemical synthesis of human insulin (Sieber et al, 1974), which was shown to be biologically equivalent to the natural hormone (Märki and Albrecht, 1977). Due to the limited availability of material, only one short-term study of the neutral, soluble synthetic human insulin was conducted in six diabetics and three patients with insulin allergy (Diem and Teuscher, 1979; Teuscher, 1979). The total synthesis method was too costly to be a source of human insulin for widespread clinical use.

1.2.3.3 Enzymatic conversion of porcine to human insulin

Shortly after the publication of the amino acid sequence of human insulin (Nicol and Smith, 1960), several chemists tried to synthesise the hormone by various methods (reviewed by Geiger, 1976; Markussen, 1977). An early unsuccessful attempt involved treating porcine insulin with a large excess of free threonine in an aqueous solution with either trypsin or carboxy-peptidase A (Bodansky and Fried, 1966). The first successful semi-synthesis was carried out by Obermeier and Geiger (1976), who used trypsin to cleave the insulin at arginine B22 yielding desoctapeptide-B (23–30)-insulin, which was eventually coupled with synthetic human octapeptide B(23–30). The overall yield of human insulin using this method was very low, approximately 6–10%.

The turning point was the discovery by Homandberg et al (1978), that proteases in mixtures of water and organic solvents were able to reverse the hydrolytic reaction they normally produce and instead bring about the formation of peptide bonds. The application of enzymes to peptide synthesis in organic solvents made the conversion of porcine into human insulin technically possible (Morihara et al, 1979; Gattner et al, 1980, Markussen, 1980). Schmitt and Gattner (1978) selectively removed the alanine B30 residue from porcine insulin resulting in des (Ala-B30)-insulin using carboxypeptidase A and an ammonium buffer to prevent cleaving off asparagine (A21). This process was employed to produce human insulin by both Morihara et al (1979) and Gattner et al (1980) (Figure 1.9).

Both porcine and human insulin have two basic amino acid residues: lysine B29 and arginine B22. Trypsin has a high specificity for positively charged side chains of basic peptides. Markussen and co-workers found that the specificity of trypsin could be controlled by reaction conditions so that no reactions occur at arginine B22. The method described by Markussen et al (1981, 1982 and

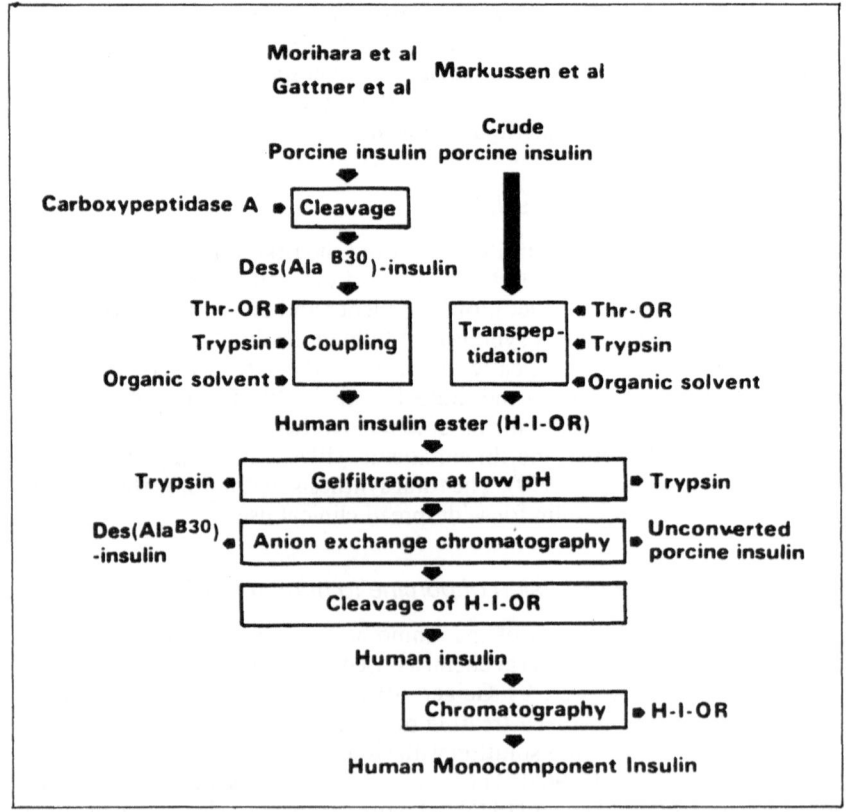

Figure 1.9 Comparison of semi-synthetic methods to human insulin (after Markussen, 1984)

Markussen (1982a, b) involves crude porcine insulin brought to react with a threonine ester by porcine trypsin in a mixture of water and organic solvents, in which the alanine residue B30 is replaced by a threonine ester (Figure 1.9).

The reaction is a transpeptidation reaction catalysed by porcine trypsin in a mixture of water and organic solvents in the presence of a large excess of the threonine ester (Markussen and Schaumburg 1982; Figure 1.10). The trypsin-catalysed transpeptidation reaction initially involves the formation of a porcine insulin–trypsin Michaelis complex. This is followed by the formation of an ester bond between the carboxyl group of lysine B29 and the hydroxyl group of the serine residue of the active site of trypsin, i.e. des (Ala-B30)-insulinyl-trypsin ester (DAI-trypsin) with the release of alanine. The hydrolysis of this intermediate to des (Ala-B30) insulin (DAI) is virtually blocked under conditions suitable for transpeptidation, i.e. 20% (v/v) water, 1 M threonine ester and 2.5 M acetic acid (Markussen and Schaumberg, 1982). Instead, aminolysis occurs with the threonine ester converting the intermediate DAI-trypsin to human insulin ester (Figure 1.10). The stability of trypsin is improved by adding calcium ions and lowering the temperature.

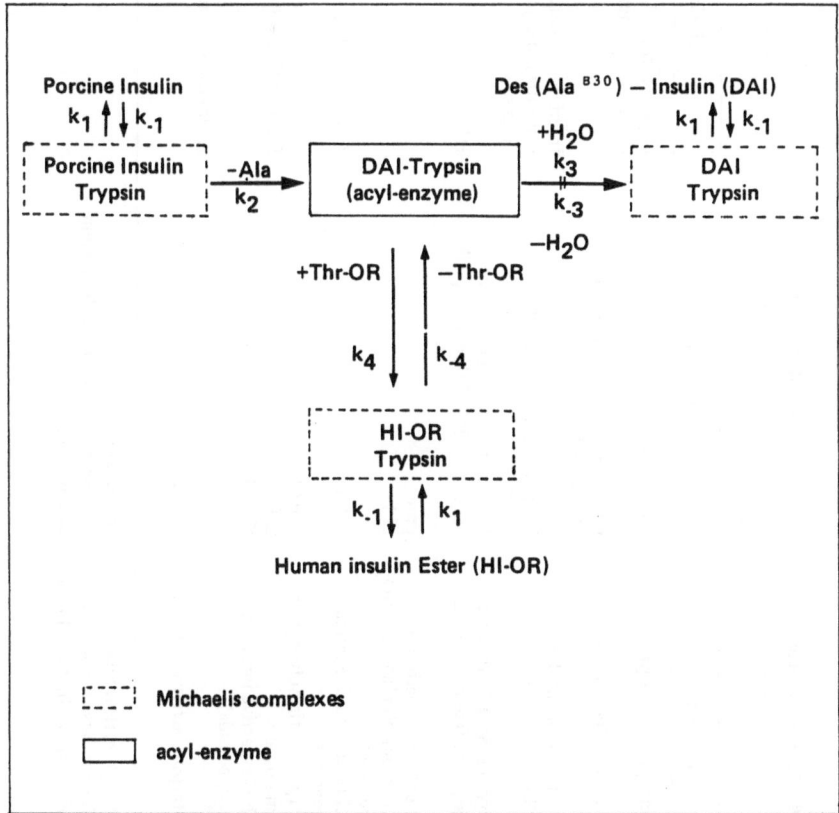

Figure 1.10 Reaction mechanism of the trypsin-catalysed transpeptidation of porcine insulin into human insulin ester (after Markussen, 1982)

Table 1.9 Purity and identity tests applied to 'semi-synthetic' human insulin

Purity tests

Test/method	Results
Disc electrophoresis at pH 8.9	One band only
HPLC, reverse phase mode	One peak only, absorbance at 280 nm > 99% of total
Absence of porcine insulin	
(a) HPLC*	No porcine insulin detectable d.l. < 3%
(b) Degradation with trypsin; analysis of free amino acids	No alanine detectable, d.l. for alanine < .1% of threonine peak
Peptides detectable with RIA:†	ppm
PLI (proinsulin like immuno-reactivity)	≤ 1
GLI (glucagon like immuno-reactivity)	≤ 0.1
PP (pancreatic polypeptide)	≤ 0.01
Somatostatin	≤ 0.01
VIP (vasoactive intestinal polypeptide)	≤ 0.01
Porcine trypsin, activity test	$< 1: 10^{22}/w/w$

Identity tests

Test/method	Results
Crystal form (2 and 4 Zn^{++}/hexamer)	Regular rhombohedra, identical with those of porcine insulin and with NHI‡
Interference pattern of X-ray exposures of crystals (Laue diagrams)	Identical with those of NHI,‡ small but significant differences with those of porcine insulin
HPLC*	Retention time coinciding with that of NHI‡ Retention time shorter than that of porcine insulin
Amino acid sequence studies	In accordance with literature (Nicol and Smith, 1960)
Degradation with trypsin	Threonine only amino acid released
Biological strength	28.5 IU/mg dry substance; 185 ± 51IU/mg N (95% confidence limits)

* HPLC: high-performance liquid chromatography
† Radioimmunoassay, ppm = parts per million by weight of the dry insulin
‡ NHI: Human insulin from human pancreas glands

Transpeptidation at arginine B22 can be virtually eliminated by increasing the water and weak acid content of the reaction mixture. The yield of human insulin ester in a process involving a water content of 20% (v/v), pH of 4.5 at 12°C is approximately 97%. The 3% loss is unconverted porcine insulin and des-heptapeptide-(B24–B30), threonine ester-(B23) insulin. During the reaction certain contaminants in crude porcine insulin, i.e. proinsulin, insulin intermediates (arginyl, diarginyl insulins), are also transpeptidised to human insulin ester together with porcine insulin. The additional yields of human insulin ester from the convertible components of crude porcine insulin compensate almost completely for the 3% loss in conversion of porcine insulin.

Following transpepidation, trypsin is deactivated and removed by gel filtration chromatography at acid pH to below the detection limit of 1 ppm (w/w). Subsequent ion exchange and crystallisation processes further reduce the trypsin content to less than 1 in 10^{22} (w/w), or less than 3 molecules of trypsin per kg of human insulin (Table 1.9). Next, unconverted porcine insulin is removed by anion exchange chromatography, followed by the cleavage of

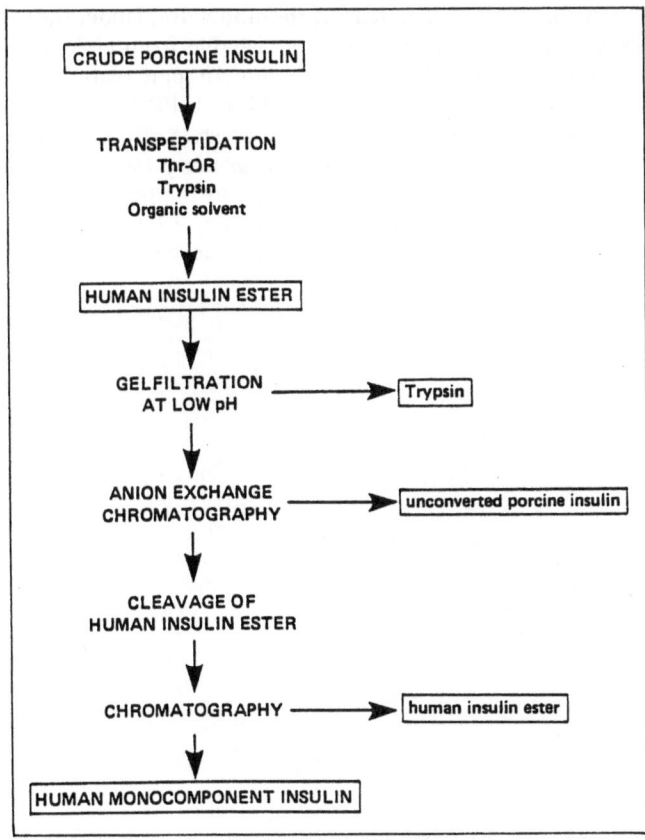

Figure 1.11 Manufacture of human monocomponent insulin from crude porcine insulin (after Markussen, 1983c)

the ester group of the threonine-(B30) residue rendering human insulin. A final ion exchange chromatographic step is included to remove any small amounts of residual human insulin ester.

The further processing of human insulin ester is illustrated in Figure 1.11.

Identity and properties of human insulin

Finally, the human insulin preparation underwent tests to confirm its purity, identity and biological potency (Markussen et al, 1982, 1983a,b,c; Markussen, 1982a,b, 1984). The results of purity and identity tests applied to the 'semi-synthetic' human insulin are summarised in Table 1.9. The purity of the 'semi-synthetic' human insulin meets the specifications of monocomponent insulin (Jørgensen et al, 1970, 1982; Schlichtkrull et al, 1974).

Crystal structure of human insulin

Human insulin co-crystallises with zinc (2 or 4 Zn^{++} per hexamer) iso-morphically to porcine insulin as perfect rhombohedra. Under the microscope the crystals are morphologically indistinguishable from crystals of porcine insulin or human insulin derived from human pancreatic glands, when prepared under the same conditions (Schlichtkrull, 1957).

X-ray crystallographic analysis of insulin crystals affords a very sensitive method of ascertaining the identity of the primary (sequence), secondary (helixes), the tertiary (spatial conformation) and the quarternary structures (association behaviour) (Blundell and Johnson, 1976). X-ray diffraction patterns of 'semi-synthetic' human insulin and porcine insulin demonstrate

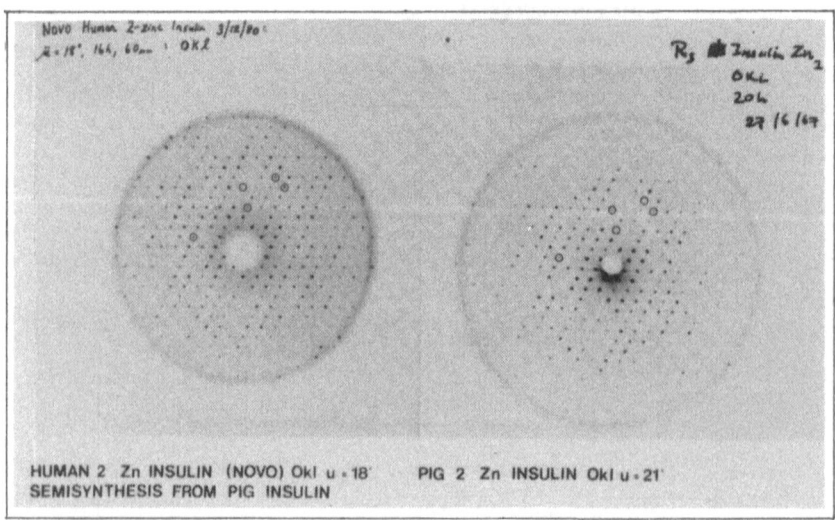

Figure 1.12 X-ray diffraction photographs of 'semi-synthetic' human insulin (Novo) and porcine insulin. Equivalent reflections showing distinct intensity changes are circled (after Chawdhury et al, 1982)

distinct differences in the intensity patterns observed in precision photographs (Chawdhury et al, 1982, 1983) (Figure 1.12).

Crystallographic analysis and refinement using the fast Fourier least squares technique (Agarwal, 1978; Baker and Dodson, 1980) of 'semi-synthetic' human insulin have shown that its spatial structure is similar to porcine insulin except at the C terminus of the B-chain. Changes in the water structure in the region of B28–B30 are also seen between human and porcine insulin crystal structures, which is consistent with the greater solubility of human insulin. The small differences between human and porcine insulin observed in the X-ray diffraction patterns has not, however, significantly altered their three-dimensional structures. The molecular structure of human insulin derived from human pancreas and 'semi-synthetic' human insulin is identical within experimental error (Chawdhury et al, 1982).

The amino acid composition of 'semi-synthetic' insulin determined after hydrolysis was in agreement with the theory for human insulin (Nicol and Smith, 1960). After oxidative sulfitolysis to split the insulin followed by gel filtration to separate the chains, amino acid analysis was undertaken (Chang et al, 1978), confirming that no alteration had occurred at the N-terminal part of either the A- or B-chain (Markussen et al, 1983a). Finally, amino acid analysis of the C-terminal residue revealed the presence of threonine, which was confirmed by thin layer chromatography (Markussen et al, 1983a).

Gel filtration and disc electrophoresis indicated an identical molecular size and charge of porcine and human insulin (Markussen, 1982a; Markussen et al, 1983a,b). The greater hydrophilicity of human insulin allows the two species to be distinguished by using isocratic reversed-phase high-performance liquid chromatography (RP-HPLC) (Terabe et al, 1979; Chance et al, 1981a,b; Kroeff and Chance, 1982; Lloyd and Corran, 1982). A single symmetrical peak confirmed the identity of human insulin of pancreatic origin and 'semi-synthetic' human insulin of porcine origin (Markussen et al, 1983a).

Comparisons of the immunoreactivity of 'semi-synthetic' and pancreatic human insulin, using a number of different insulin antibodies, did not demonstrate any difference in antigenicity (Markussen et al, 1983a; Heding, 1983). Immunisation studies in rabbits with monocomponent porcine and human insulin revealed a similar low level of immunogenicity (Markussen et al, 1983a,b). Differences between human and porcine insulin have been documented previously with other antisera (Yalow and Berson, 1961).

The potency of human insulin is similar to porcine/bovine insulin, i.e. 185 IU/mgN when using the 4th International Standard (154 IU/mgN) (Bangham and Mussett, 1959) or monocomponent porcine insulin (185 IU/mgN), in a variety of bioassays (British Pharmacopoeia 1980; European Pharmacopoeia 1975; United States Pharmacopoeia 1980).

1.2.3.4 Recombinant DNA technology

Advances in molecular biology and synthetic nucleotide chemistry have led to the preparation of several mammalian polypeptide hormones by micro-biological fermentation (Gilbert and Villa-Komaroff, 1980; Wetzel, 1980). The

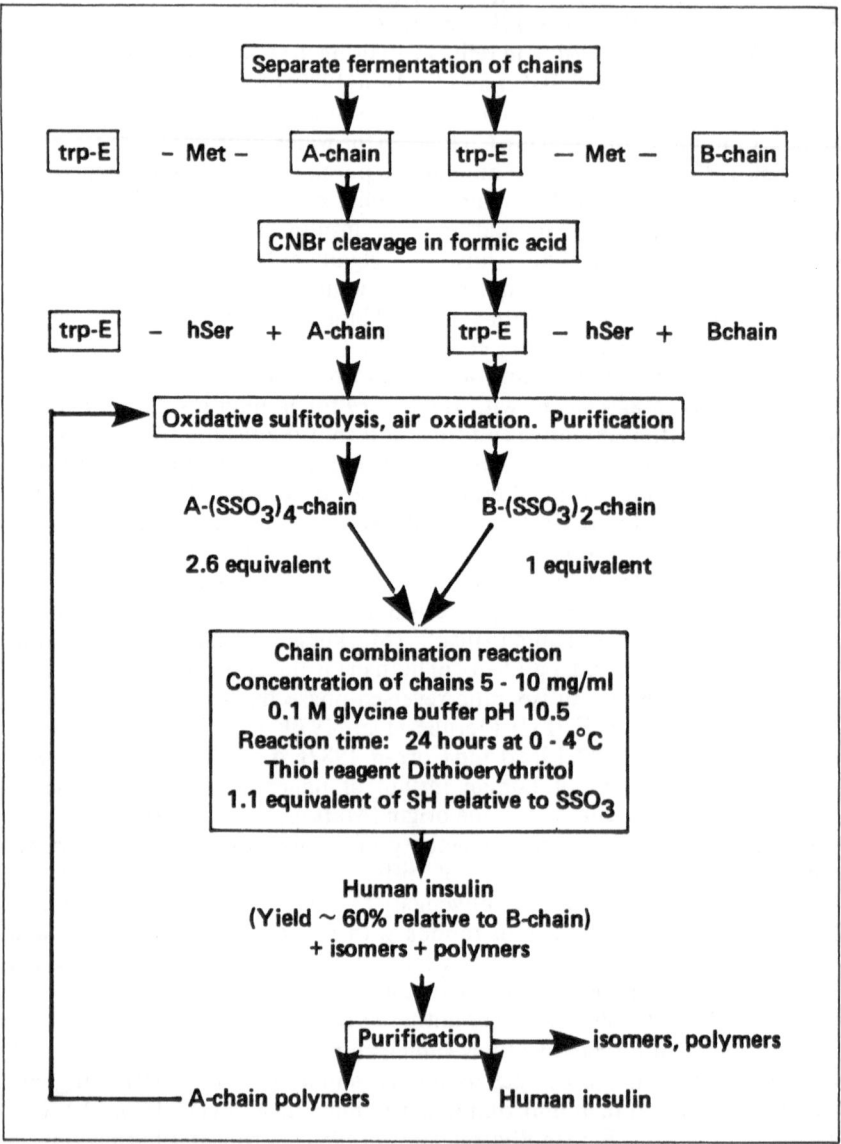

Figure 1.13 Production of 'biosynthetic' human insulin from the production of the individual A- and B-chains of human insulin by *E. coli*, followed by a chain combination reaction (Chance et al, 1981b)

basis of the recombinant DNA technology involves isolating the organism's plasmid DNA, cleaving with restriction enzymes, and inserting the appropriate gene structure and re-introducing the desired plasmid DNA into micro-organisms by means of vectors and then cloning (Goeddel et al, 1979; Miller and Baxter, 1980; Ross, 1981).

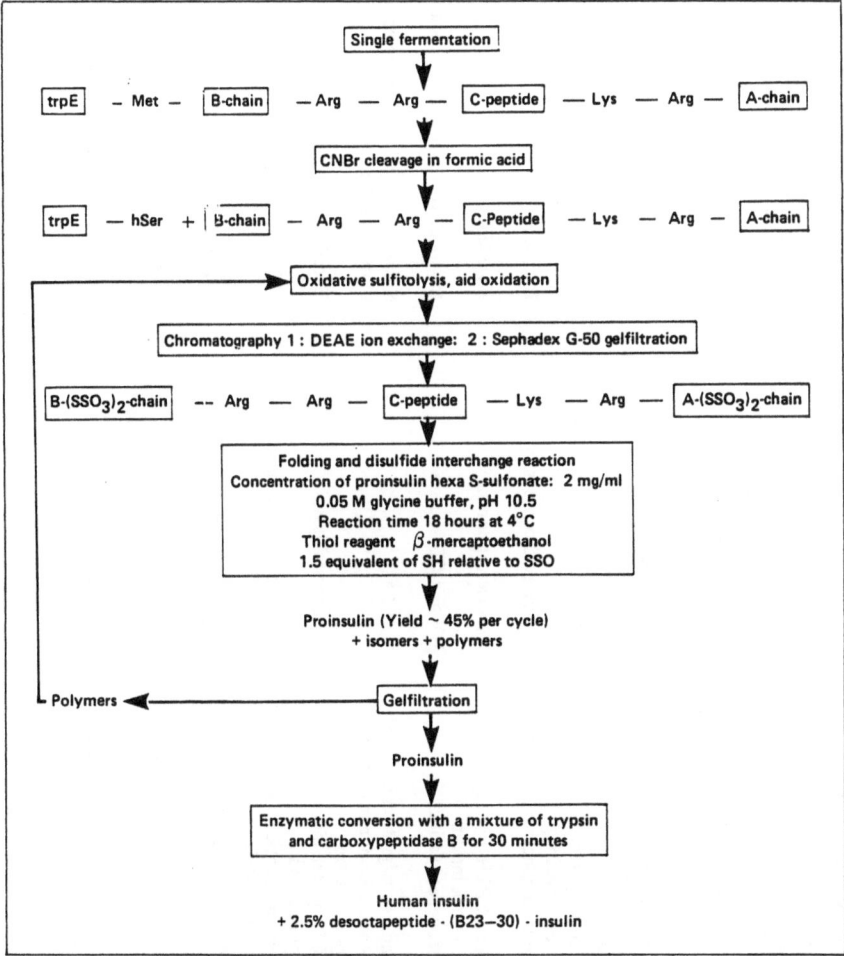

Figure 1.14 Production of 'bio-synthetic' human insulin from the chimerically-bound linear sequence of human proinsulin (after Frank et al, 1981)

Human insulin – 'biosynthetic' human insulin – produced by recombinant DNA methods can be prepared by either (a) A- and B-chain combination (Goeddell et al, 1979; Chance et al, 1981a,b,c; Figure 1.13) or (b) conversion of proinsulin (Frank et al, 1981; Johnson, 1982; Figure 1.14).

The A- and B-chain genes have been prepared by synthetic nucleotide chemistry (Crea et al, 1978), while the proinsulin gene was derived semi-synthetically (Villa-Komaroff et al, 1978). A codon for methionine was introduced, linking the synthetic A- and B-chains to the original promoter β-galactosidase, and latterly tryptophane synthetase (Trp E). The constructed genes are then inserted into plasmids and cloned in *Escherichia coli* (*E. coli*). Fermentation of the bacteria results in the production of the promoter-linked product of A- or B-chain (Figure 1.13) or proinsulin-chimeric proteins (Figure

Table 1.10 Biosynthetic human insulin (recombinant DNA): purity and identity tests applied to 'biosynthetic' human insulins

Derived by chain combination		Derived from human proinsulin	
Test	Results	Test	Results
†USP rabbit hypoglycaemia assay	27.5 ± 1.7 U/mg ($p \leq 0.05$)	†USP rabbit hypoglycaemia assay (144 rabbits)	28.0 ± 2.2 U/mg
Insulin radioimmunoassay	Relative immunopotency 98 ± 22% of pancreatic human insulin ($p \leq 0.05$)	Insulin radioimmunoassay	106 ± 10% of pancreatic human insulin standard
Insulin radioreceptor assay	Relative potency 98 ± 7% of purified pork insulin ($p \leq 0.05$)	Insulin radioreceptor assay	96 ± 3% of pancreatic human insulin standard
Amino acid composition	Comparable to pancreatic human insulin	Amino acid composition	Excellent
Quantitative NH_2 terminal analysis by Edman degradation	PTH-Gly and PTH-Phe equivalent to purified pork insulin	Gel electrophoresis	Excellent
Amino acid sequence of A- and B-chains used to make insulin.	Correct sequences verified	UV and CD spectra	Identical to pork insulin standard
Polyacrylamide gel electrophoresis	Electrophoretic migration identical with pancreatic human insulin and purified pork insulin	HPLC*	Same retention time as pancreatic human insulin
Absorption and circular dichroic spectra	UV and CD spectra identical to purified pork insulin	Zinc crystallisation	Excellent
HPLC*	Peak retention identical to pancreatic human insulin	Limulus assay for bacterial endotoxin	< 0.1 ng/mg
Zinc insulin crystallisation	Excellent	†USP rabbit pyrogen test	Non-pyrogenic
Limulus amebocyte lysate test for pyrogenic bacterial endotoxin	< 0.6 ng/mg	‡BP proteolytic activity assay	Satisfactory
†USP rabbit pyrogen test	Satisfactory	Proinsulin radioimmunoassay	11.3 ppm
		C-peptide radioimmunoassay	< 1 ppm
		E. coli peptide radioimmunoassay	< 4 ppm

*HPLC: high-performance liquid chromatography
†USP: United States Pharmacopeia
‡BP: British Pharmacopoeia

1.14). The methionine linkage facilitates the eventual chemical cleavage of the polypeptide chains from the promoter protein by cyanogen bromide, which cleaves specifically at methionine. In the current method for producing 'biosynthetic' human insulin the A- and B-chains are converted to stable S-sulphonate salts by oxidative sulfitolysis, purified and combined in the presence of excess A-chains to yield human insulin which is then submitted to further purification (Figure 1.13). This method of producing human insulin is regarded as a forerunner to even better future methodologies (Chan et al, 1981).

The alternative approach to human insulin via proinsulin, involves plasmids into *E. coli* K12 (Frank et al, 1981). The preparation of human insulin from human proinsulin is illustrated in Figure 1.14. The steps leading to the proinsulin hexa-S-sulphonate derivative are similar to those for the individual A- and B-chains. The proinsulin S-sulphonate is then treated with a thiol reagent, beta-mercaptoethanol, which allows the proinsulin molecule to fold and form the disulphide bonds.

After purification the proinsulin is enzymatically converted using a mixture of trypsin and carboxypeptidase B (Kemmler et al, 1971) to yield human insulin which is then purified by gel filtration and ion-exchange chromatography (Figure 1.14).

The properties and characteristics of 'biosynthetic' human insulin derived by the two routes have been well described (Chance et al, 1980, 1981a,b; Johnson, 1982; Ross et al, 1982; Table 1.10).

X-ray diffraction patterns of crystals of the two 'biosynthetic' human insulins are indistinguishable from the 'semi-synthetic' and natural human insulin (Chawdhury et al, 1982, 1983; Figure 1.15).

'Biosynthetic' human insulin could contain contaminants derived from the production organism *E. coli*, including bacterial endotoxins that act as pyrogens and *E. coli* polypeptides (ECPs) that could act as antigens. Therefore, from a safety point of view, several screening tests are carried out. The *Limulus* amebocyte lysate method – the most sensitive *in vitro* endotoxin assay – shows the bacterial endotoxin content of 'biosynthetic' human insulin at the lower limit of detection, and not detectable in the USP rabbit pyrogen tests or endogenous pyrogen tests (Johnson, 1982; Ross et al, 1982). Immunoradiometric assays for a heterogeneous mixture of *E. coli* contaminants in 'biosynthetic' human insulin indicate a level of 4 ppm (Baker et al, 1981; Johnson, 1982; Ross et al, 1982). In a small number of subjects, no difference in ECP antibody levels (IgG, IgE) has been seen between patients treated for 6 months on biosynthetic human insulin and normal controls (Baker et al, 1981; Ross et al, 1982). Biosynthetic human insulin has also been found to be safe and non-reactive in skin tests in humans (Keen et al, 1980; Federlin et al, 1981).

Human insulin, derived by recombinant DNA methodology, has the advantage that contamination with other hormones such as glucagon and somatostatin is ruled out. It is still very necessary, however, to develop more sensitive assay systems to ensure the near absence of ECPs from the final preparations (Baker et al, 1981; Johnson, 1982; Ross et al, 1982).

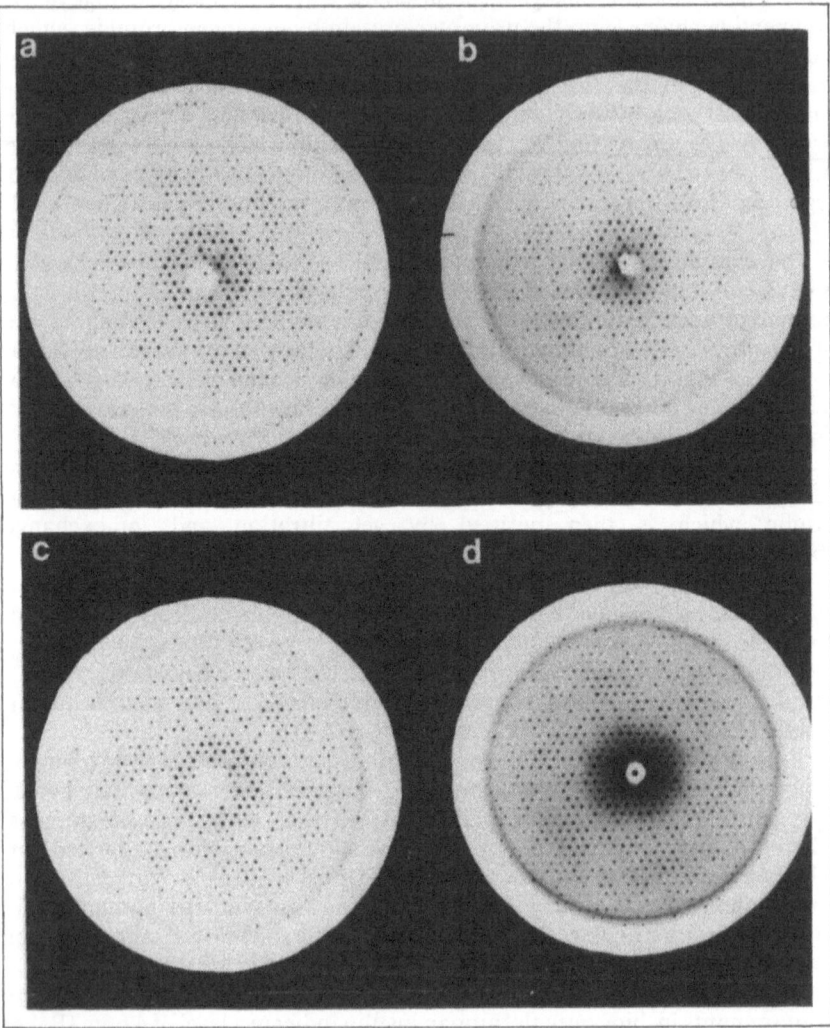

Figure 1.15 X-ray diffraction photographs of human insulin derived from different sources: (a) bacterial production of the separate chains, (b) bacterial production of pro-insulin, (c) semi-synthesis from porcine insulin, and (d) human pancreas

1.2.4 SUMMARY

Since the discovery and availability of insulin for the treatment of diabetes in 1922, a number of advances have been made influencing the development of insulin preparations for the treatment of the diabetic patient. These developments can be grouped together into three major achievements.

The first was the *modification of insulin* (Table 1.11) to vary its timing of hypoglycaemic action (onset, peak and duration), thereby making available

Table 1.11 Modification of insulin to prolong its duration of action

Hagedorn et al	1936	Protamine insulin
Scott and Fisher	1936	Protamine zinc insulin (PZI)
Umber et al	1938	Surfen insulin
Bauman and Reiner	1939	Globin insulin
Krayenbühl and Rosenberg	1946	Isophane insulin (NPH)
Hallas-Møller et al	1951	Lente insulins
Schlichtkrull et al	1959	Biphasic insulin

insulin preparations described as 'short-', 'intermediate-' or 'long-acting'.

The second major advance was, and continues to be, the increasing *purification of insulin* (Table 1.12). The scientific achievements in this area have immeasurably improved the tolerance and efficacy of insulin preparations.

Table 1.12 Purification of insulin

Abel	1926	Crystallisation of insulin
Berson, Yalow et al	1956	Radioimmunoassay
Mirsky and Kawamura	1966	Heterogeneity of insulin
Schlichtkrull et al	1969	Monocomponent insulin

The third major achievement was the *production of human insulin* (Tables 1.13, 1.14).

Table 1.13 Preparation of human insulin

Mirsky et al	1963	Isolation and crystallisation of human insulin
Kung et al	1966	Total chemical synthesis of bovine insulin
Sieber et al	1974	Total chemical synthesis of human insulin
Obermeier and Geiger	1976	'Semi-synthesis' of human from porcine insulin
Gattner et al } Morihara et al }	1979	'Semi-synthesis' of human from porcine insulin

During the late 1970s and early 1980s two techniques, developed in parallel, have made human insulin available in sufficient quantities for the treatment of insulin-requiring diabetic patients (Table 1.14).

Table 1.14 Production of human insulin for therapy

Goeddel et al; Chance et al	1979–1981	'Biosynthetic' human insulin* derived via recombinant DNA technology
Markussen	1980	'Semi-synthetic' human insulin† from porcine insulin

Nomenclature The term '*human insulin*', applies to a protein having the normal structure of the natural antidiabetic principle produced by the human pancreas. Human insulin produced by artificial means bears an approved code indicative of the method of production, e.g. *crb** – produced by the chemical combination of the A- and B-chains of the protein, each chain having been obtained from bacteria genetically modified by recombinant DNA technology; †*emp* – produced by the enzymatic modification of insulin obtained from the pancreas of the pig.

2
Objectives of Investigations

The availability of human insulin in large amounts has resulted in the formulation of a range of highly purified human insulin ('short-', 'inter-mediate-' and 'long-acting') preparations for use in the management of diabetes mellitus.

This book encompasses the first clinical pharmacological studies on each of the highly purified human insulin (emp) preparations produced by the enzymatic conversion of porcine insulin (Novo Industri A/S, Copenhagen). The studies in normal man were designed and conducted primarily to assess the safety and comparative hypoglycaemic effects, other metabolic and hormonal responses and plasma insulin profiles for the new range of 'semi-synthetic' human insulins (Table 2.1) and their porcine and bovine counterparts.

Table 2.1 Human insulin (emp)

Insulin preparations		
Actrapid®	HM	(neutral soluble insulin)*/†/††
Monotard®	HM	(insulin zinc suspension – Lente insulin)*
Protaphane®	HM	(NPH)*
Actraphane®	HM	(Actrapid® HM: Protaphane® HM – 30 : 70)*
Ultratard®	HM	(insulin zinc suspension – Ultralente insulin)*

Route of administration
Subcutaneous* Intramuscular† Intravenous††

Subjects
Normal male volunteers

In addition to considering the relevance of pharmaceutical formulation and species of insulin on subcutaneous absorption, the influence of additional factors such as the site of injection, aprotinin, insulin concentration, admixing of 'short-' and 'intermediate-acting' preparations and 'within' and 'between' subject variation on the absorption of human insulin, has been examined (Table 2.2).

Table 2.2 Factors influencing subcutaneous absorption of human (emp) insulin

---

Insulin
  pharmaceutical formulation
  concentration
  admixing

Site of injection and local factors

'Within' and 'between' subject variation

Therefore studies have been carried out to characterise the absorption of various insulin preparations under certain conditions which are pertinent to the day-to-day care of insulin-requiring diabetic patients.

3
Investigational Procedures

3.1 CLINICAL

The studies were carried out in accordance with guidelines for the conduct of studies in normal subjects (Declaration of Helsinki, WHO, 1976). All of the studies were approved by the local Ethical Committee and written informed consent obtained from each volunteer.

3.1.1 Subjects

Male volunteers only were entered into the studies following satisfactory clinical and laboratory (haematological, biochemical) screening. The subjects were aged between 18 and 40 years and within 20% of their ideal body weight (Metropolitan Life Insurance Co, 1960). Only one out of a total of 46 normal volunteer subjects had a family history of diabetes. The presence of carbohydrate intolerance in this subject was excluded with a 75 g oral glucose tolerance test. The individual subjects were allowed to participate in up to three separate studies, the number of studies per subject dependent on type, number and duration of the experimental study days. Full haematological and biochemical screenings were conducted at the end of each study, with serial checks of haematological parameters during studies involving four or more study days.

Each study period was preceded by a 10h overnight fast, all subjects being advised not to take alcohol during the previous 24h. For studies of 12h or longer the volunteers were advised to take a high-carbohydrate diet for the preceding 2 days. For some studies a standard diet high in carbohydrate content was provided on the previous day. At the end of each experiment the individual subjects were fed and discharged only following clinical assessment. Transportation of subjects to and from studies was arranged as deemed necessary. More specific details of the subjects (age, weight, etc.) will be included with the individual studies.

3.1.2 Materials

The insulin preparations used in the studies were as follows:

'Short-acting' insulins (neutral, soluble):

human (emp)	Actrapid® HM	40 and 100 IU/ml
human (crb)	Humulin® S	40 IU/ml
porcine	Actrapid® MC	40 IU/ml
bovine	Actrapid® MC	40 IU/ml

'Intermediate-acting' insulins (insulin suspensions):

Insulin zinc suspensions:		
human (emp)	Monotard® HM	40,100 IU/ml
porcine	Monotard® MC	40,100 IU/ml

Isophane (NPH) insulins:		
human (emp)	Protaphane® HM	40,100 IU/ml
human (crb)	Humulin I®	40 IU/ml
porcine	Protaphane® MC	40 IU/ml

'Biphasic' insulin:

human (emp)	Actraphane® HM	100 IU/ml

'Long-acting' insulins (insulin zinc suspensions):

human (emp)	Ultratard® HM	100 IU/ml
bovine	Ultratard® MC	100 IU/ml
porcine	Ultratard® MC	100 IU/ml

The 'semi-synthetic' human insulin preparations were produced by Novo Industri A/S, Copenhagen, Denmark, and the 'biosynthetic' human insulins by Eli Lilly and Company, Indianapolis, USA.

With each study, details relating to the insulin preparations will include nitrogen content and potency estimations and contents of excipients when necessary.

Nomenclature adopted

The family of human (emp) insulin preparations will be referred to as *'semi-synthetic' human insulins*, with the suffix HM after the registered name, e.g. Actrapid® HM, Monotard® HM, etc. The human (crb) insulins will be designated *'biosynthetic' human insulins* (BHI).

3.1.3 Methods

The studies were conducted in a four-bedded Diabetes and Metabolism Investigations Unit in the Department of Medicine, University of Wales College of Medicine. The unit was familiar with the requirements of intensive care during investigational procedures involving both normal subjects and diabetic patients. All the studies were carried out in fasting normal male volunteer subjects.

Each study was commenced about 0800 h with the siting of an intravenous cannula (Venflon) into a median cubital fossa vein attached via a three-way tap to a slow-running saline (0.154 mmol/l) infusion to facilitate blood sampling and avoid the need for oral fluids. At each of the sampling time points the saline infusion was stopped, and 2 ml of blood was withdrawn and discarded prior to obtaining the sample for subsequent analysis. The volume and frequency of the samples varied between the studies. Common to all the studies, aliquots were taken into fluoride for glucose, and lithium heparin for immunoreactive insulin (IRI) and C-peptide estimations. According to the requirements of the study, additional samples were taken (0.5 ml) into 2 ml 3% (w/v) perchloric acid for intermediary metabolites (lactate, alanine, glycerol and 3-hydroxybutyrate) and lithium heparin for glucagon, growth hormone and cortisol determinations. All heparin bottles contained the freeze-dried residue from 0.6 ml aprotinin (Trasylol, Bayer AG), with the addition of reduced glutathione as preservative for analysis of adrenaline. All samples were taken onto ice, centifuged at +4°C within 5 min of sampling and the supernatants stored at –20°C until assay. Plasma samples for insulin antibody determinations were taken at the end of each study day.

Depending on the study design, a second intravenous infusion of somatostatin (or saline) was given into the opposite arm. The insulin preparations and diluting medium (control), were administered either subcutaneously, intra-muscularly or intravenously. The order of the 'treatments' was according to a randomisation schedule.

During each study the subjects remained rested in the supine position. No smoking was allowed during the studies and the room temperature was kept constant at 22°C. The subjects were carefully monitored clinically and biochemically (capillary blood glucose) during each study. Injection sites were specifically examined immediately after injection, during and at the end of each experimental period.

In view of the different study protocols employed, specific details relating to the subjects (age, weight, numbers), frequency and total number of experimental days, duration of basal and post-treatment periods, insulin dose, site, route, method of preparation, and administration of test materials and the use of concomitant therapy will be described separately for each study or group of similar studies.

3.2 LABORATORY METHODS

The parameters (response variables) measured and assay methods used in the course of the investigations are summarised in Tables 3.1 and 3.2.

Summary of assay procedures

3.2.1 Glucose assays

Plasma glucose was estimated using one of two methods:

(i) *Hexokinase method* (Auto-analyser, Technicon).

INVESTIGATIONAL PROCEDURES

Table 3.1 Laboratory assays

Parameters	Assay methods
*Glucose	hexokinase[1]
	glucose oxidase[2]
Insulin	Heding (1972)[1]
(Immunoreactive)	double antibody RIA[2]
C-peptide	Heding (1975)[1]
	double antibody RIA[2]
Glucagon	Heding (1971)[1]
	Alford et al (1977)[2]
Growth hormone	Boden and Soeldner (1976)
Cortisol	Baum et al (1974)
Adrenaline	Da Prada and Zürcher (1976)
Insulin antibody	Reeves and Kelly (1980)
†Lactate, alanine, glycerol, 3-hydroxybutyrate	Lloyd et al (1978)

*Plasma, †blood

Table 3.2 The Institutes/Departments and personnel involved in performing the various laboratory assays

Novo Research Institute, Copenhagen, Denmark.	Dr. L. G. Heding	Insulin[1], C-peptide[1] and glucagon[1]
Dept. of Medicine, Royal Postgraduate Medical School, London.	Professor S. R. Bloom	Glucagon[2]
Dept. of Clinical Biochemistry and Metabolic Medicine, Royal Victoria Infirmary, Newcastle upon Tyne.	Professor K. G. M. M. Alberti	Growth hormone, cortisol and metabolites
Dept. of Immunology and Medicine, University Hospital, Nottingham.	Professor W. G. Reeves	Insulin antibody
Dept. of Medicine, Kantonsspital Basel, Switzerland.	Dr. U. Keller	Adrenaline
Dept. of Clinical Biochemistry, University Hospital of Wales, Cardiff.	Professor G. Elder Dr. S. Woodhead	Growth hormone
Department of Medicine, University of Wales College of Medicine, Cardiff.	Professor R. Hall Dr. T. M. Hayes Mr. S. Luzio	Glucose[1,2,] insulin[2] and C-peptide[2]

The measurement of glucose was based on the following reactions:

$$\text{glucose} + \text{ATP} \xrightarrow{\text{hexokinase}} \text{glucose-6-phosphate} + \text{ADP}$$

$$\text{glucose-6-phosphatase} + \text{NADP}^+ \xrightarrow[\text{dehydrogenase}]{\text{glucose-6-phosphate}} \text{6-phosphogluconate} + \text{NADPH} + \text{H}^+$$

(ii) *Glucose oxidase method* (23AM glucose analyser: Yellow Springs Instrument Co. Inc. Ohio, USA).

This analyser uses an oxidase enzyme hydrogen peroxide sensor which is highly specific for glucose. The determination of glucose is based on the following reactions:

(1) $\quad$ D-glucose + O_2 $\xrightarrow[\text{oxidase}]{\text{glucose}}$ gluconic acid + H_2O_2

(2) $\qquad\qquad$ H_2O_2 $\xrightarrow{\hspace{2cm}}$ $2H^+ + O_2 + 2^e$

(3) $\qquad$ $4H^+ + O_2$ $\xrightarrow{\hspace{2cm}}$ $2H_2O - 4^e$

Glucose and oxygen are converted to gluconic acid and hydrogen peroxide by means of glucose oxidase (1). A platinum anode in the analyser oxidises a constant portion of the hydrogen peroxide, the current created being directly proportional to the glucose concentration in the sample (2). The circuit is completed by a silver cathode in which oxygen is reduced to water (3).

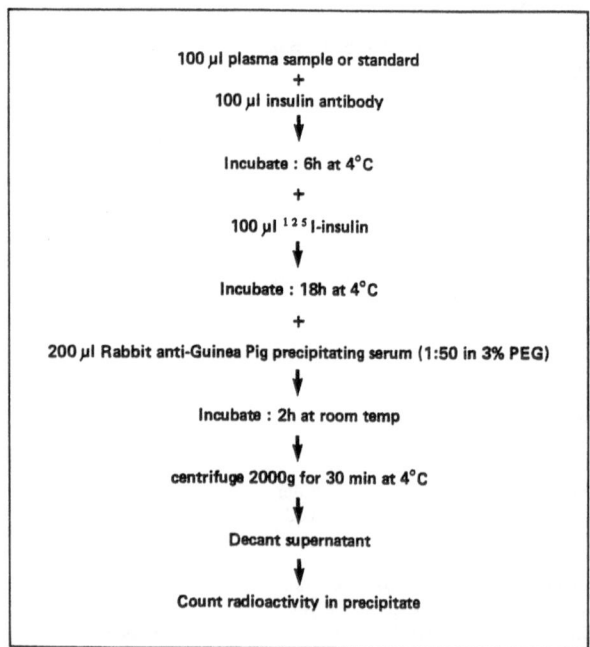

100 μl plasma sample or standard
+
100 μl insulin antibody
↓
Incubate : 6h at 4°C
+
100 μl ^{125}I-insulin
↓
Incubate : 18h at 4°C
+
200 μl Rabbit anti-Guinea Pig precipitating serum (1:50 in 3% PEG)
↓
Incubate : 2h at room temp
↓
centrifuge 2000g for 30 min at 4°C
↓
Decant supernatant
↓
Count radioactivity in precipitate

Figure 3.1 $\quad$ Double-antibody insulin radioimmunoassay

For the analysis of glucose 25 μl of plasma is pipetted directly into the glucose analyser. The instrument was calibrated after every 10 samples.

3.2.2 Insulin radioimmunoassays

Immunoreactive insulin (IRI) was measured according to the method of Heding (1972), and a modification of this method using a second antibody to separate the free and antibody-bound ^{125}I-insulin. Two specific insulin antibodies, M8170 and M8309 (Novo Research Institute, Copenhagen) were used in the assays.

The procedure for the double antibody radioimmunoassay (RIA) can be seen in the flow diagram (Figure 3.1). Plasma sample or standard was incubated for 6h at 4°C with the specific anti-insulin antibody (M8309). ^{125}I-insulin (Amersham International plc, Amersham) was added and the

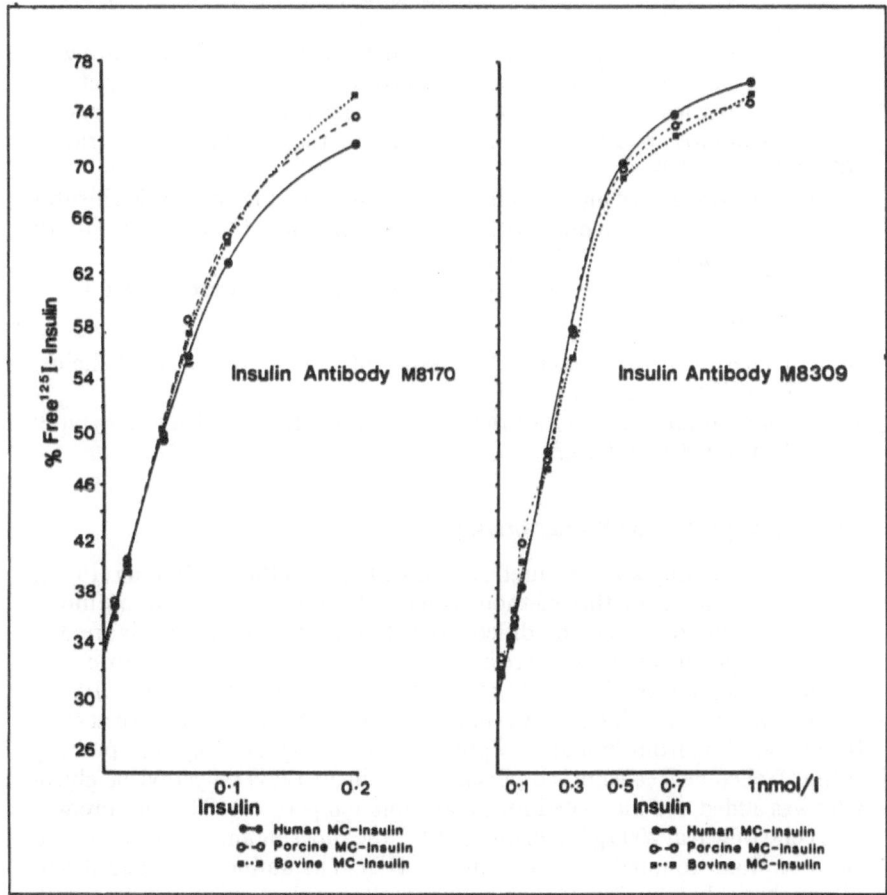

Figure 3.2 Insulin radioimmunoassay: standard curves of human, porcine and bovine insulin using two different antisera

mixture incubated for a further 18h at 4°C. Free and bound insulin were separated by adding rabbit anti-guinea pig precipitating serum (Wellcome Reagents Ltd., Beckenham) made up in 3% (w/v) polyethylene glycol 6000 (BDH Chemicals Ltd., Poole). The mixture was incubated for 2h at room temperature and then centrifuged at 2000 g for 30 min at 4°C. The tubes were decanted and the precipitate counted on a Minigamma counter (LKB Instruments Ltd., Croydon).

The concentration of insulin (IRI) in the plasma was calculated from a standard curve prepared with human insulin standard (Novo Research Institute, Copenhagen), diluted in plasma stripped of insulin by charcoal, in a range from 0 to 1.55 nmol/l, which was included in every assay. Human, porcine and bovine insulin reacted identically with the anti-porcine-insulin antibodies M8170 and M8309 in the insulin radioimmunoassay (Figure 3.2). Dilution of the antibody and ^{125}I-insulin for use in the assay was made in phosphate buffer pH 7.4 and the samples assayed in duplicate. Non-specific binding was <5%. Quality control samples were included at the beginning and end of each assay. The within and between batch coefficient of variation was determined as 4.6% and 7.3%, respectively. The detection limit of immunoreactive insulin was 0.022 nmol/l and the sensitivity (SD within-assay) was 0.009 nmol/l, based on the initial part of the standard curve (range 0.022–0.093 nmol/l).

The detection limit of immunoreactive insulin, using the unmodified insulin radioimmunoassay of Heding (1972), was 0.0062 nmol/l and the sensitivity (SD within-assay) was 0.0025 nmol/l.

The radioimmunoassays of insulin for different studies were carried out in two laboratories:

(a)   Department of Medicine, University of Wales College of Medicine, Cardiff, using the modified RIA.
(b)   Immunological Laboratories of Dr. L. G. Heding, Novo Research Institute, Copenhagen.

3.2.3   C-peptide radioimmunoassays

The C-peptide assay was measured according to the method of Heding (1975), and a modification of this method using a PEG assisted second antibody separation procedure. The modified procedure is represented in Figure 3.3. Plasma samples or standards were incubated for 6h at room temperature with the anti-C-peptide antibody M1230. ^{125}I-labelled synthetic human Tyr-C-peptide solution was added and the mixture incubated for a further 18h at 4°C. To separate free from bound C-peptide, rabbit anti-guinea pig precipitating serum (Wellcome Reagents Ltd., Beckenham) in 3% (w/v) polyethylene glycol 6000 was added and incubated for 2h at room temperature. The mixture was then centrifuged at 2000 g for 30 min at 4°C, the supernatant decanted off and the precipitate counted in a γ-counter (LKB). The antibody, standard and ^{125}I-synthetic human Tyr-C-peptide were all supplied by Novo Research Institute, Copenhagen.

A standard curve was freshly made and included in every assay, using

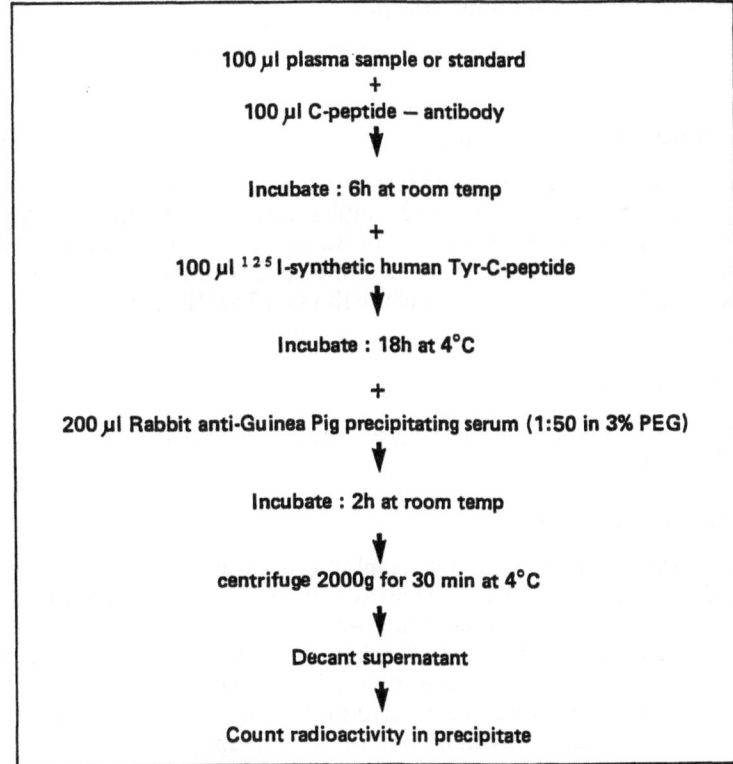

100 µl plasma sample or standard
+
100 µl C-peptide — antibody
↓

Incubate : 6h at room temp

+

100 µl ^{125}I-synthetic human Tyr-C-peptide
↓

Incubate : 18h at 4°C

+

200 µl Rabbit anti-Guinea Pig precipitating serum (1:50 in 3% PEG)
↓

Incubate : 2h at room temp
↓

centrifuge 2000g for 30 min at 4°C
↓

Decant supernatant
↓

Count radioactivity in precipitate

Figure 3.3   Double antibody C-peptide radioimmunoassay

synthetic human C-peptide in the range 0–2.5 nmol/l in charcoal-treated plasma. All other reagents were diluted in phosphate buffer pH 7.4 and the samples were assayed in duplicate.

Quality control samples were included at the beginning and end of each assay. The within and between assay coefficient of variation was calculated at 5.4 and 8.8%, respectively. The non-specific binding was 2.5%. The detection limit of the assay was 0.035 nmol/l and the sensitivity (SD within assay) 0.015 nmol/l. Using the unmodified C-peptide assay of Heding (1975), the detection limit was 0.01 nmol/l and the sensitivity 0.004 nmol/l.

The radioimmunoassays of C-peptide for different studies were carried out in two laboratories:

(a)   Department of Medicine, University of Wales College of Medicine, Cardiff, using the modified RIA described above.

(b)   Immunological Laboratories of Dr. L. G. Heding, Novo Research Institute, Copenhagen.

The cross-reactivity of the anti-C-peptide antisera (M1230, M1221) with proinsulin was approximately 10%, therefore no prior separation of proinsulin was felt necessary in the context of the studies (Faber et al, 1978).

3.2.4 Glucagon radioimmunoassays

Glucagon was assayed according to the methods described by Heding (1971) and Alford et al (1977).

3.2.5 Growth hormone assays

Growth hormone was measured by a sensitive double antibody radioimmunoassay (Boden and Soeldner, 1976). The samples were assayed against standards derived from a reference preparation of human growth hormone (66/217 – National Institute of Biological Standards and Control, London). The procedure is fully automated by use of the Kemtek 3000 (Kemble Instruments, Burgess Hill).

3.2.6 Cortisol assay

Plasma cortisol was measured using a simple competitive protein binding assay (Baum et al, 1974).

3.2.7 Adrenaline assay

A radiometric-enzymatic assay was employed to measure plasma adrenaline (Da Prada and Zürcher, 1976). The assay is based on the 3-o-methylation of catecholamines by the enzyme catechol-o-methyl-transferase (COMT), in the presence of labelled S-adenosyl-methionine (^{3}H-SAM) which acts as a methyl donor. Sodium tetraphenylborate is used as a complexing agent for the labelled o-methylated products extracted into diethyl ether. The products of the reaction are separated by thin-layer chromatography.

3.2.8 Intermediary metabolite assays

Perchloric acid extracts of blood were assayed for lactate, alanine, glycerol and 3-hydroxybutyrate according to the enzymatic fluorometric automated analysis of Lloyd et al (1978).

Lactate assay

The lactate measurements were based on the reaction:

$$\text{Lactate} + \text{NAD}^+ \xrightleftharpoons[\text{dehydrogenase}]{\text{Lactate}} \text{pyruvate} + \text{NADH} + \text{H}^+$$

Buffer: 0.5M glycine buffer, pH 0.6, was prepared containing 0.2 mol of hydrazine and 2g of disodium ethylenediaminetetracetate per litre. The enzyme–coenzyme reagent was prepared with 20 mg of NAD and 400 U of lactate dehydrogenase in 10 ml of 0.1 mol/litre phosphate buffer, pH 7.5.

Alanine assay

The assay uses L-alanine dehydrogenase which catalyses the reversible reaction:

$$\text{L-alanine} + NAD^+ + H_2O \rightleftharpoons \text{pyruvate} + NADH + NH_4^+$$

Buffer: 40 mol/litre tris (hydroxymethyl) methylamine buffer, pH 10, was made up containing 1 mol of hydrazine and 500 mg of disodium ethylene-diaminetetracetate per litre. The enzyme–coenzyme reagent was prepared with 20 mg of NAD^+, and 15 or 45 U of L-alanine dehydrogenase in 10 ml 0.1 mol/litre phosphate buffer, pH 7.4.

Glycerol assay

The assay for plasma glycerol levels is based on the reactions:

$$\text{L-glycerol} + ATP \xrightarrow{\text{glycerokinase}} \text{L-glycerol-l-phosphate} + ADP$$

$$\text{L-glycerol-l-phosphate} + NAD^+ \underset{\text{dehydrogenase}}{\overset{\text{glycerol-3-phosphate}}{\rightleftharpoons}} \text{hydroxyacetone phosphate} + NADH + H^+$$

Buffer: 0.2 M glycine buffer was prepared and 1 mol of hydrazine, and 0.01 ml of magnesium chloride per litre were added. The enzyme–coenzyme reagent was prepared by dissolving 20 mg of NAD^+, 20 mg of ATP, 20 U of glycerokinase and 30 U of glycerol-3-phosphate dehydrogenase in 10 ml of 0.4 M triethanolamine buffer, pH 7.4

3-hydroxybutyrate assay

The assay is based on the following reaction catalysed by 3-hydroxybutyrate dehydrogenase:

$$\text{3-hydroxybutyrate} + NAD^+ \rightleftharpoons \text{acetoacetate} + NADH + H^+$$

Buffer: 0.1 M tris (hydroxymethyl) methylamine buffer, pH 9.0, was prepared containing 500 mg/l of disodium ethylenediaminetetracetate. The enzyme-coenzyme reagent was prepared by dissolving 20 mg of NAD^+ and 1.5 U of 3-hydroxybutyrate dehydrogenase in 10 ml 0.1 M phosphate buffer, pH, 7.4.

3.2.9 Insulin antibody assay

The determination of insulin antibody levels was made according to the method described by Reeves and Kelly (1980).

4
Clinical–Pharmacological Studies

4.1 'SHORT-ACTING' INSULIN PREPARATIONS

Introduction

During 1979 sufficient amounts of 'semi-synthetic' human insulin produced by enzymatic conversion of porcine insulin (Markussen, 1980) became available for pre-clinical toxicity and general pharmacological studies in animals. No real difference was found between the effects of human and porcine insulin (Gamst-Andersen et al, 1983; Jørgensen et al, 1983). Following the satisfactory completion of these studies, human insulin prepared to monocomponent specifications (Schlichtkrull et al, 1970, 1974) became available for clinical evaluation during August 1980.

The first series of clinical–pharmacological studies were therefore primarily conducted for the purpose of assessing the safety and efficacy of 'semi-synthetic' human insulin in man following subcutaneous (sc), intravenous (iv) and intramuscular (im) administration. For comparative purposes, equivalent formulations of porcine and bovine insulin were also included in the studies, which were conducted both with and without the concomitant use of somatostatin.

Study Ref Nos.	Insulin Species			Dose (U/kg)			Route of admin			Concomitant somatostatin
	H	P	B	0.05	0.075	0.15	sc	im	iv	
4.1.1	x	x			x		x			x
4.1.2	x	x	x		x		x			x
4.1.3	x	x			x		x			0
4.1.5	x	x	x	x	x	x	x			0
4.1.6	x				x			x	x	x
4.1.7	x	x	x		x			x	x	0
4.1.8	x*	x					x		x*	0

H = 'Semi-synthetic' human; * + 'biosynthetic' human; P = porcine; B = bovine neutral, soluble insulin

Figure 4.1 Schematic summary of studies involving 'short-acting' insulin preparations

The initial studies of the 'short-acting' insulins allowed the influence of species, route of administration, and somatostatin on the metabolic and hormonal responses to exogenous insulin in man to be examined. The studies are summarised with respect to insulin species, dosage, route of administration and the use or not of somatostatin, in Figure 4.1.

4.1.1 Study of safety and efficacy of human insulin in normal man

The main purpose of this first clinical–pharmacological study was to assess the safety of 'semi-synthetic' human insulin relative to its porcine counterpart (Actrapid MC), and to see if it possessed any advantages over porcine insulin following subcutaneous administration to normal man.

Subjects, materials and methods

Six male subjects aged 28–37 years within 10% of ideal body weight were entered into the study (Table 4.1).

Table 4.1

Subjects No./initials		Age (years)	Height (cm)	Weight (kg)	*Percentage of ideal body weight	Insulin dose U	U/kg
1	KJ	31	183	78	103	6	0.077
2	DO	37	179	72.6	102	6	0.083
3	GJ	31	178	75	107	6	0.080
4	JB	29	180	79.4	106	6	0.076
5	CB	36	165	59	102	5	0.085
6	CD	28	175	69.5	101	6	0.086

*Metropolitan Life Insurance Company Tables (1960)

Materials

The two highly purified insulins used in the study were (i) neutral, soluble 'semi-synthetic' human insulin (Actrapid HM): and (ii) neutral, soluble porcine insulin (Actrapid MC) (Table 4.2). Actrapid diluent was used in the control studies. Cyclic somatostatin (Bachem, Los Angeles, USA) was used to suppress endogenous insulin secretion (Alberti et al, 1973; Mortimer et al, 1974; Giustina et al, 1975; Guillemin and Gerich, 1976).

Table 4.2

	Actrapid HM (human)	Actrapid MC (porcine)	Actrapid diluent	Somatostatin
Nitrogen (mg/ml)	0.190	0.217	—	—
Potency[a] (IU/ml)	35.2	40.15	—	—

[a]Theoretical potency: 185 IU/mgN

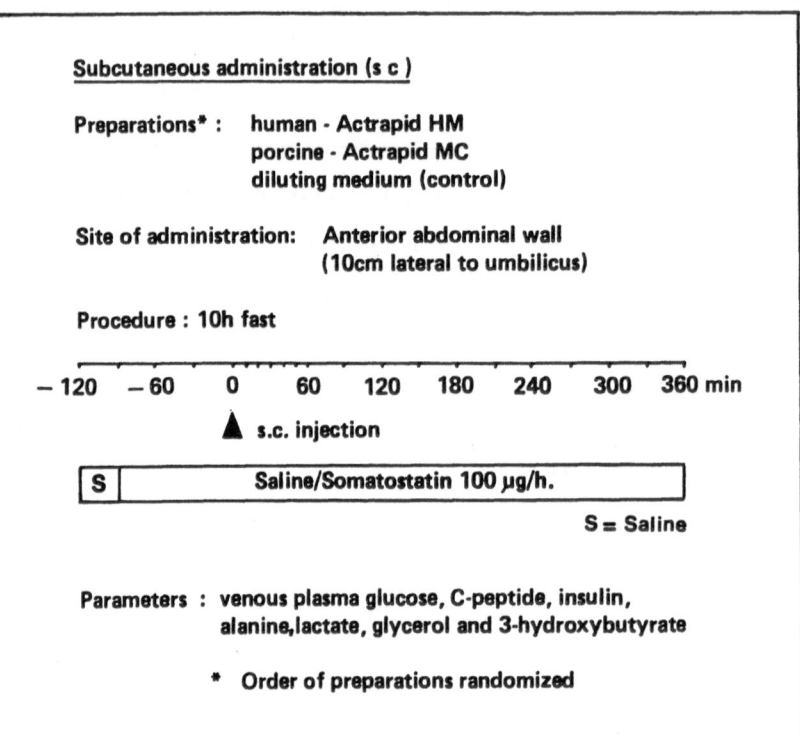

Figure 4.2 Study protocol

Methods

Each volunteer subject was studied on three separate occasions with an interval of 3–14 days between successive tests. On the study day, following a 10 h overnight fast, a cannula was sited into an antecubital vein kept patent by a slow running infusion of N saline (0.154 mmol/l). A second intravenous cannula was inserted into the opposite arm and after 30 min somatostatin infusion (100 μg/h) was commenced (−90 min) and continued throughout the study (Figure 4.2). At the end of a 2h basal period, either human insulin, porcine insulin or diluting medium was administered by bolus subcutaneous injection, using a Plastipak SFP 1 ml syringe (Becton-Dickinson), into the anterior abdominal wall midway between the umbilicus and anterior superior iliac spine. The dose of the insulins was 5 or 6 U, i.e. approximately 0.075 U/kg body weight, with an equal volume of diluting medium being used during the control days. Venous blood samples were obtained half-hourly during the basal period, every 10 min for the first hour after subcutaneous injection, and thereafter every 30 min up to 360 min.

At each time point aliquots were taken into fluoride for plasma glucose determination (hexokinase), and also heparin for the measurement of

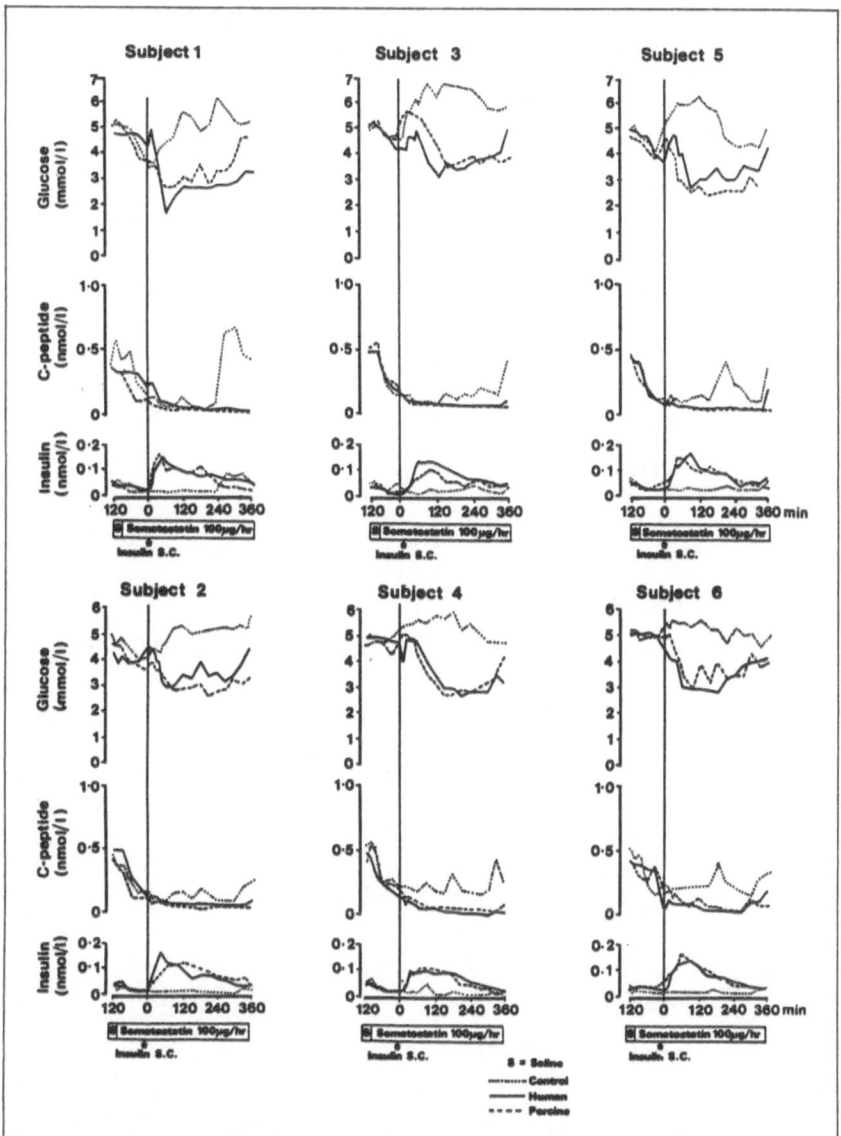

Figure 4.3   Effect of human and porcine insulins on plasma glucose, C-peptide and insulin (IRI) concentrations in each of the six volunteer subjects. Somatostatin infused from –90 to 360 min. Insulin (~0.075 U/kg) or diluent given subcutaneously (sc) at time 0

immunoreactive insulin (IRI) (Heding, 1972) and C-peptide (Heding, 1975), and 0.5 ml into 2 ml 3% (w/v) perchloric acid for the estimation of lactate, alanine, glycerol and 3-hydroxybutyrate concentrations (Lloyd et al, 1978). Within 5 min of sampling the samples were centrifuged and the supernatants stored at –20°C until assay.

Statistical methods

The results are expressed as means ±SE except where stated otherwise. Concentrations of 3-hydroxybutyrate were log transformed to normalise

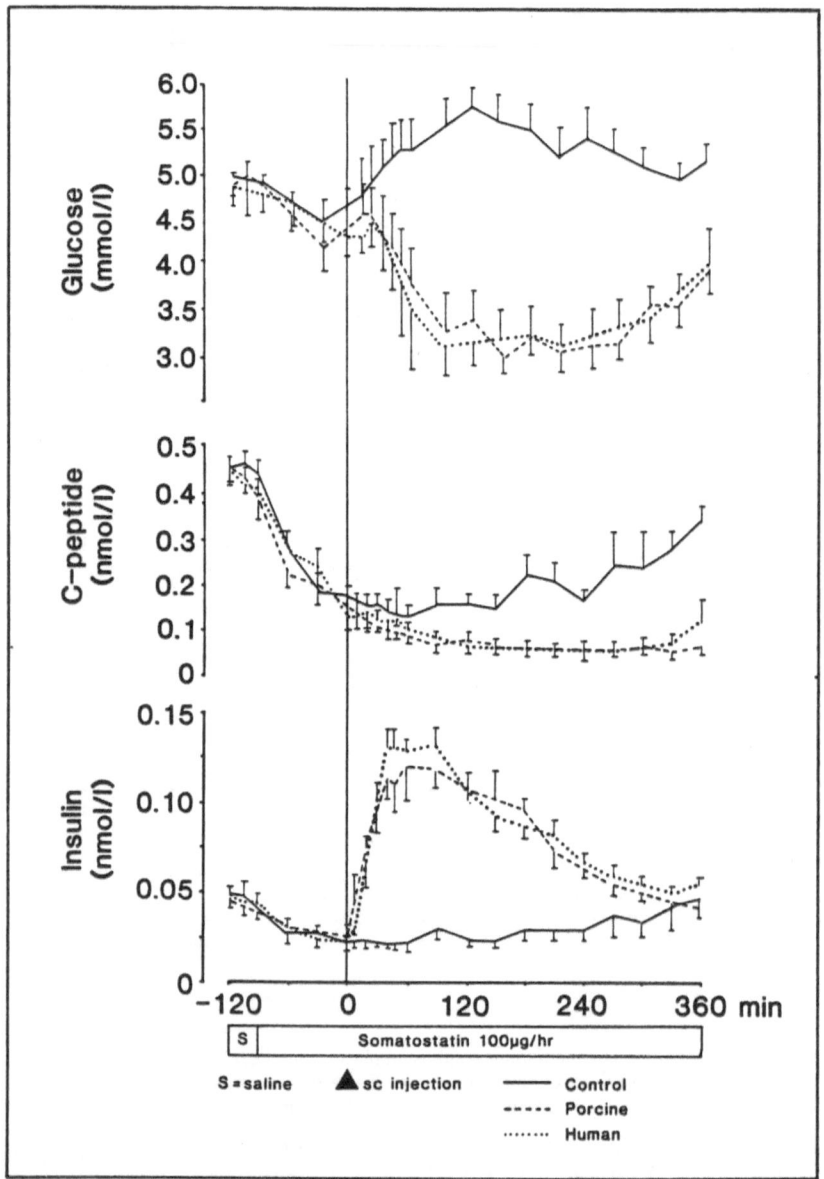

Figure 4.4 Effect of human and porcine insulins on plasma glucose, C-peptide and insulin (IRI) concentrations (means ± SE) in six subjects. Somatostatin infused from −90 to 360 min. Insulin (∼0.075 U/kg) or diluent (control) given subcutaneously (sc) at time 0

distribution (Foster et al, 1978). Individual pairs of treatments were compared using paired analysis of variance. The computer program used was the Statistical Package for the Social Sciences.

Results

None of the subjects experienced any adverse local or systemic reactions to either insulin preparation or the diluting medium.

Figure 4.3 shows the plasma glucose, C-peptide and insulin levels for each subject when infused with somatostatin and given subcutaneous bolus injections of diluent (control preparation), human insulin and porcine insulin. The individual curves demonstrate occasional interruptions in the somatostatin infusion due to pump malfunction. The mean ± SEM plasma glucose, C-peptide and insulin values for the six subjects are shown in Figure 4.4. Comparison of the effect of human and porcine insulins on plasma glucose, C-peptide and insulin (IRI) are represented in Figure 4.5 as means of differences (with 95% confidence limits) between responses to the two insulins.

The basal fasting plasma glucose levels were similar in the three study periods. During this pre-insulin period somatostatin caused a fall in plasma glucose of approximately 0.4 mmol/l. In the control study day this initial fall was followed by a rise to 5.8 ± 0.2 mmol/l at 120 min followed by a slow decline to 5.1 ± 0.1 mmol/l by the end of the study (Figure 4.3). Approximately 30 min after subcutaneous administration of human and porcine insulin the plasma glucose level started to fall rapidly, reaching a nadir of 3.1 ± 0.3 and 2.9 ± 0.1 mmol/l at 90 and 150 min, respectively. Over the remainder of the study the plasma glucose levels slowly recovered to within 1.5 mmol/l of control values at 360 min. From 30 min after injection of both insulins the glucose levels were significantly lower than controls ($p<0.05$–0.001). There was no difference, however, in the glucose response to human and porcine insulin throughout the study period (Figure 4.5).

The C-peptide concentration decreased from 0.45 ± 0.05 nmol/l to 0.15 ± 0.03 nmol/l during the first 90 min of the somatostatin infusion (Figure 4.4). During the control study the C-peptide level continued to fall, reaching a nadir of 0.13 ± 0.03 nmol/l at 60–90 min, followed by a gradual increase reaching a value of 0.34 ± 0.03 nmol/l by the end of the study. This later response may be partly due to the interruption of the somatostatin infusion in two of the subjects. The plasma C-peptide concentrations after insulin were significantly lower than after the diluent, from 30 min with porcine insulin and 120 min with human insulin. The C-peptide values remained between 0.04 and 0.06 nmol/l from 120 to 330 min during the insulin studies (Figure 4.4). There was no significant difference between the plasma C-peptide concentrations after human and porcine insulin (Figure 4.5).

During the control study the initial plasma insulin concentration of 0.04 ± 0.003 nmol/l fell to 0.022 ± 0.001 nmol/l after 90 min of somatostatin. Thereafter the values remained low (0.02 ± 0.001 – 0.027 ± 0.05 nmol/l) up to 270 min before reverting to fasting values at 360 min. Subcutaneous injection of human insulin resulted in a rapid rise in plasma insulin concentrations, from a pre-injection level of 0.02 ± 0.002 nmol/l reaching a peak of about 0.132

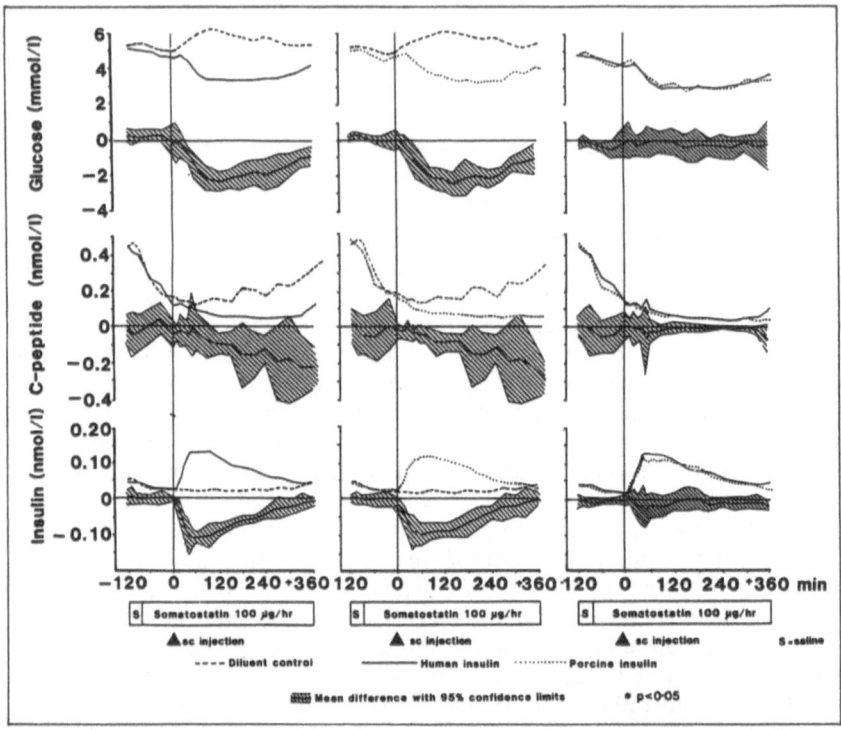

Figure 4.5 Comparison of effect of human and porcine insulins and diluent (control) on plasma glucose, C-peptide and insulin (IRI) concentrations in six subjects. Somatostatin infused from –90 to 360 min. Insulin (~0.075 U/kg) or diluent (control) given subcutaneously (sc) at time 0. Results shown as means and means of differences (with 95% confidence limits) between responses to the two insulins and diluent (human minus control, porcine minus control and porcine minus human)

nmol/l after 90 min, and then decreasing slowly to a value of 0.052 ± 0.005 nmol/l at the end of the study (Figure 4.4). The plasma insulin levels were significantly higher than controls from 10 min onwards ($p<0.05$–0.001). In comparison, after porcine insulin, peak insulin concentrations of approximately 0.12 nmol/l were reached between 40 and 120 min after injection. The values were also significantly higher than controls from 10 min after insulin administration. The peak insulin concentration observed with porcine insulin was 0.118 ± 0.01 nmol/l at 60 min. A significant difference ($p<0.05$) in the plasma insulin values between the two species of insulin was observed at 360 min only, with a higher concentration after human insulin (Figure 4.5).

There was considerable intra- and inter-individual variations in the intermediary metabolite values. In general, the blood 3-hydroxybutyrate and glycerol concentrations increased during the somatostatin infusion prior to insulin injections. During the control study the 3-hydroxybutyrate concentrations continued to rise, whereas after each insulin the concentrations promptly fell, reaching a nadir at 180 min (Table 4.3; Figure 4.6), with no consistent differences between the two insulins. Thereafter, a pronounced post-hypoglycaemic rise in 3-hydroxybutyrate levels was observed. The increased blood glycerol concentrations fell reaching minimum values at 40–90 min and 60–180 min with porcine and human insulin, respectively. Subsequently, in contrast to 3-hydroxybutyrate, there was no marked post-hypoglycaemic rise in blood glycerol levels (Table 4.3; Figure 4.6).

Table 4.3 Intermediary metabolite values in normal man given highly purified human and porcine insulin (n = 6)

	3-Hydroxybutyrate (mmol/l)		Glycerol (mmol/l)	
	Porcine	Human	Porcine	Human
Basal				
mean	0.020	0.065	0.045	0.088
range	0.005–0.055	0.020–0.175	0.005–0.085	0.010–0.225
Pre-injection				
mean	0.170	0.305	0.115	0.185
range	0.025–0.390	0.045–0.735	0.050–0.165	0.130–0.325
Nadir*				
mean	0.020	0.075	0.045	0.055
range	0.005–0.050	0.020–0.20	0.020–0.090	0.030–0.085
360 min				
mean	0.395	0.370	0.115	0.095
range	0.045–1.060	0.080–0.615	0.075–0.170	0.055–0.140

* 3-Hydroxybutyrate: porcine insulin 150–180 min; human insulin 180 min
* Glycerol: porcine insulin 40–90 min; human insulin 60–180 min

Discussion

In this study the reference neutral, soluble porcine insulin and the new human insulin preparation (Markussen, 1980) were well tolerated, with no unwanted local or systemic effects observed. The experimental model used to assess the response to insulin involved a low-dose intravenous infusion of somatostatin (100 μg/h) to suppress endogenous insulin secretion (Alberti et al, 1973; Mortimer et al, 1974; Guillemin and Gerich, 1976). Suppression was achieved as demonstrated by the C-peptide response. A further lowering of C-peptide concentrations was observed following insulin injection, suggesting either an additional direct suppression of insulin secretion (Schatz and Pfeiffer, 1977) or, more likely, that endogenous pancreatic beta-cell secretion was further depressed due to the associated hypoglycaemia (Horwitz et al, 1975). Therefore, with the use of somatostatin, the plasma insulin profiles reflected more precisely the absorption and elimination characteristics of the injected insulins.

After subcutaneous administration of human and porcine insulin into the anterior abdominal wall the plasma insulin concentrations increased rapidly, becoming significantly higher than control values from 10 min onwards and reaching peak levels between 90 and 120 min. The plasma insulin profiles for the two insulins were similar, suggesting similarities in local (absorption) and systemic clearance rates. The plasma glucose lowering effect was also identical

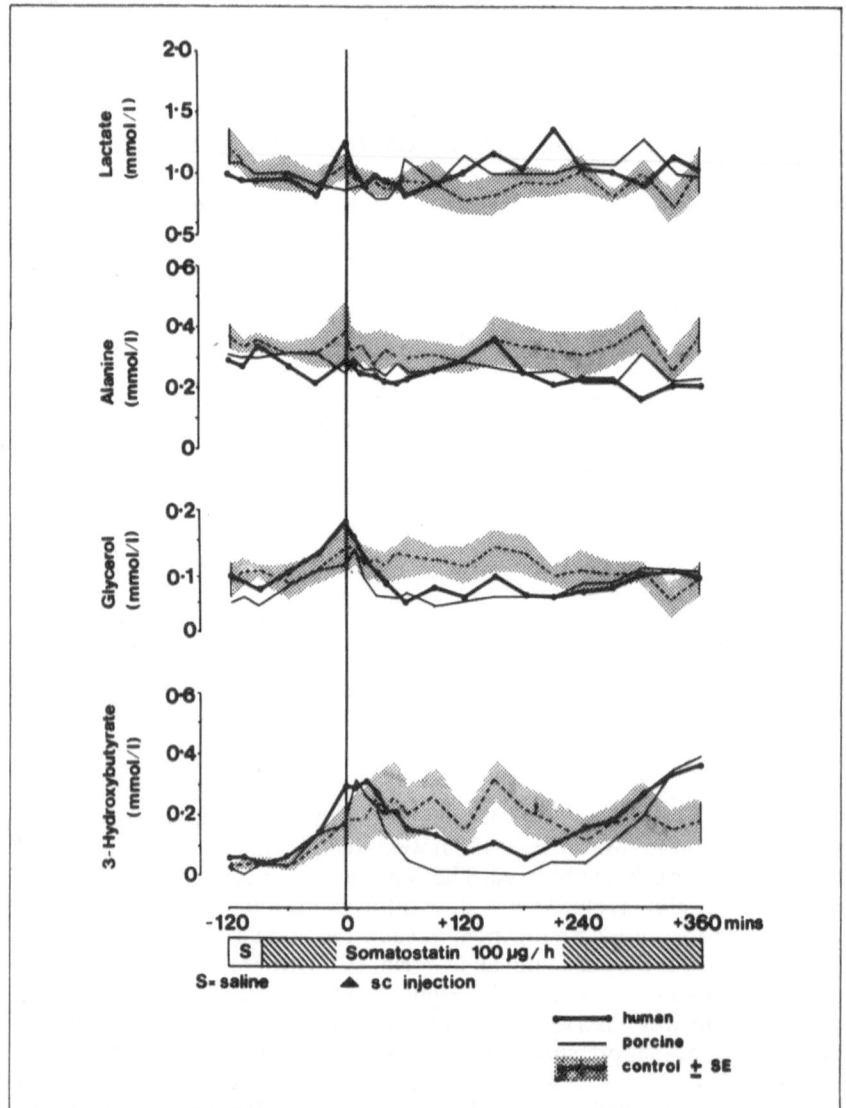

Figure 4.6 Effect of human and porcine insulin on blood lactate, alanine, glycerol and 3-hydroxybutyrate concentrations (means) in six subjects. Somatostatin infused from –90 to 360 min. Insulin (~0.075 U/kg) or diluent (control) given subcutaneously at time 0. Results for control shown as means ± SE

for the two species of insulin. In view of the fact that somatostatin can influence the secretion of other hormones (Assan, 1976; Gerich, 1981) and diminish splanchnic blood flow (Felig and Wahren, 1976), no firm physiological extrapolations can be made. Laube and co-workers (1981a, b) also observed similar plasma insulin profiles in normal subjects following subcutaneous injections into the abdominal region of porcine and 'semi-synthetic' human Actrapid insulin, although they observed an earlier and more pronounced hypoglycaemic effect with human insulin. In contrast, significantly higher plasma insulin levels and a greater hypoglycaemic response have been observed with 'semi-synthetic' human Actrapid insulin than its porcine counterpart following injections into the thigh (Sundermann et al, 1981).

Using *E. coli*-derived human insulin in normal man, Keen et al (1980) also failed to show any real differences in the plasma glucose lowering effect of porcine and human insulins following subcutaneous injection into the anterior abdominal wall.

It is seen that, under the experimental conditions described, the hypoglycaemic 'potency' and timing of effect of 'semi-synthetic' human insulin is similar to its porcine counterpart when administered by subcutaneous bolus injection into the anterior abdominal wall in normal male subjects (Owens et al, 1981a).

The first study of 'semi-synthetic' human insulin in man confirmed its short-term safety and biological efficacy, thereby providing the basis upon which to explore the metabolic and hormonal response to human insulin in clinical–pharmacological studies employing different experimental models, routes and sites of administration and other pharmaceutical formulations.

4.1.2 Comparison of subcutaneous human, porcine and bovine insulin in man

Introduction

The initial study with 'semi-synthetic' human insulin involved a comparison with the equivalent pharmaceutical formulation of porcine insulin as the reference insulin (Owens et al, 1981a). Relatively recently, high-performance liquid chromatography (HPLC) has proved to be an invaluable technique for analysis of insulins (Biemond et al, 1980; Kasama et al, 1980; Szepesi and Gazdag 1981; Kroeff and Chance, 1982). The separation of bovine and porcine insulin by HPLC was achieved by Beimond et al (1979), Damgaard and Markussen (1979) and Dinner and Lorenz (1979). Terabe et al (1979) then separated human insulin from the other two species of insulin, demonstrating differences in the physicochemical behaviour of the three species of insulin used clinically. Reversed-phase high-performance liquid chromatography (RP-HPLC) can rapidly separate these and other species of insulin, even though they differ structurally by only one or two amino acid residues (Figure 4.7).

The purpose of this study, which was an extension of the first study, was to compare the glucose-lowering effect, the C-peptide response and the insulin levels, following the subcutaneous administration of the three species of neutral, soluble insulins formulated in the same way and administered at the same dose level of 6 U ($\sim$ 0.075 U/kg body weight).

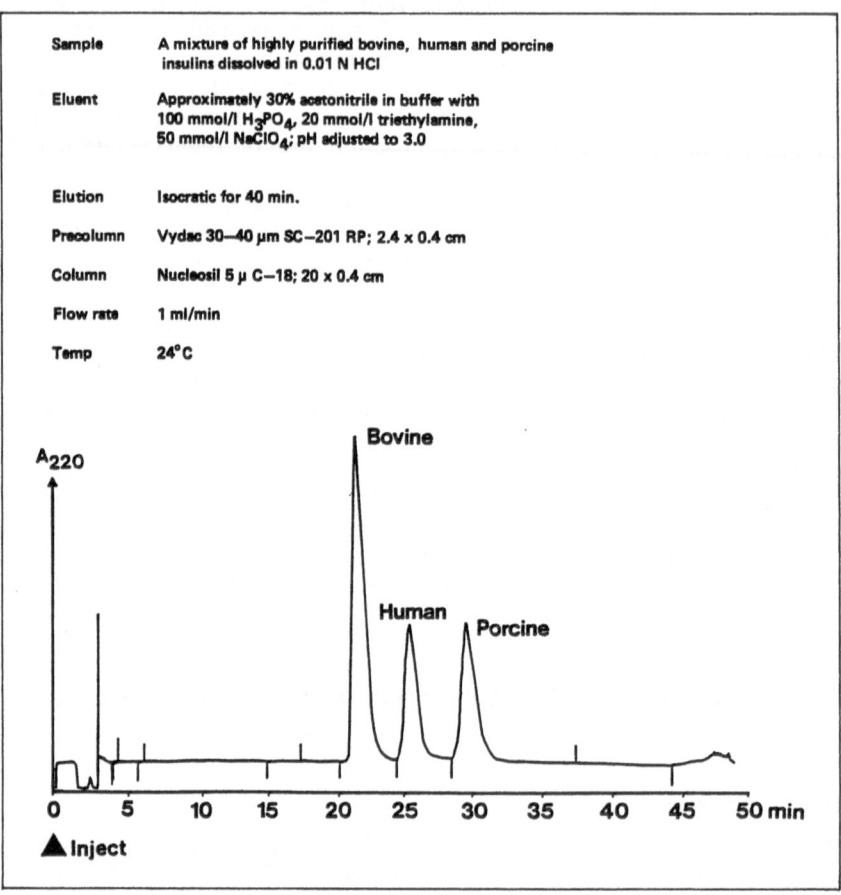

Sample	A mixture of highly purified bovine, human and porcine insulins dissolved in 0.01 N HCl
Eluent	Approximately 30% acetonitrile in buffer with 100 mmol/l H_3PO_4, 20 mmol/l triethylamine, 50 mmol/l $NaClO_4$; pH adjusted to 3.0
Elution	Isocratic for 40 min.
Precolumn	Vydac 30—40 µm SC–201 RP; 2.4 x 0.4 cm
Column	Nucleosil 5 µ C–18; 20 x 0.4 cm
Flow rate	1 ml/min
Temp	24°C

Figure 4.7 High-performance liquid chromatography (HPLC) separation of bovine, human and porcine insulins

Subjects, materials and methods

This study involved the same six subjects entered into the first study. There was an interval of 6 to 12 weeks between the two studies, during which time none of the volunteers had gained weight or taken any other medication.

Bovine insulin was prepared as a neutral, soluble preparation, purified to monocomponent specifications: nitrogen content 0.215 mg/ml, with a potency of 39.8 IU/ml (theoretical potency 185 IU/mgN).

The study protocol was exactly as for the first study (cf. 4.1.1).

Results

The mean plasma glucose, C-peptide and insulin concentrations for the bovine, porcine and human insulin study days are shown in Figure 4.8. The

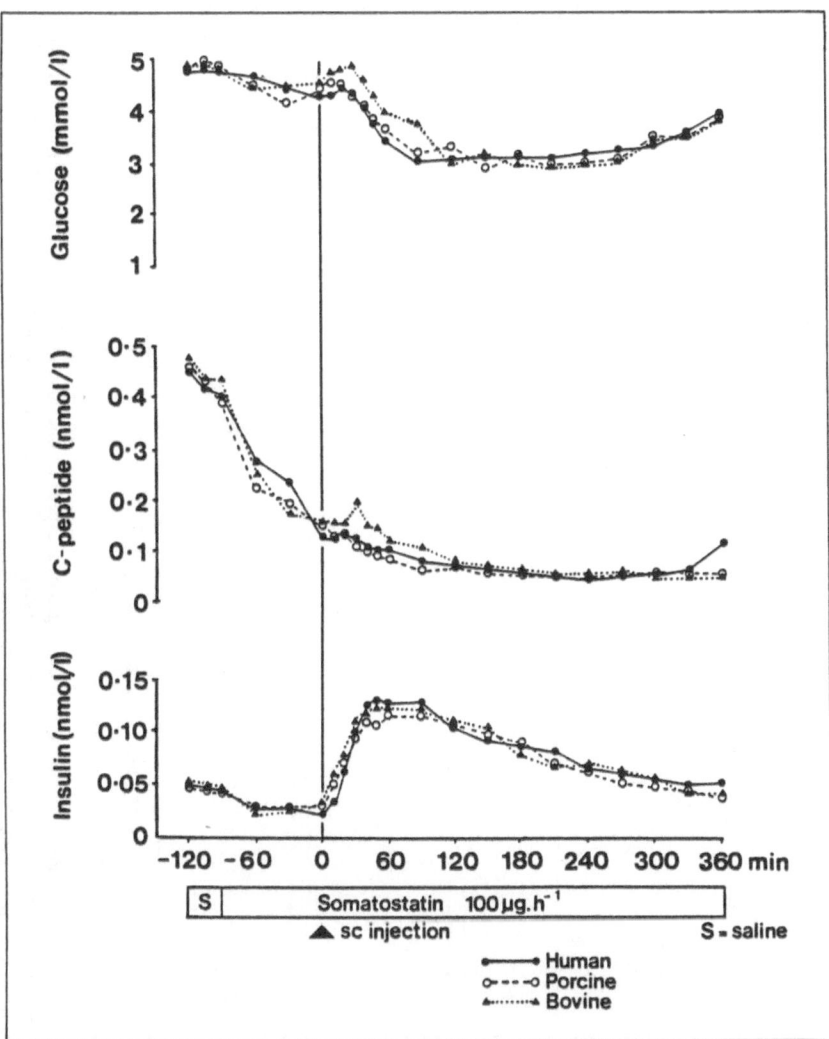

Figure 4.8 Effect of human, porcine and bovine insulins on plasma glucose, C-peptide and insulin (IRI) concentrations (means) in six subjects. Somatostatin infused from –90 to 360 min. Insulin (~0.075 U/kg) injected subcutaneously (sc) at time 0

mean basal (pre-somatostatin) plasma glucose value (–120 to –90 min) was similar for each of the comparative study periods, i.e. about 4.9 mmol/l. The somatostatin infusion lowered the plasma glucose by approximately 0.4 mmol/l after 90 min. After the injection of porcine and human insulin the expected secondary rise in glucose levels was halted between 10 and 20 min after administration, with the glucose lowered below pre-injection levels by 30 and 40 min, respectively. After bovine insulin, however, the plasma glucose continued to increase from 4.6 ± 0.3 mmol/l reaching 4.9 ± 0.2 mmol/l at 30 min,

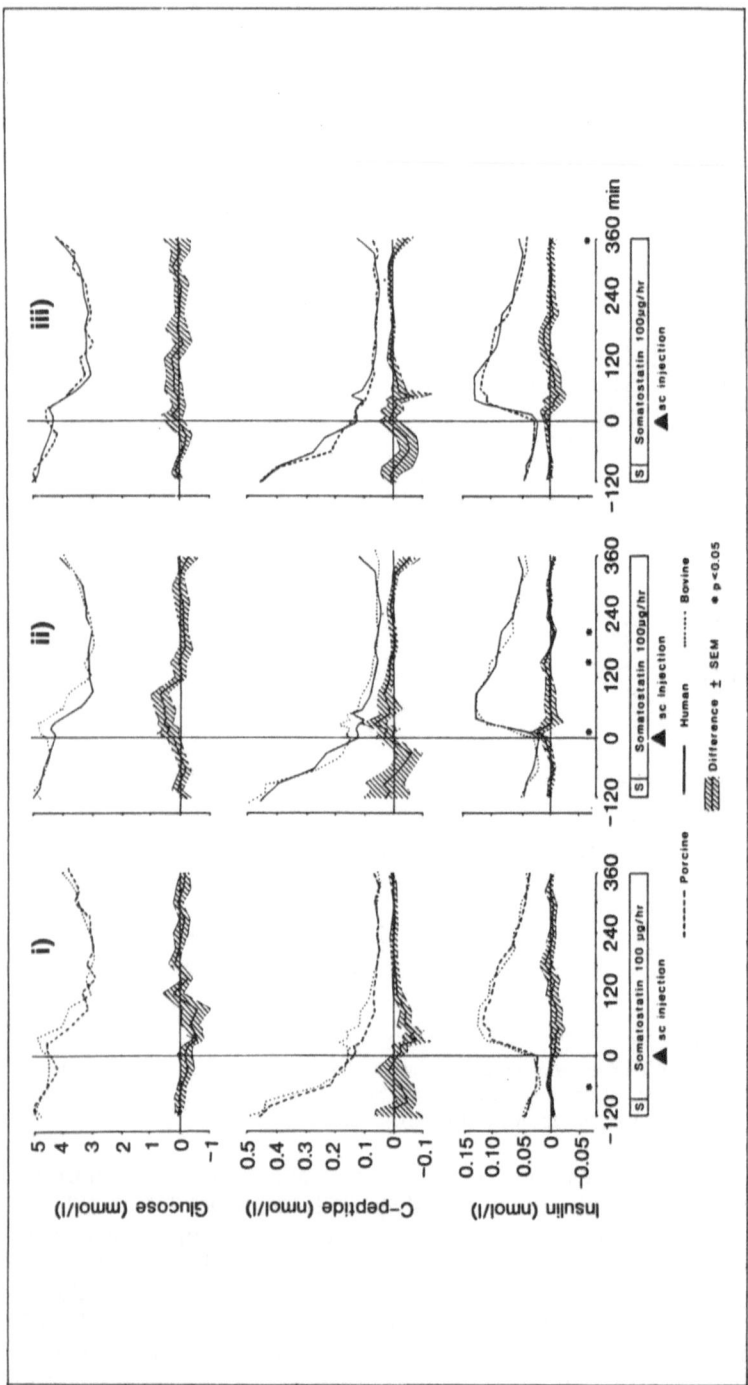

Figure 4.9 Comparison of effect of human, porcine and bovine insulins on plasma glucose, C-peptide and insulin (IRI) concentrations in six subjects. Somatostatin infused from −90 to 360 min. Insulin (~0.075 U/kg) injected subcutaneously (sc) at time 0. Results shown as means and means of differences ± 1 SE between responses to the three insulins ((i) porcine minus bovine, (ii) bovine minus human, (iii) porcine minus human)

i.e. an increment of 0.32 mmol/l, compared to 0.12 and 0.18 mmol/l following porcine and human insulin, respectively. The mean plasma glucose level remained higher on bovine than porcine or human insulin up to 120 min after subcutaneous administration. The difference only reached significance between bovine and human insulin at 30 min post-injection ($p<0.05$: Figure 4.9). Subsequently, the rate of fall of plasma glucose was similar for the three insulins, with nadir values of 2.9 ± 0.1, 3.1 ± 0.3 and 3.0 ± 0.1 mmol/l at 150, 90 and 210 min for porcine, human and bovine insulin, respectively.

Prior to insulin during the somatostatin infusion, the plasma C-peptide concentration fell from 0.44 ± 0.023 nmol/l at –90 min to 0.17 ± 0.02 nmol/l immediately prior to subcutaneous injection, i.e. a fall of approximately 60%. After insulin administration a further significant reduction in C-peptide concentration was observed from 30, 40 and 60 min onwards with porcine, human and bovine insulin, respectively. Similar nadir C-peptide levels of 0.048 ± 0.004, 0.047 ± 0.003 and 0.05 ± 0.01 nmol/l for porcine, human and bovine insulin (about 10% of basal values) were reached between 210 and 240 min after administration. There was no significant difference in the plasma C-peptide response between the three species of insulin at any time-point throughout the study (Figure 4.9).

The plasma insulin levels, after 90 min of somatostatin infusion, were similar at about 0.025 nmol/l in the three comparative groups (Figure 4.8). The subsequent injection of porcine, human and bovine insulin resulted in similar peak levels of 0.12 ± 0.01, 0.13 ± 0.01 and 0.13 ± 0.01 nmol/l at 60, 90 and 90 min, respectively. Bovine insulin gave significantly higher plasma insulin concentrations than human insulin at 10 and 150 min ($p<0.05$), and lower than human insulin at 210 min ($p<0.05$; Figure 4.9).

There was considerable intra- and inter-individual variation in the intermediary metabolite values observed in the three comparative study periods. The mean blood lactate, alanine, glycerol and 3-hydroxybutyrate concentrations are represented in Figure 4.10. No consistent change was observed in the blood lactate and alanine levels following the three insulins. In contrast, blood glycerol and 3-hydroxybutyrate levels increased during the somatostatin infusion and promptly fell with each insulin, followed by a moderate post-hypoglycaemic rise in glycerol levels and a more marked increase in 3-hydroxybutyrate levels. The glycerol and 3-hydroxybutyrate levels after porcine, human and bovine insulin are summarised in Table 4.4.

Discussion

Differences in amino acid sequence between bovine, porcine and human insulin give rise to different physicochemical properties (Biemond et al, 1979; Damgaard and Markussen, 1979; Terabe et al, 1979; Hansen et al, 1982; Kroeff and Chance, 1982). As all three species of insulin are used therapeutically, it is important to compare the response to identical formulations of these insulins.

Bioassay remains the basis for pharmacopoeial methods for determining insulin 'potency' relative to an International Standard, using different methodologies which include (i) the rabbit blood sugar twin cross-over assay

Table 4.4 Intermediary metabolite values in normal man given highly purified porcine, human and bovine insulin ($n = 6$)

	3-Hydroxybutyrate (mmol/l)			Glycerol (mmol/l)		
	Porcine	Human	Bovine	Porcine	Human	Bovine
Basal						
mean	0.020	0.065	0.085	0.045	0.088	0.107
range	0.005–0.055	0.020–0.175	0.010–0.220	0.005–0.085	0.010–0.225	0.055–0.200
Pre-injection						
mean	0.170	0.305	0.282	0.115	0.185	0.196
range	0.025–0.390	0.045–0.735	0.030–0.500	0.050–0.165	0.130–0.325	0.160–0.235
Nadir*						
mean	0.020	0.075	0.040	0.045	0.055	0.062
range	0.005–0.050	0.020–0.20	0.020–0.085	0.020–0.090	0.030–0.090	0.040–0.095
360 min						
mean	0.395	0.370	0.207	0.115	0.095	0.118
range	0.045–1.060	0.080–0.615	0.135–0.295	0.075–0.170	0.055–0.140	0.075–0.180

* 3-hydroxybutyrate: porcine insulin 150–180 min; human insulin 180 min; bovine insulin 60 min.
* Glycerol: porcine insulin 40–90 min; human insulin 60–180 min; bovine insulin 60 min

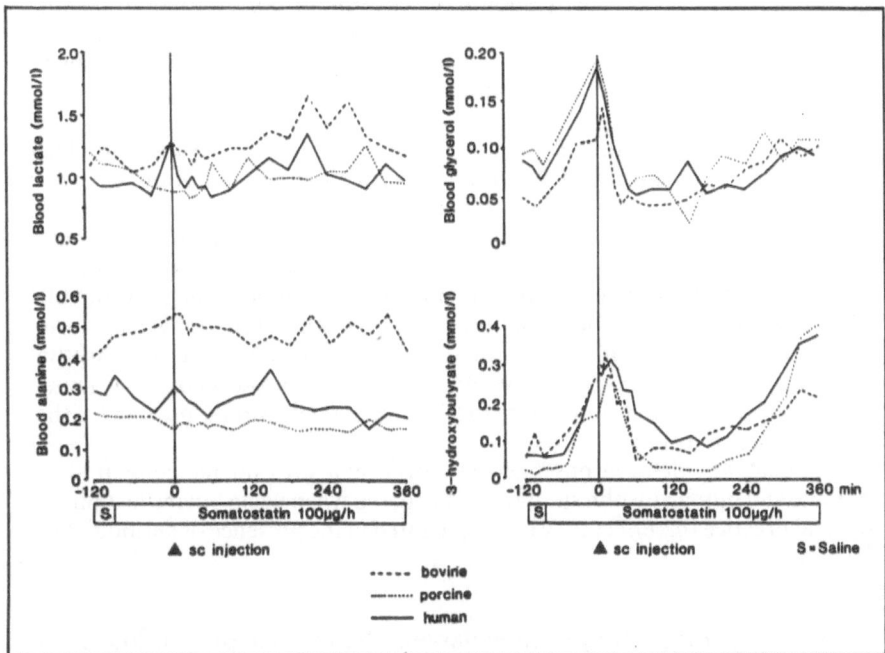

Figure 4.10 Effect of human, porcine and bovine insulins on blood lactate, alanine, glycerol and 3-hydroxybutyrate (means) in six subjects. Somatostatin infused from –90 to 360 min. Insulin (~0.075 U/kg) injected subcutaneously (sc) at time 0

accepted by the International Pharmacopoeia 1967, European Pharmacopoeia 1975, and the US Pharmacopoeia 1980; (ii) the two-dose quantal response mouse convulsion assay, European Pharmacopoeia 1975, British Pharmacopoeia 1980; and (iii) the twin cross-over blood glucose assay in mice, British Pharmacopoeia 1980. The assessment of insulin 'potency', using either the rabbit or mouse blood glucose assay, depends on the blood sampling times (Vølund et al, 1982). More recently, however, due to the high purity of insulin, it has become possible to assess 'potency' using chemical methods minimising the variation in 'potency' estimations (Pingel et al, 1982).

The results from this study in man indicate that the relative hypoglycaemic 'potency' of bovine, human and porcine neutral, soluble insulin is dependent on the sampling times, supporting earlier findings in the rabbit bioassay system (Vølund et al, 1982). Both porcine and human insulin have a quicker hypoglycaemic effect than bovine insulin, the difference reaching significance between porcine and bovine insulin at 30 min after subcutaneous injection. There was no corresponding difference in the duration of action.

Gray et al (1984) did not observe a difference in the glucose disposal rates between intravenous infusions of bovine and 'biosynthetic' human insulin using the euglycaemic clamp technique in normal subjects. The early response was not, however, specifically considered by this group. Only one previous study has compared the 'potency' of bovine and human or porcine insulins, demonstrating a more rapid response to intravenous porcine than to bovine insulin in insulin-dependent diabetics (Nosadini et al, 1981). This difference may be related to the presence of antibodies to insulin, although the binding of bovine and porcine insulin by the antibodies was not significantly different in the patients studied.

The data suggest a time-dependent 'potency' variation between porcine, human and bovine insulin in man following subcutaneous injection, whereas in the classical pharmacopoeial methods, porcine and bovine insulins have been assumed to exert similar hypoglycaemic effects. It is therefore pertinent to lend support to the concerns expressed about the validity of the rabbit bioassay method for determining the 'potency' of porcine, human or bovine insulin relative to a reference standard such as the 4th International Standard, which contains approximately an equal mixture of porcine and bovine insulin (Bangham and Mussett, 1959). Therefore, further studies are necessary in man ('human bioassay'), to fully explore the relative hypoglycaemic 'potency' of the three species of insulin.

The relatively delayed onset of hypoglycaemia with bovine compared to porcine and human insulin should be considered when using bovine insulin. In clinical practice this effect may be exaggerated in the presence of antibodies to insulin.

4.1.3 Comparative study of subcutaneous human and porcine insulin in man, without the concomitant use of somatostatin

Introduction

In the initial study (cf. 4.1.1) no differences either in bioavailability or biological effects were observed between neutral, soluble porcine and 'semi-synthetic' human monocomponent insulins in an experimental model that involved the suppression of endogenous insulin secretion by somatostatin (Owens et al, 1981a). Other investigators, also using normal subjects but without the concomitant administration of somatostatin, noted a more potent hypoglycaemic response to 'semi-synthetic' human insulin, associated either with (Sundermann et al, 1981) or without (Laube et al, 1981a, b) significantly higher plasma insulin levels.

The use of somatostatin attempts to overcome the considerable difficulties in the interpretation of in vivo studies owing to endogenous insulin release (Frost et al, 1973; Tranberg and Dencker, 1978). In normals, however, it results in a biphasic plasma glucose response consisting of an initial fall, followed by a secondary rise (Devane et al, 1974; Lins and Efendič, 1976; Sherwin et al, 1977a, b; Blauth et al, 1977). In addition, pharmacological levels of somatostatin can inhibit the secretion of a number of hormones involved in glucose counterregulation (Assan, 1976; Sherwin et al, 1977a, b), thereby enhancing insulin-induced hypoglycaemia (Gerich et al, 1974a, 1979a; Harano et al, 1977, Liljenquist et al, 1977). Somatostatin can also cause a decrease in splanchnic blood flow (Wahren and Felig, 1976), which may delay insulin degradation.

In view of the above considerations a further study was carried out to compare human and porcine insulin without the concomitant use of somatostatin.

Subjects, materials and methods

Six healthy male subjects aged 22–30 years were entered into the study which comprised three separate study days, 1–4 weeks apart.

Materials

The preparations used in the study are shown in Table 4.5. The dose of the insulin was 6 U (~0.075 U/kg body weight), with an equal volume of the Actrapid diluent being used during the control days. The preparations were administered using a Plastipak SFP 1 ml syringe (Becton–Dickinson).

Table 4.5

	Actrapid MC (porcine)	Actrapid HM (human)	Actrapid diluent
Nitrogen (mg/ml)	0.215	0.216	—
Potency[a] (IU/ml)	39.8	40.0	—

[a]Theoretical potency: 185 IU/mgN

Methods

After a 2 h basal period, human insulin, porcine insulin or diluting medium were administered (at time 0) in random order as a bolus subcutaneous injection into the anterior abdominal wall, mid-way between the umbilicus and anterior superior iliac spine. Blood samples were taken every 30 min throughout the 8 h study period with additional samples taken every 10 min during the first hour. Venous blood samples were placed in fluoride for plasma glucose estimation (hexokinase), heparin for plasma insulin (immuno-reactive) (Heding, 1972) and C-peptide determinations (Heding, 1975). For the measurement of lactate, alanine, glycerol and 3-hydroxybutyrate concentration, aliquots (0.5 ml) were taken into 2 ml 3% (w/v) perchloric acid (Lloyd et al, 1978).

Statistical methods

The results are expressed as means ± SE unless stated otherwise. The Student's paired t-test was used to determine significant differences at each time point between individual pairs of treatment. The 3-hydroxybutyrate levels were log transformed to normalise distribution (Foster et al, 1978).

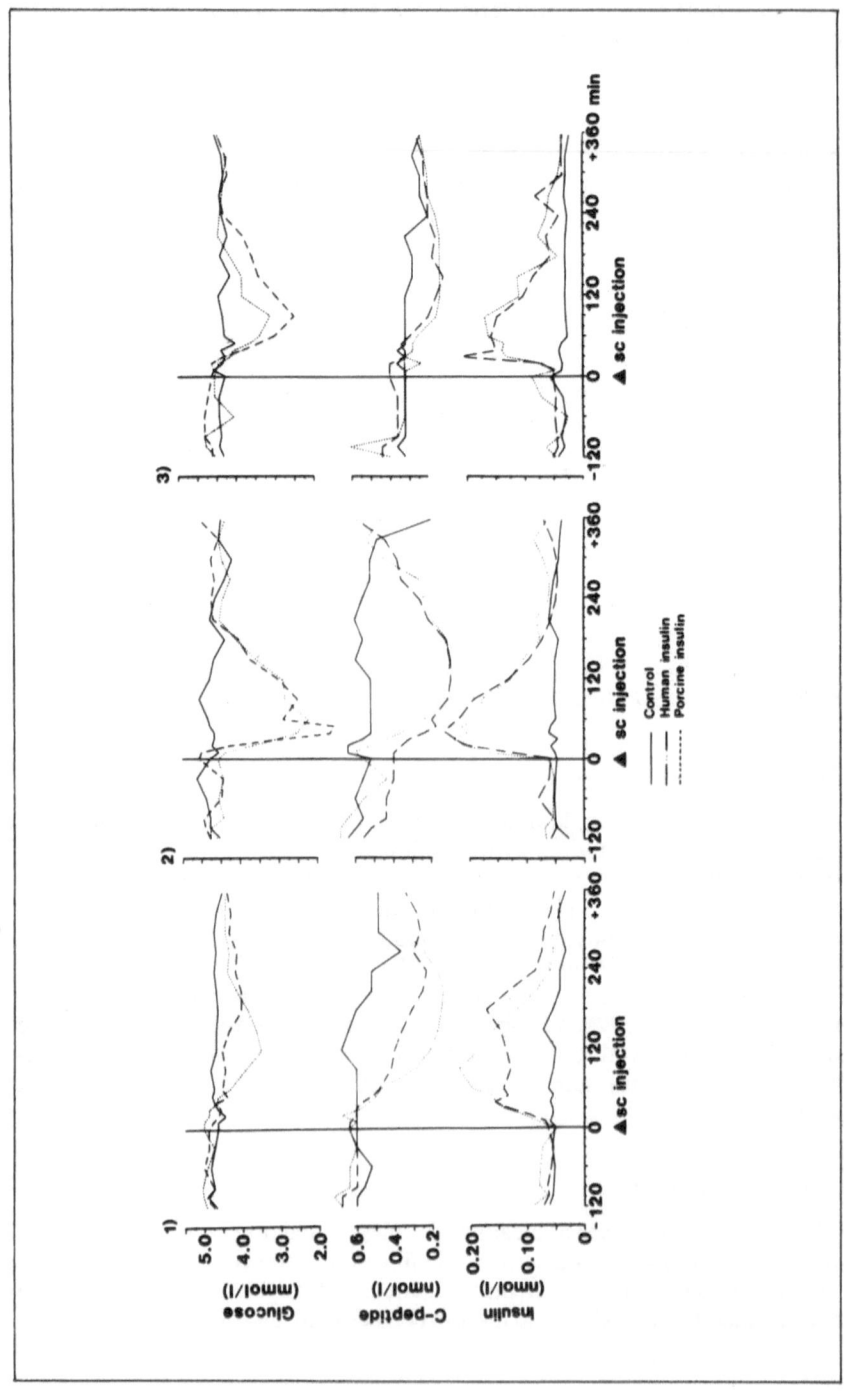

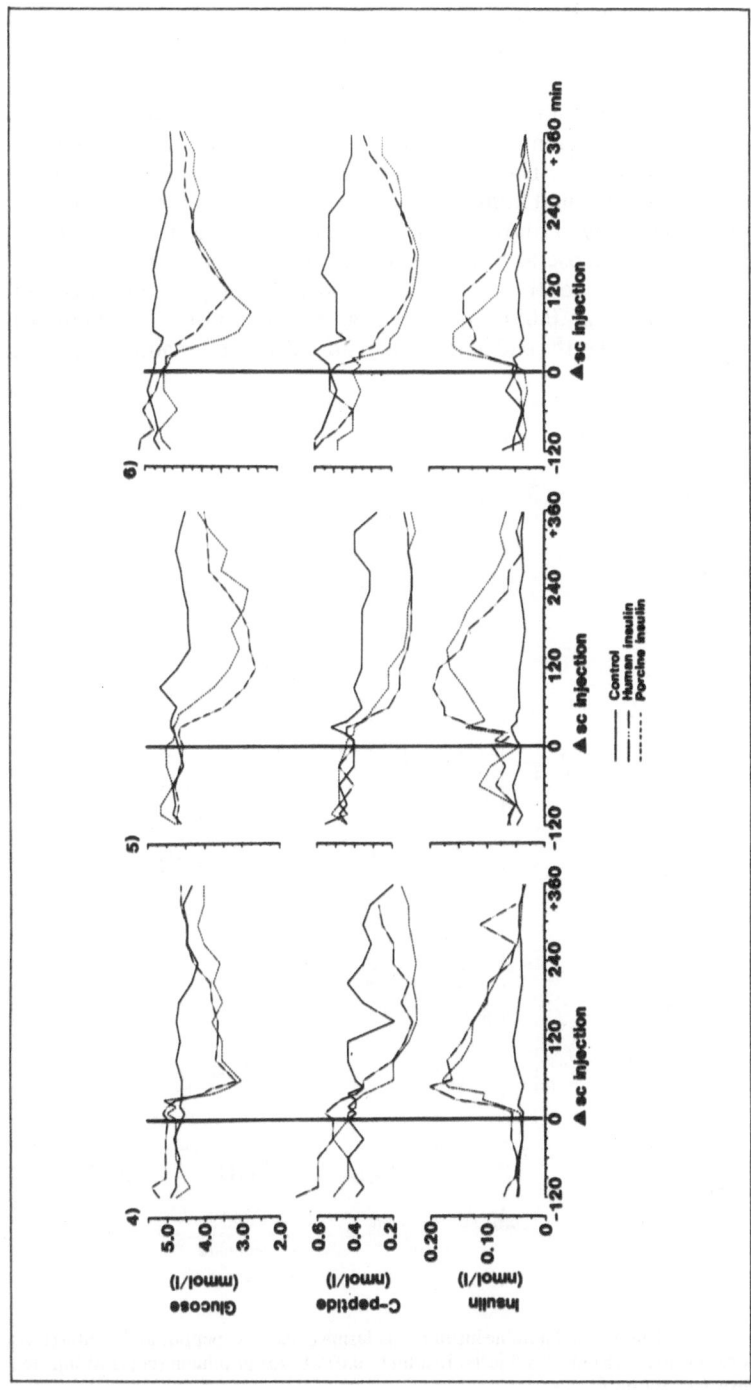

Figure 4.11 Effect of human and porcine insulins on plasma glucose, C-peptide and insulin (IRI) concentrations in the six subjects. Insulin (~0.075 U/kg) or diluent (control) injected subcutaneously (sc) at time 0

Results

The individual plasma glucose, C-peptide and insulin levels are illustrated in Figure 4.11 with the means ± SE values shown in Figure 4.12. During the control day there was a gradual fall in the plasma glucose concentration from 4.7 ± 0.1 mmol/l at the beginning (−120 min) to 4.5 ± 0.03 mmol/l at the end of the 480 min study period. The plasma glucose levels prior to injection of diluent (control), porcine and human insulin were 4.7 ± 0.1, 4.9 ± 0.1 and 4.8 ± 0.1 mmol/l, respectively. Following the subcutaneous injection of porcine insulin, the plasma glucose level began to fall after 20 min, with the levels significantly lower than controls between 50 and 180 min ($p<0.05$–0.01) and from 270 min onwards ($p<0.05$). The plasma glucose nadir of 3.3 ± 0.2 mmol/l was reached at 90 min. By the end of the study, i.e. 360 min after administration

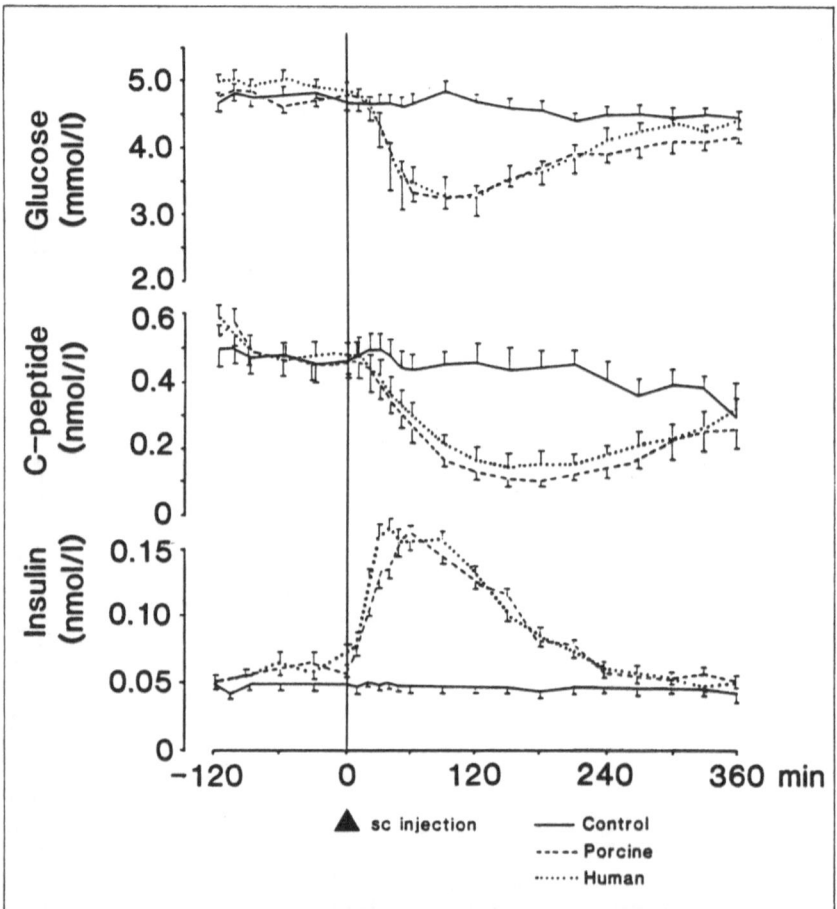

Figure 4.12 Effect of human and porcine insulins on plasma glucose, C-peptide and insulin (IRI) concentrations (means ± SE) in six subjects. Insulin (~0.075 U/kg) or diluent (control) injected subcutaneously (sc) at time 0

of porcine insulin, the glucose had returned to within 0.5 mmol/l of the pre-injection value (Figure 4.12). A similar rapid fall in plasma glucose was observed, with human insulin becoming significantly lower than controls ($p<0.05-0.01$) from 60 to 210 min reaching a nadir of 3.2 ± 0.3 mmol/l at 120 min after administration. By the end of the study the plasma glucose level had returned to 4.5 ± 0.1 mmol/l. There was no statistically significant difference in the plasma glucose levels between porcine and human insulin.

The plasma insulin level during the control day gradually decreased from 0.052 ± 0.004 nmol/l at -120 min to 0.031 ± 0.002 nmol/l at 360 min. After the subcutaneous administration of both porcine and human insulin, a steep rise in plasma insulin levels was observed after 20 to 30 min, with the values remaining significantly higher than controls for both insulins between 30 and 210 min ($p<0.05-0.001$). Similar peak insulin levels of 0.163 ± 0.007 nmol/l and 0.165 ± 0.023 nmol/l were observed with porcine and human insulin at 60 and 50 min post-injection, respectively. The plasma insulin profiles were similar for both species of insulin throughout the study period.

In parallel to the gradually falling plasma glucose and insulin values during the control day, the C-peptide levels decreased from 0.50 ± 0.053 nmol/l to 0.30 ± 0.058 nmol/l. Following the administration of porcine and human insulin, the C-peptide levels fell rapidly reaching minimum levels of 0.11 ± 0.015 nmol/l and 0.15 ± 0.043 nmol/l at 180 and 150 min, respectively, i.e. a reduction of approximately 70–75% of basal values. The C-peptide levels were significantly lower than the controls from 40 to 300 min ($p<0.05 \pm 0.001$) for porcine insulin, and from 60 to 330 min ($p<0.05 \pm 0.001$) after human insulin. There was no significant difference in the degree of C-peptide suppression between porcine and human insulin.

The mean blood lactate, alanine, glycerol and 3-hydroxybutyrate values are represented in Figure 4.13. During the control day the mean lactate, alanine and glycerol levels remained relatively constant, in contrast to 3-hydroxybutyrate concentrations which started to increase after 150 min from a level of 0.056 ± 0.02 mmol/l to 0.228 ± 0.7 mmol/l at 360 min. No significant change in blood lactate levels occurred with human insulin, whereas after porcine insulin the levels were significantly higher than controls from 90 to 150 min ($p<0.05$). The difference in blood lactate levels between porcine and human insulin reached significance at 10 to 20 min after injection ($p<0.05$). There was no change in alanine levels with either insulin. The injection of porcine and human insulin resulted in a fall in glycerol levels, reaching a nadir at 120 min followed by a moderate post-hypoglycaemic rise (Figure 4.13). The blood glycerol concentrations were significantly lower than controls following porcine insulin between 90 and 120 min ($p<0.05-0.01$) and human insulin at 150 min ($p<0.05$). The level was significantly lower with porcine than human insulin from 90 to 120 min ($p<0.05-0.01$). Initially, after insulin administration, there was a significant fall in 3-hydroxybutyrate levels between 90 and 180 min ($p<0.05$) followed by a steep post-hypoglycaemic rise (Figure 4.13). There was no significant difference in the blood 3-hydroxybutyrate levels between the two species of insulin.

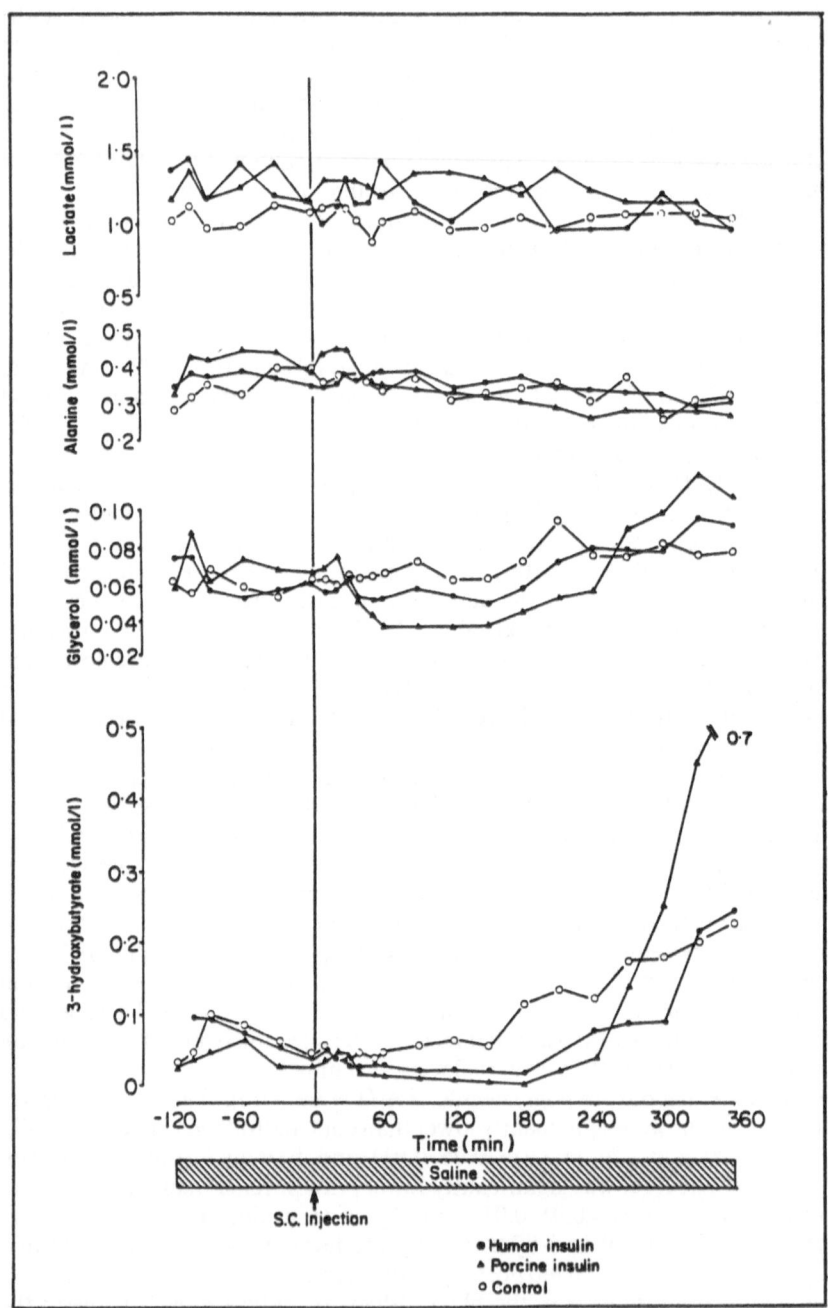

Figure 4.13 Effect of human and porcine insulins on blood lactate, alanine, glycerol and 3-hydroxybutyrate concentrations (means) in six subjects. Insulin (~0.075 U/kg) or diluent (control) injected subcutaneously (sc) at time 0

Discussion

Different experimental procedures, number of subjects, degrees of 'within' and 'between' subject variation and assay methodologies may account for the inconsistent findings in the plasma insulin profiles and metabolic responses between subcutaneously administered neutral, soluble porcine and human insulin in normal man. Laube and co-workers (1981a, b, 1982), observed that 'semi-synthetic' human insulin when administered subcutaneously into the anterior abdominal wall, at a dose level of 0.1 U/kg, resulted in a greater fall in plasma glucose 30 to 60 min after injection compared to porcine insulin. This difference could not be explained by the plasma insulin profiles which were identical for the two species of insulin. In comparison, Sundermann et al (1981) and Sonnenberg et al (1983) after the subcutaneous injection of 10 U into the thigh region, demonstrated that 'semi-synthetic' human insulin achieved a higher plasma insulin level and an earlier and more prolonged hypoglycaemic effect than porcine insulin.

Ebihara et al (1983), in a study comparing subcutaneous 'semi-synthetic' human and porcine insulin injected into the anterior abdominal wall at two dose levels (0.05 and 0.1 U/kg), found that there were no species differences in the resulting plasma insulin levels. The area under the insulin curve (AUC_{0-6h}), however, was significantly greater ($p < 0.05$) on human insulin at the low dose. The hypoglycaemic response to porcine and human insulin differed in opposite directions for the two dose levels, being greater on human insulin at 0.05 U/kg (120 min; $p < 0.05$) and on porcine insulin at 0.10 U/kg body weight (60 min; $p < 0.05$) (Ebihara et al, 1983). Similar findings have emerged from human volunteer studies involving 'biosynthetic' human insulin (BHI). Whereas Keen et al (1980) did not detect a true difference in the hypoglycaemic effect between 'biosynthetic' human and porcine insulin following subcutaneous injection into the anterior abdominal wall, they suggested that human insulin was slightly more potent than porcine insulin at 4.8 U and slightly less at 9.6 U. Botterman and co-workers (1981) stated that 'biosynthetic' human insulin was absorbed quicker than Des-Phe-insulin, when comparing their recent data with human insulin to previous results with the Des-Phe-insulin. Federlin et al (1981) observed significantly higher plasma insulin levels and lower glucose values with 'biosynthetic' human insulin compared to purified porcine insulin following subcutaneous injection into the upper arm region. In contrast, others have found that subcutaneous 'biosynthetic' human insulin and purified porcine insulins are equipotent in lowering plasma glucose in normal subjects who were either fasting (Galloway et al, 1981a, b) or undergoing the Gerritzen test involving regular carbohydrate feeds (Gerritzen, 1952; Weinges et al, 1981).

It is difficult to equate the above findings due to fundamental differences between the studies. Different sites of administration have been used, including the upper arm region (Galloway et al, 1981b; Federlin et al, 1981), abdomen (Keen et al, 1980; Owens et al, 1981a, 1982; Laube et al, 1981a, b; Ebihara et al, 1983), thigh region (Sundermann et al, 1981) and unspecified (Bottermann et al, 1981; Weinges et al, 1981).

It is documented that human insulin is preferentially absorbed following subcutaneous injection into the thigh region, compared to porcine insulin, resulting in an earlier hypoglycaemic response (Sundermann et al, 1981). Studies involving regions associated with a more rapid rate of absorption are equally divided between those showing no difference between human ('biosynthetic' and 'semi-synthetic') and porcine insulin (Keen et al, 1980; Galloway et al, 1981b; Owens et al, 1981a, 1982), and those demonstrating significantly lower plasma glucose values after human insulin (Federlin et al, 1981; Laube et al, 1981a, b; Ebihara, 1983). Unfortunately, only two studies have attempted to refer to the 'potencies' of the insulins employed (Keen et al, 1980; Owens et al, 1981a, 1982). This is very important for such comparative studies, especially in view of the relatively low plasma insulin profiles recorded by some investigators following the administration of porcine insulin (Federlin et al, 1981; Sundermann, 1981). Other differences include the subjects themselves and their metabolic status before and especially during the period of investigation, as the normal volunteers are either fasting (Keen et al, 1980; Federlin et al, 1981; Galloway et al, 1981b; Laube et al, 1981a, b; Sundermann et al, 1981; Owens et al, 1982; Ebihara et al, 1983) or being fed regularly (Weinges et al, 1981).

Thus the studies demonstrate either no difference or minimal differences between neutral, soluble human ('semi-synthetic' and 'biosynthetic') and purified porcine insulin following subcutaneous absorption in normal subjects. Differences are more likely to occur when using sites associated with a relatively slower rate of absorption. It is also relevant to note that significantly higher insulin levels with one species of insulin relative to another, do not necessarily mean a difference in the hypoglycaemic response, and vice-versa. The influence of dose is another important variable when assessing the relative pharmacokinetic and potency differences between insulin preparations.

4.1.4 The influence of somatostatin on the metabolic and hormonal responses to subcutaneous human and porcine insulin

Introduction

In 1972, Guillemin and co-workers first isolated somatostatin as a growth-hormone release-inhibitory factor from the hypothalamus (Vale et al, 1975; Schally et al, 1976), a tetradecapeptide (Burgus et al, 1973), which was later produced synthetically (Rivier, 1974). It was found to be widely distributed in the nervous system and other tissues, including the D-cells of the pancreatic islets (Arimura et al, 1975; Brownstein et al, 1975; Orci et al, 1975; Polak et al, 1975; Kronheim et al, 1976; Patel and Reichlin 1978). Dependent on its site of elaboration, somatostatin may therefore function either as a neurohormone, neurotransmitter and/or a parahormone, resulting in a wide spectrum of biological events in addition to its inhibition of growth hormone and insulin secretion (Guillemin and Gerich, 1976; Luft et al, 1978; Pimstone et al, 1978; Gerich, 1981).

In addition to its potent inhibition of growth hormone secretion in humans (Hall et al, 1973; Hansen et al, 1973; Siler et al, 1973; Giustina et al, 1975), somatostatin can also inhibit basal and TRH, stimulated TSH release (Hall et al, 1973; Weeke et al, 1974), the secretion of insulin (Alberti et al, 1973; Christensen et al, 1974; Mortimer et al, 1974), glucagon (Gerich et al, 1974a, b, 1975c; Iversen 1974; Hansen and Lundbaek, 1976) and various gastrointestinal hormones (Bloom et al, 1974; Barros D'Sa et al, 1975; Gomez-Pan et al, 1975). Amongst the most extensively studied actions of somatostatin has been its inhibition of pancreatic islet hormone secretion (Guillemin and Gerich, 1976; Hansen and Lundbaek, 1976).

Pharmacological doses of somatostatin can accentuate insulin-induced hypoglycaemia (Liljenquist et al, 1977; Harano et al, 1977; Rizza et al, 1979) by inhibiting the secretion of several glucose counterregulatory hormones (Mortimer et al, 1974; Assan, 1976) and possibly also by reducing splanchnic blood flow (Wahren and Felig, 1976), which may slow hepatic insulin degradation. Somatostatin may also have glucoregulatory actions independent of glucagon and insulin availability (Sacca et al, 1980).

In patients with insulin-dependent diabetes, short-term infusion of somatostatin has the ability to decrease both fasting (Gerich et al 1974a; Del Geurcio et al, 1976) and post-prandial hyperglycaemia (Gerich et al, 1975a), in addition to preventing the development of severe ketoacidosis following acute withdrawal of insulin (Gerich et al, 1975b). Consequently, it has been suggested that somatostatin may be useful as an adjunct to insulin therapy (Gerich et al, 1977).

The two studies comparing subcutaneous human and porcine insulin (cf. 4.1.1 and 4.1.3), identical in all other respects apart from the concomitant use of somatostatin in one (cf. 4.1.1), allow the influence of a low-dose infusion of

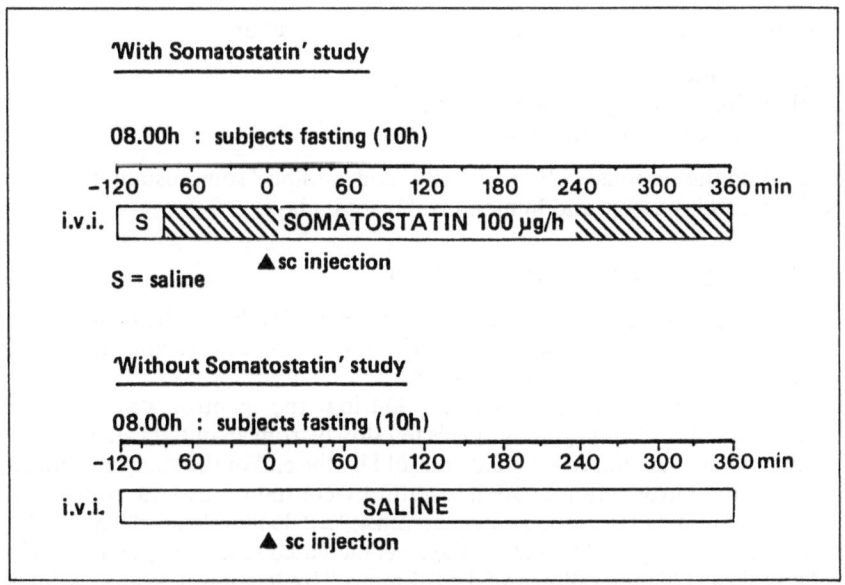

Figure 4.14 Experimental designs. Parameters: plasma glucose; C-peptide; insulin (IRI); growth hormone; glucagon; blood intermediary metabolites: lactate, alanine, glycerol, 3-hydroxybutyrate

somatostatin (100 μg/h) on the metabolic and hormonal responses to insulin-induced hypoglycaemia and insulin kinetics to be evaluated.

Subjects, materials and methods

Details of the subjects and materials for the 'with' and 'without' somatostatin studies are included with each individual study, i.e. 4.1.1 and 4.1.3, respectively. The designs of the two studies are summarised in Figure 4.14. In addition to the assays quoted earlier in the individual studies, for the purpose of this evaluation the samples were also assayed for glucagon (Alford et al, 1977) and growth hormone (Boden and Soeldner, 1976).

Statistical methods

The results are expressed as means ± SE except where stated otherwise. The significance of the differences between the individual pairs of data was assessed using the Student's unpaired t-test. The comparisons for the glucose, C-peptide and insulin were carried out on both the raw data and the Δ values (derived by subtracting the mean pre-somatostatin value from all subsequent levels having adjusted for the control day). For the intermediary metabolites, glucagon and growth hormone, the values were not corrected for the control day levels, due to the large 'within' and 'between' subject variation observed for these parameters.

Results

The results will be presented under the following sections:

1. plasma glucose, C-peptide and insulin,
2. blood intermediary metabolites, and
3. counterregulatory hormones,

comparing the responses observed 'with' and 'without' somatostatin for each of the control, porcine and human insulin study days.

1.   Plasma glucose, C-peptide and insulin

The mean plasma glucose, C-peptide and insulin levels for the control and insulin study days, 'with' and 'without' the concomitant administration of somatostatin are shown in Figures 4.15a, b.
(a)   *Control study (Figure 4.15a).* During the control day without somatostatin the plasma glucose levels fell slowly from an initial value of 4.7 ± 0.1 mmol/l at –120 min to 4.5 ± 0.03 mmol/l by the end of the study period. In contrast, the introduction of somatostatin by constant intravenous infusion caused an initial fall in plasma glucose from 4.9 ± 0.05 mmol/l at –90 min to 4.5 ± 0.2 mmol/l, 1 h later. Thereafter, the level increased reaching a peak of 5.8 ± 0.2 mmol/l at 120 min, falling to 5.1 ± 0.1 mmol/l by 360 min. The glucose level was significantly higher with somatostatin than without from 120 min onwards ($p < 0.05$–0.001)

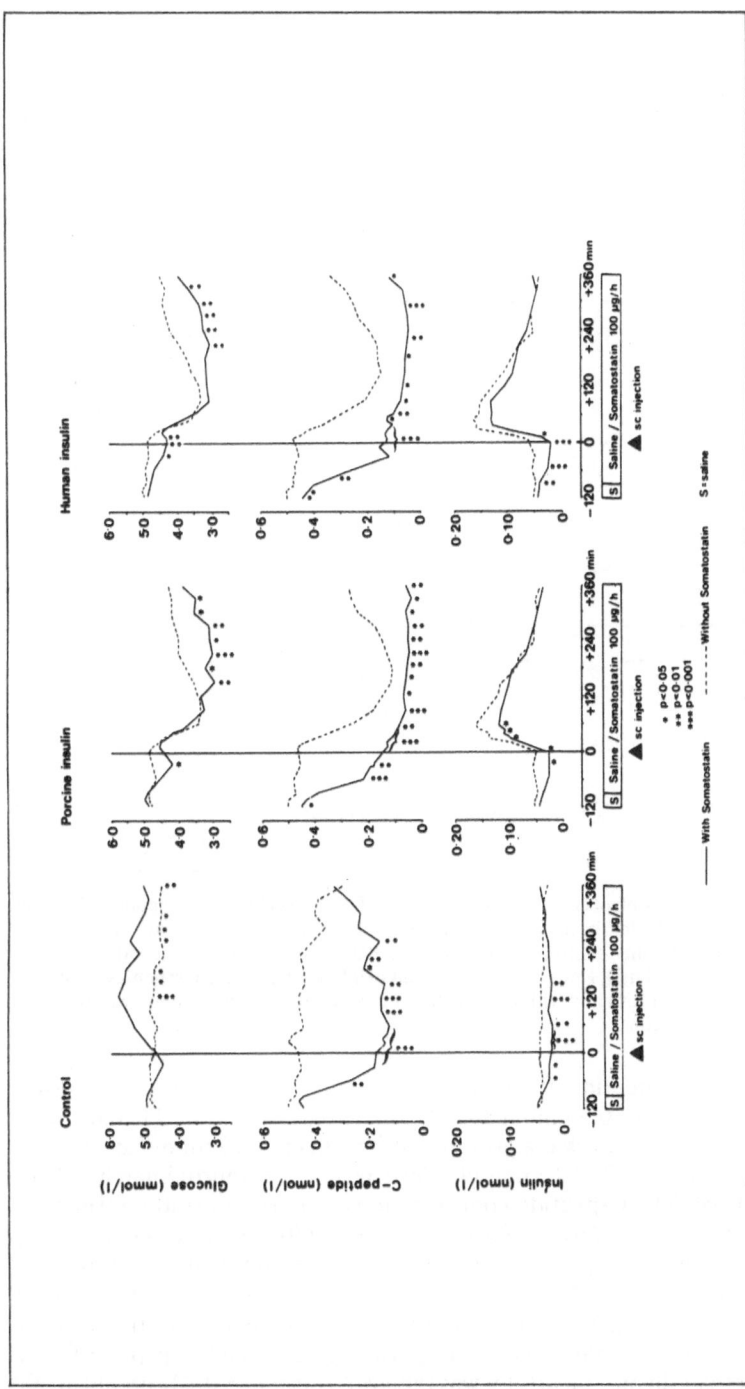

Figure 4.15a Comparison of effect of somatostatin on the plasma glucose, C-peptide and insulin (IRI) levels (means) before and after the injection of diluent (control), porcine and human insulins in six normal subjects. Saline or somatostatin infused from −90 to 360 min. Insulin (~0.075 U/kg) or diluent (control) injected subcutaneously (sc) at time 0

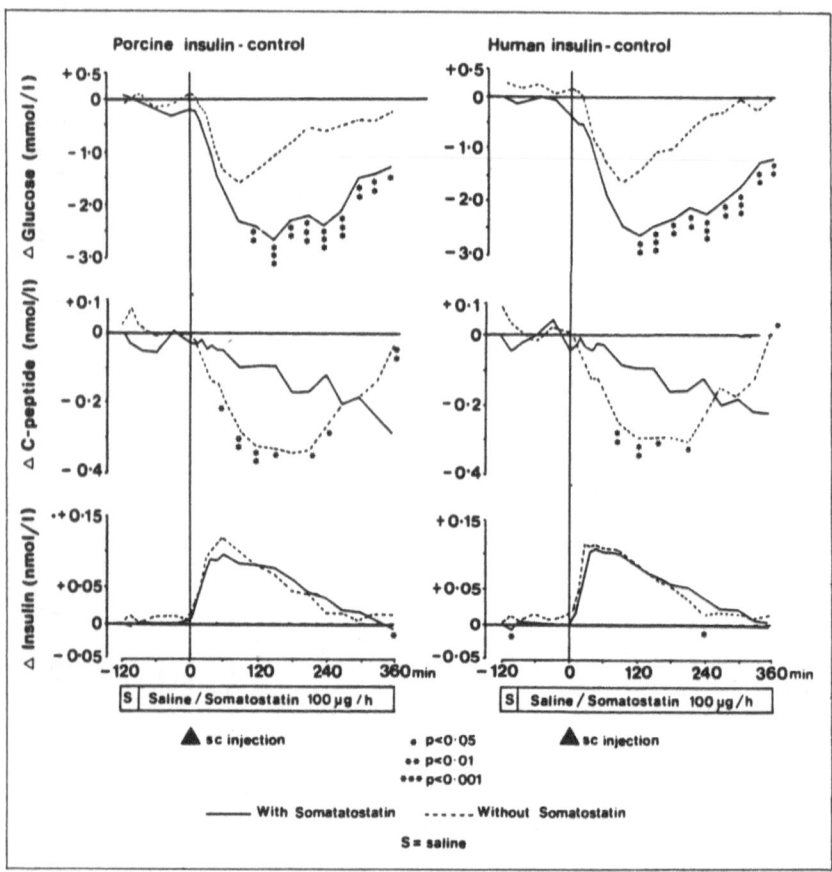

Figure 4.15b Comparison of effect of somatostatin on the plasma glucose, C-peptide and insulin (IRI) levels before and after the injection of porcine and human insulins in six subjects. Saline or somatostatin infused from –90 to 360 min. Insulin (~0.075 U/kg) or diluent (control) injected subcutaneously (sc) at time 0. Results shown as means of differences between responses to porcine insulin (minus control) with and without somatostatin, and human insulin (minus control) with and without somatostatin

The plasma C-peptide level on the control day without somatostatin decreased from 0.50 ± 0.5 nmol/l at –120 min to 0.30 ± 0.05 nmol/l at 360 min. With somatostatin there was a prompt fall from 0.44 ± 0.02 nmol/l at –90 min, reaching a nadir of 0.13 ± 0.03 nmol/l at 50 to 60 min, i.e. approximately 25% of the basal level. The C-peptide concentrations were significantly lower with somatostatin between –60 and 240 min ($p < 0.05$–0.001). By the end of the study period, however, the C-peptide levels were similar in both control studies.

During prolonged fasting the insulin level fell from 0.052 ± 0.004 nmol/l at the beginning to 0.031 ± 0.002 nmol/l at the end of the control day, in agreement with the small decrease in plasma glucose and C-peptide levels. With somatostatin plasma insulin was reduced from 0.04 ± 0.003 nmol/l at –90 min to a nadir of 0.02 ± 0.002 nmol/l at 50 min. The levels were significantly lower with somatostatin from -60 to 150 min ($p < 0.05$–0.001).

(b) *Porcine insulin (Figures 4.15a, b)*. In the absence of somatostatin and within 10 min of the subcutaneous administration of porcine insulin, the glucose began to fall from a pre-injection level of 4.8 ± 0.1 nmol/l (time 0 min), reaching a nadir of 3.3 ± 0.2 mmol/l at 90 min. While a similar fall in plasma glucose was observed during the initial 120 min with somatostatin, the level continued to fall reaching a lower minimum value of 2.9 ± 0.1 mmol/l at 150 min. The glucose was significantly lower with somatostatin from 150 to 330 min ($p < 0.05 \pm 0.001$). The recovery towards normoglycaemia also started later at 270 min with somatostatin, compared to 120 min without.

Insulin without somatostatin resulted in a rapid reduction in the plasma C-peptide level from 0.47 ± 0.05 (time 0 min) to 0.11 ± 0.02 nmol/l at 180 min. In the comparative study, as somatostatin had already lowered the plasma C-peptide level from 0.39 ± 0.05 nmol/l to 0.15 ± 0.02 nmol/l, only a small additional fall occurred in the C-peptide concentrations, reaching a nadir of 0.05 ± 0.004 nmol/l at 270 min after the addition of insulin. The plasma C-peptide concentrations were significantly lower during the somatostatin study from -60 min onwards ($p < 0.05$–0.001).

Compared to the without somatostatin study, where the insulin levels were relatively constant during the pre-insulin period at about 0.045 nmol/l, the levels became significantly lower ($p < 0.05$) with somatostatin at -30 and 0 min. At 60 min, after insulin, peak mean levels of 0.12 ± 0.01 nmol/l and 0.16 ± 0.01 nmol/l were observed in the 'with' and 'without' somatostatin studies, respectively. The plasma insulin concentrations were lower in the presence of somatostatin during the first hour at 30, 50 and 60 min ($p < 0.05$).

For the Δ values the hypoglycaemic effect was significantly greater 'with' somatostatin from 120 min onwards ($p < 0.01$–0.001; Figure 4.15b). The concomitant use of somatostatin did not alter the incremental plasma insulin profile with porcine insulin.

(c) *Human insulin (Figures 4.15a, b)*. Somatostatin caused a significant reduction in plasma glucose levels between -30 and 0 min ($p < 0.05$–0.01) during the pre-insulin period. Without somatostatin human insulin lowered the plasma glucose level from 4.9 ± 0.1 mmol/l, to a nadir of 3.3 ± 0.3 mmol/l at 90 min. The corresponding values with somatostatin were 4.3 ± 0.2 and 3.1 ± 0.3 mmol/l, respectively. Subsequently, somatostatin caused a delay in the recovery of plasma glucose towards normoglycaemia, with the levels remaining lower between 210 and 330 min ($p < 0.01$–0.001).

Somatostatin lowered the basal C-peptide level from 0.41 ± 0.03 nmol/l at -90 min to 0.13 ± 0.02 nmol/l at 0 min, a reduction of about 70%. With the addition of insulin, it fell further to 0.047 ± 0.003 nmol/l at 240 min, i.e. about 10% of the pre-injection level with no subsequent recovery. In comparison, without somatostatin there was no real change in plasma C-peptide during the equivalent basal period (-90 to 0 min), whereas after insulin it fell rapidly from a normal fasting level of 0.48 ± 0.04 nmol/l to 0.15 ± 0.04 nmol/l at 150 min, returning to 0.33 ± 0.07 nmol/l at 360 min. The C-peptide level was significantly lower ($p < 0.01$–0.001) with somatostatin from -60 min onwards.

Inhibition of endogenous beta-cell secretion by somatostatin was also

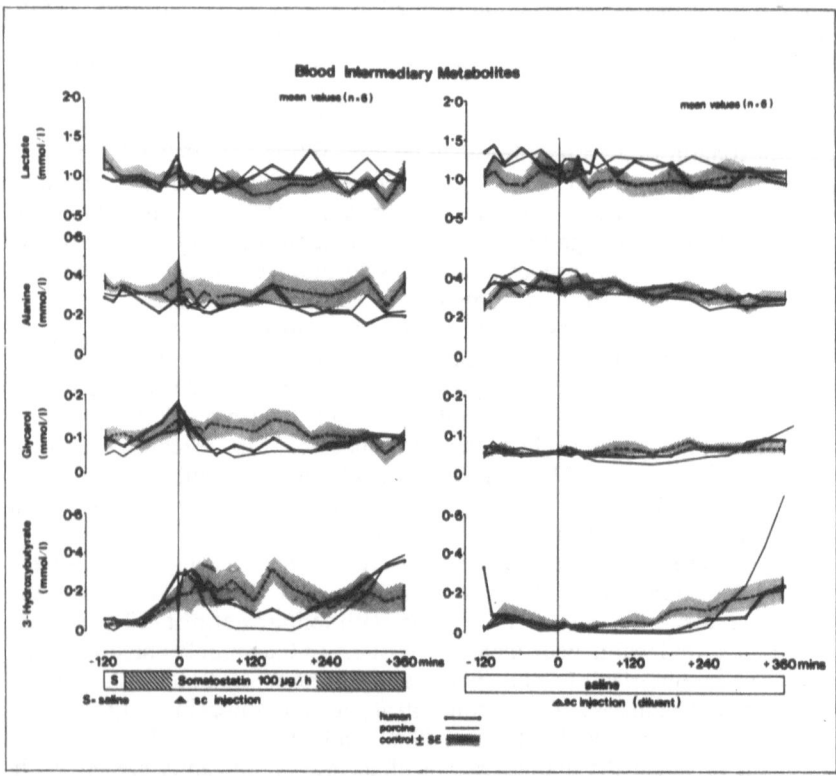

Figure 4.16a Effect of human and porcine insulin on the blood lactate, alanine, glycerol and 3-hydroxybutyrate levels (means) (i) with or (ii) without somatostatin in six subjects. Somatostatin infused from –90 to 360 min. Insulin (~0.075 U/kg) or diluent (control) injected subcutaneously (sc) at time 0. Results for the control days shown as means ± SE

reflected in the significantly lower plasma insulin levels from –60 to 10 min ($p < 0.05$–0.001). After insulin in the 'with' and 'without' somatostatin studies, the levels increased from 0.02 ± 0.002 and 0.06 ± 0.006 nmol/l, reaching peak levels of 0.13 ± 0.01 and 0.17 ± 0.02 nmol/l at 90 and 50 min, respectively.

Whereas somatostatin did not influence the incremental plasma insulin values, the hypoglycaemic response to human insulin was accentuated by somatostatin from 120 min onwards ($p < 0.01$–0.001; Figure 4.15b).

2. Blood intermediary metabolites (Figures 4.16a, b)

The mean blood lactate, alanine, glycerol and 3-hydroxybutyrate levels during the control and insulin study days, both with and without somatostatin, are shown in Figure 4.16a. Comparison of the Δ values between the 'with' and 'without' somatostatin studies for the control, porcine and human insulin study days are illustrated in Figure 4.16b.

(a) *Control study.* During the comparative control days the blood lactate

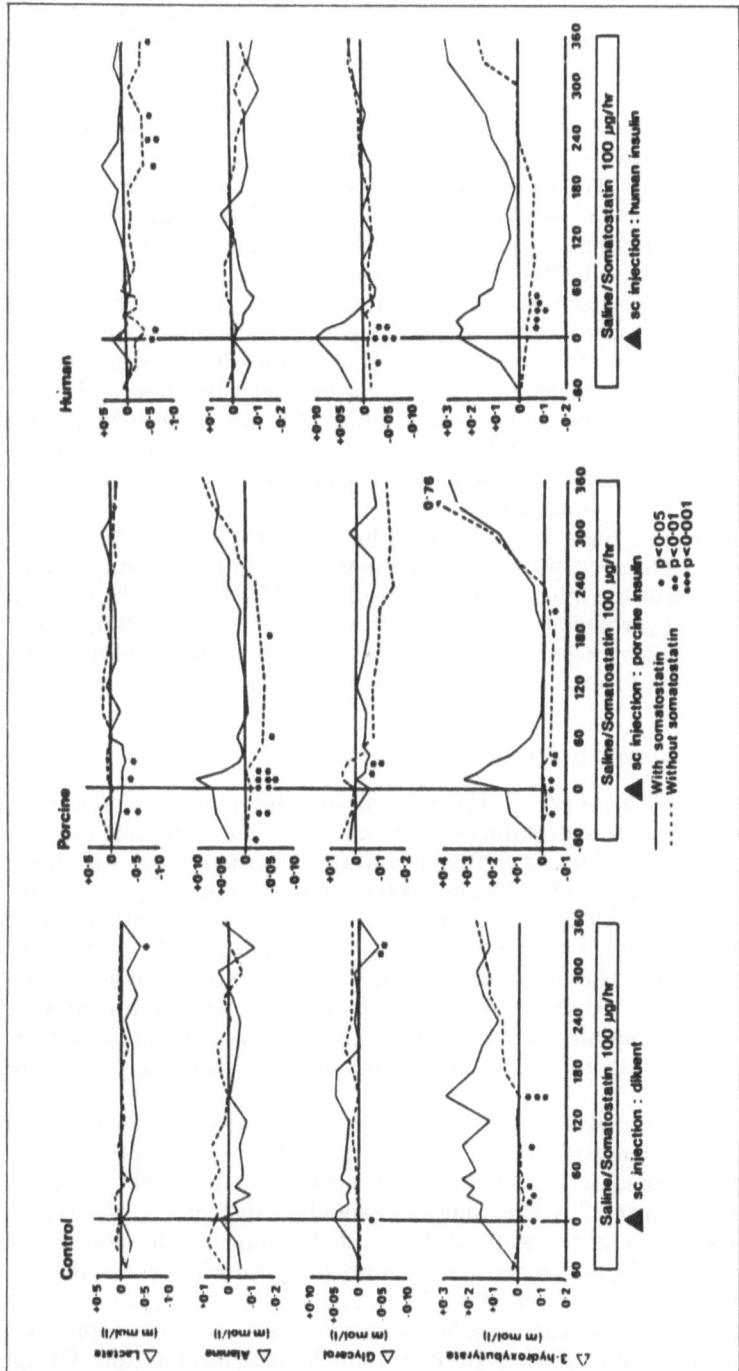

Figure 4.16b Comparison of effect of somatostatin on the blood lactate, alanine, glycerol and 3-hydroxybutyrate levels before and after the injection of diluent (control), porcine and human insulin in six subjects. Somatostatin infused from –90 to 360 min. Insulin (~0.075 U/kg) or diluent (control) injected subcutaneously (sc) at time 0. Results shown as mean Δ values

levels were similar, remaining relatively constant throughout the studies, and there was no real difference either 'within' or 'between' the studies for blood alanine levels. Soon after the commencement of somatostatin, however, there was an increase in blood glycerol and 3-hydroxybutyrate levels. The 3-hydroxybutyrate levels were significantly higher with somatostatin compared to without from 0 to 150 min ($p<0.05$–0.001).

(b) *Porcine insulin*. The blood lactate and alanine levels were lower ($p<0.05$–0.01) in the presence of somatostatin at –30, 10, 30 min and 20, 30 min, respectively. Somatostatin resulted in a significantly higher glycerol level from –60 to 20 min ($p<0.05$–0.001). From 10 min after the insulin injection a fall in blood glycerol occurred reaching a nadir at 90 min, followed by a small post-hypoglycaemic rise in both the 'with' and 'without' somatostatin studies.

Somatostatin caused the blood 3-hydroxybutyrate levels to increase rapidly, becoming significantly higher than the values observed with saline from –30 to 40 min ($p<0.05$). Subsequently, the injection of insulin in the somatostatin study caused a dramatic fall in levels followed by a marked post-hypoglycaemic rise. An even more pronounced post-hypoglycaemic rebound was observed without somatostatin.

(c) *Human insulin*. Significantly higher blood glycerol and 3-hydroxybutyrate levels were observed 'with' somatostatin within the first 150 min from the commencement of the infusion. Whilst insulin rapidly lowered the elevated glycerol and 3-hydroxybutyrate levels during the first 60 to 120 min after injection, the post-hypoglycaemic rise in blood glycerol and 3-hydroxybutyrate levels observed from 180 min onwards were similar in both studies.

3. Counterregulatory hormones

(a) *Glucagon (Figures 4.17a–c)*. The mean plasma glucagon levels for both the 'with' and 'without' somatostatin control, porcine and human insulin studies are shown in Figure 4.17a. An analysis of variance was carried out on the basal glucagon values (–120, –150, –90 min) as they showed rather large variations. The levels were significantly lower in the group who subsequently received somatostatin, compared to the group who received only saline ($p<0.05$–0.01). During this basal period there was a tendency in both studies to decreasing levels, which makes it difficult to define an appropriate baseline for studying the subsequent variation. The means of the three basal sampling times have, however, been used in the analyses which, for the above reasons, are subject to criticism.

In the somatostatin study there was a general tendency to higher incremental glucagon levels after insulin than in the control study, the difference reaching statistical significance at 150 min ($p<0.01$) and 180 min ($p<0.05$) for porcine insulin only (Figure 4.17b). The values were significantly higher ($p<0.05$) with porcine than to human insulin at 180 and 360 min. In the absence of somatostatin even higher glucagon levels were observed with porcine insulin, compared to controls at 150, 180, 210, 270, 330, 360, min ($p<0.05$–0.01), whereas no such differences were seen with human insulin. The glucagon levels were significantly higher after porcine than human insulin from 90 min onwards ($p<0.05$–0.01; Figure 4.17b).

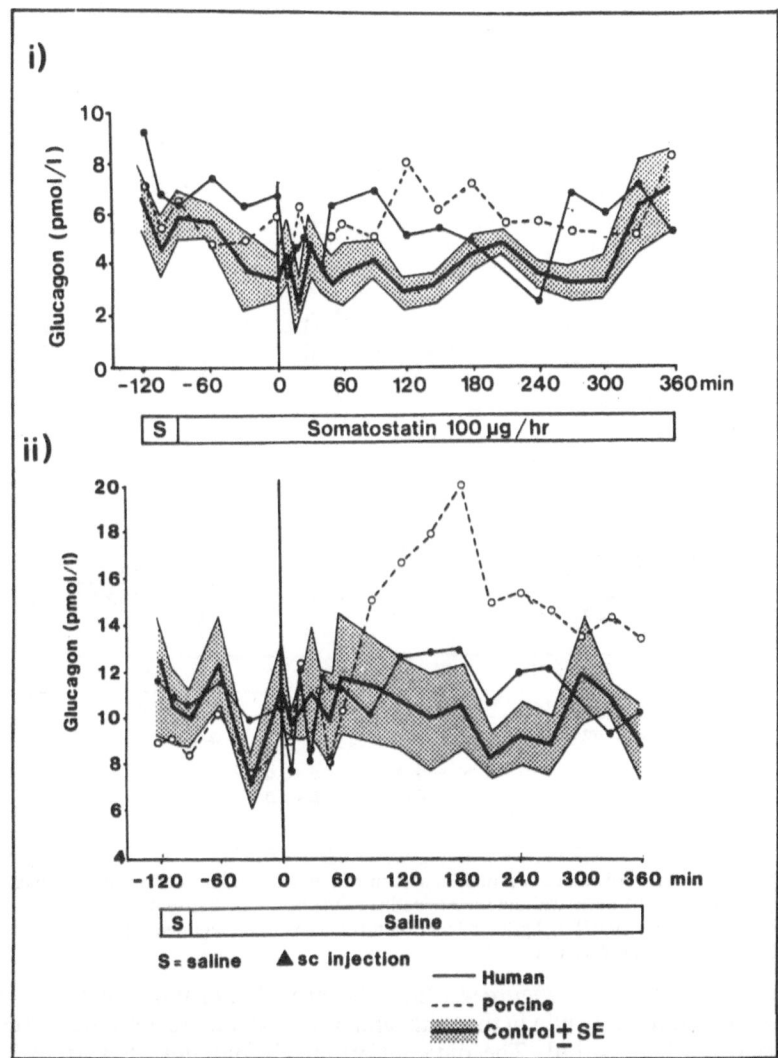

Figure 4.17a Effect of human and porcine insulins on plasma glucagon levels (means) (i) with or (ii) without somatostatin in six subjects. Somatostatin infused from –90 to 360 min. Insulin (~0.075 U/kg) or diluent (control) injected subcutaneously (sc) at time 0. Results for the control shown as means ± SE

Comparing the 'with' and 'without' somatostatin control days, there was a tendency to lower values with somatostatin from 0 to 150 min, although the difference was not statistically significant (Figure 4.17c). The glucagon response to hypoglycaemia was significantly less in the presence of somatostatin with porcine insulin at 90, 150 to 270, 330 min ($p<0.05$–0.001) and human insulin at 180 and 240 min ($p<0.05$–0.01). Somatostatin infusion therefore decreased the difference between the two species of insulin.

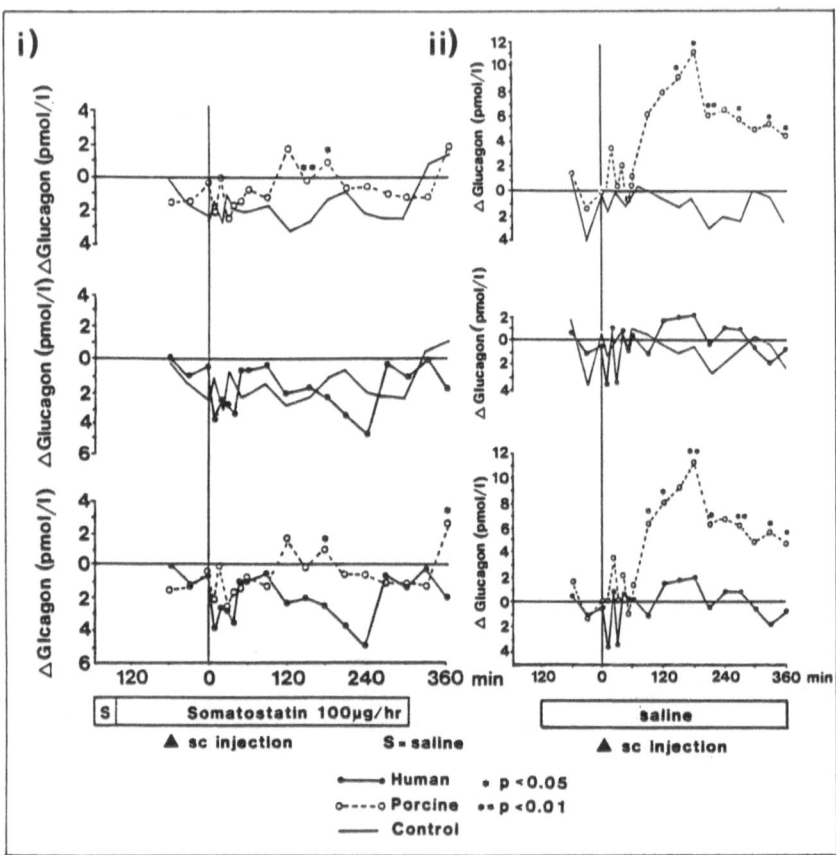

Figure 4.17b Comparison of effect of diluent (control), human and porcine insulins on plasma glucagon levels, **(i)** with or **(ii)** without somatostatin in six subjects. Somatostatin infused from –90 to 360 min. Insulin (~0.075 U/kg) or diluent (control) injected subcutaneously (sc) at time 0. Results shown as mean Δ values

(b) *Growth hormone (Figure 4.17d).* The growth hormone responses to human and porcine insulin in the 'with' and 'without' somatostatin studies can be seen in Figure 4.17d. The data unfortunately did not alow statistical analysis as most post-insulin values were >50mU/l with the samples lost for re-assay. However, there appears to be a more consistent earlier elevation of growth hormone with porcine than human insulin in the 'without' somatostatin study.

Discussion

The results clearly demonstrate that somatostatin, when given as a low-dose (100 μg/h) continuous intravenous infusion in fasting normals, results in an initial decrease in fasting glucose levels during the first hour, followed by a secondary increase. This confirms earlier observations of a biphasic glucose response with prolonged somatostatin infusion in non-diabetic subjects (Lins

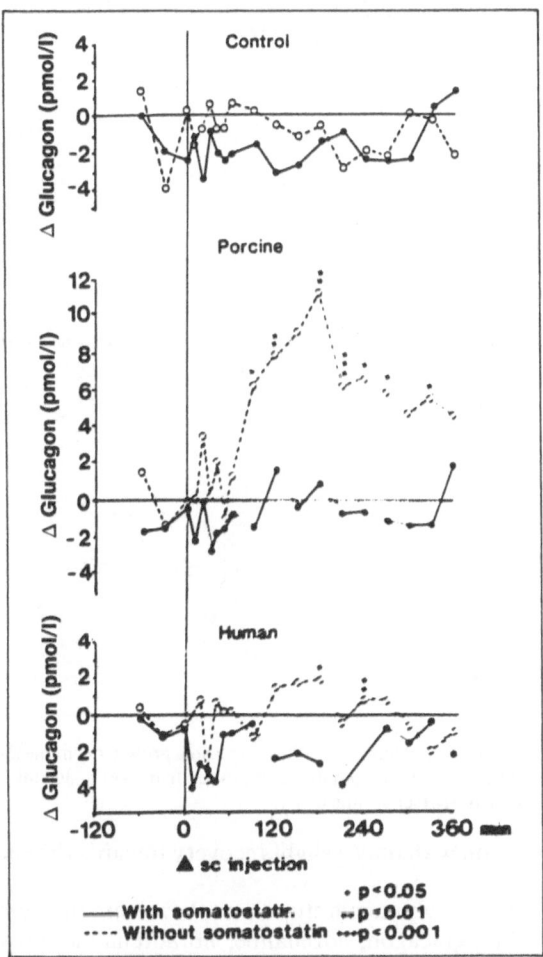

Figure 4.17c Comparison of effect of somatostatin on plasma glucagon levels before and after the injection of diluent (control), porcine and human insulins in six subjects. Somatostatin infused from –90 to 360 min. Insulin (~0.075 U/kg) or diluent (control) injected subcutaneously (sc) at time 0. Results shown as mean Δ values

and Efendič, 1976; Blauth et al, 1977; Sherwin et al, 1977a, b; Liljenquist et al, 1977). Experimental evidence from somatostatin infusion studies with replacement amounts of glucagon and insulin suggests that the initial decline in plasma glucose is primarily related to a relative glucagon lack, with the secondary hyperglycaemic phase resulting from the suppression of insulin secretion (Alford et al, 1974; Sherwin et al, 1977a). In the 'with' somatostatin study the fasting glucagon levels fell during the first 90 min of the infusion, remaining relatively stable for the following 300 min, before increasing to basal levels. In addition, the endogenous insulin secretion, as depicted by the C-peptide level, was reduced to 25% of fasting levels 150 min after the start of the

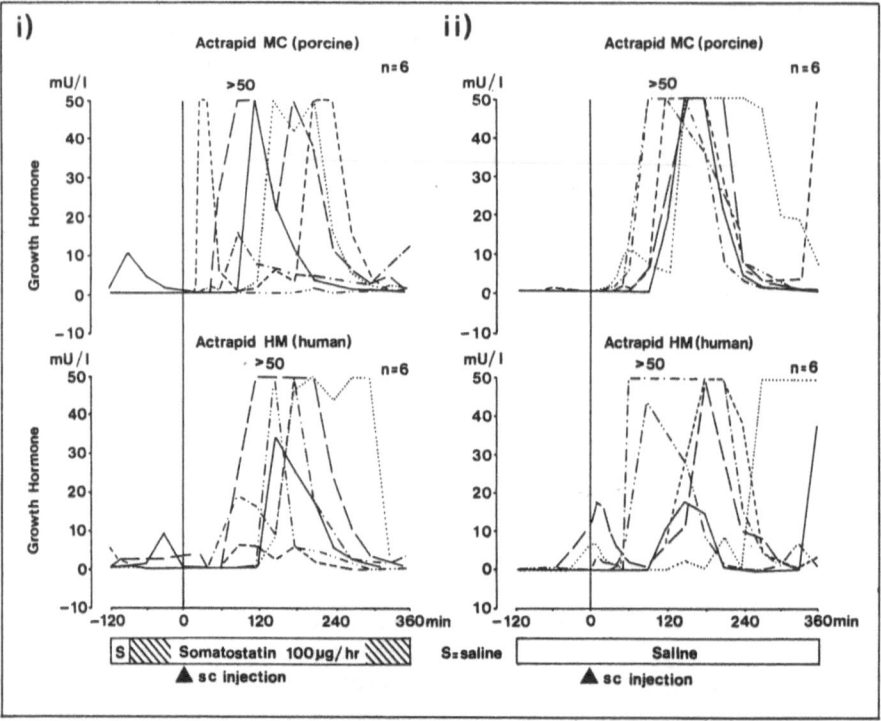

Figure 4.17d Effect of porcine and human insulins on plasma growth hormone levels (**i**) with or (**ii**) without somatostatin in six subjects. Somatostatin infused from –90 to 360 min. Insulin (~0.075 U/kg) injected subcutaneously (sc) at time 0

somatostatin infusion with only a slight recovery towards the end of the study period.

Insulin-induced hypoglycaemia stimulates the release of counterregulatory hormones including glucagon, adrenaline, noradrenaline, growth hormone and cortisol (Hall et al, 1974; Garber et al, 1976), although the relative contribution of the individual hormones to the restoration or normoglycaemia is not entirely clear. Glucagon, however, appears to have a primary role in the early recovery period, adrenaline occupying a secondary role (Gerich et al, 1979a, b; Rizza et al, 1979). The later secretion of growth hormone and cortisol may also facilitate normal recovery (Debodo and Altszuler, 1958; Santiago et al, 1980, Cryer, 1981), although their precise physiological role remains undefined (Feldman et al, 1975).

The findings from these studies clearly demonstrate that somatostatin potentiates insulin-induced hypoglycaemia and delays recovery confirming previous studies (Harano et al, 1977; Liljenquist et al, 1977; Gerich et al, 1979a, b; Rizza et al, 1979). It has been suggested that this is predominantly due to the inhibition of glucagon (Chideckel et al, 1977; Gerich et al, 1979a, b; Sacca et al, 1980) and adrenaline secretion (Rizza et al, 1979), and the consequent decrease in hepatic glucose production (Wahren et al, 1977), exceeds the concomitant decrease in glucose utilisation (Sherwin et al, 1977a, b). The glucagon response to porcine and human insulin-induced hypoglycaemia was partly suppressed by somatostatin, which also reduced the apparent difference between the two insulins. As previously observed, somatostatin impairs but does not prevent recovery from hypoglycaemia (Peracchi et al, 1974; Chideckel et al, 1975; Christensen et al, 1975). With lowered glucagon secretion, partial compensation is achieved by enhanced adrenaline secretion (Sacca et al, 1980; Gerich et al, 1979a, b; Rizza et al, 1979). The incremental plasma insulin levels following either insulin were not altered by somatostatin, suggesting that at the low-dose level used somatostatin did not affect the local or systemic clearance of subcutaneously administered insulin. This does not obviate the possibility that at a higher dose level somatostatin could decrease subcutaneous and splanchnic blood flow delaying both insulin absorption and degradation, respectively.

Somatostatin has previously been shown to have a variable influence on other substrates (Guillemin and Gerich, 1976; Hansen and Lundbaek, 1976). Results from studies 4.1.1 and 4.1.3 show that somatostatin had little or no effect on plasma lactate and alanine levels (Chideckel et al, 1977; Sherwin et al, 1977a, b). There was, however, a marked increase in blood glycerol and 3-hydroxybutyrate levels with somatostatin, due to accelerated lipolysis and ketogenesis with increasing insulin deficiency (Mahler et al, 1964; Cahill, 1971; Owen and Reichard, 1975). Insulin administration then resulted in a rapid fall in blood glycerol and 3-hydroxybutyrate levels, demonstrating its potent anti-lipolytic (Ball and Jungas, 1963) and anti-ketogenic action (Haft and Miller, 1958; Foster, 1967).

Therefore, a 'longer-acting' and more selective analogue of somatostatin may be a useful adjunct to insulin, due to its ability to reduce both fasting and post-prandial glucose levels, and to prevent the development of severe ketoacidosis upon acute insulin withdrawal in insulin-dependent diabetics (Gerich et al, 1975b). Short-term studies with somatostatin have demonstrated improvement in diurnal glycaemic control compared to insulin alone (Meissner et al, 1975; Gerich et al, 1977; Raskin and Unger, 1978). The present studies (cf. 4.1.1 and 4.1.3) show that somatostatin, at a dose level that inhibits the glucagon response to hypoglycaemia, does not alter the kinetics of subcutaneous insulin in normal subjects, which may be of relevance to the insulin-dependent diabetic. Long-term studies, however, would be necessary to ascertain any influence on diabetic control resulting from factors such as better plasma glucagon and growth hormone profiles (Burday et al, 1968; Hansen and Johansen, 1970; Johansen and Hansen, 1971; Lundbaek et al, 1971; Gerich et al, 1975a; Unger et al, 1977; Hansen et al, 1981) and altered responsiveness to cortisol, epinephrine or glucagon (Shamoon et al, 1980). In non-insulin-dependent diabetics, not on insulin, somatostatin is likely to exacerbate hyperglycaemia due to the suppression of an already inadequate insulin secretory capacity (Tamborlane et al, 1977; Waldhäusl et al, 1977).

4.1.5 Dose-response study of human, porcine and bovine insulin

This study was designed to explore further the possibility of a time-dependent variation in hypoglycaemic potency of the three species of insulin used clinically. Therefore the plasma glucose and insulin responses to subcutaneously administered neutral, soluble human, porcine and bovine insulin were examined at three dose levels (0.05, 0.075 and 0.15 U/kg body weight) in the same normal male subjects.

Subjects, materials and methods

Six healthy male volunteers were entered into the study. All were within 10% of their ideal body weight.

Details of the study preparations are included in Table 4.6.

Table 4.6

	Actrapid MC (porcine)	Actrapid HM (human)	Actrapid MC (bovine)	Actrapid diluent
Nitrogen (mg/ml)	0.217	0.216	0.215	—
Potency[a] (IU/ml)	40.1	40.0	39.8	—

[a]Theoretical potency: 185 IU/mgN

Methods

The six subjects were each involved in 10 study days 1–3 weeks apart. The subjects received, according to a randomisation schedule, bolus subcutaneous injections of human, porcine and bovine Actrapid insulin at the three dose levels of 0.05, 0.075 and 0.15 U/kg body weight and Actrapid diluent as control. After a 120 minute basal period the test preparations were administered by subcutaneous bolus injection using a Plastipak 1 ml syringe (Becton–Dickinson) into the left or right side of the anterior abdominal wall, mid-way between the umbilicus and anterior superior iliac spine. Venous blood samples were taken at half-hourly intervals throughout the 8 hour study period, with samples taken every 10 min during the first hour after injection.

The blood samples were assayed for plasma glucose by the hexokinase method and insulin (IRI) according to the method of Heding (1972).

Statistical methods

The results are presented as means ±SE except where otherwise stated. Individual pairs of treatments were compared using the Student's paired t-test for the Δ values, derived by adjusting for the control day and then subtracting the mean basal value (–120 to 0 min) from all subsequent levels on each study day. The data were also analysed in order to define suitable responses for subsequent dose–response analyses. The relation between response and log-dose could be described by parallel lines for the three species of insulin. The relative 'potency' and 'bioavailability' of the three insulins were determined by means of new multivariate statistical methods (Vølund, 1980). The statistical analyses were carried out using specially developed APL computer programs.

Results

The mean plasma glucose and insulin concentrations for the three comparative insulin preparations, human, porcine and bovine Actrapid at the three dose levels of 0.05, 0.075 and 0.15 U/kg body weight are shown in Figure 4.18. The mean Δ glucose and insulin levels for the three insulin preparations, according to species and dose, can be seen in figures 4.19a and 4.19b. The data are presented as follows:
(a) paired comparisons,
(b) analysis of dose–response relationships:
    (i) plasma glucose (biological 'potency'),
    (ii) plasma insulin ('bioavailability'),
    (iii) comparison of hypoglycaemic 'potency' and 'bioavailability'.

(a) Paired comparisons

The plasma glucose and insulin responses to the three species of insulin at each dose level were compared as follows: (i) human vs porcine, (ii) human vs bovine, and (iii) porcine vs bovine (Figures 4.20a, 4.20b and 4.20c, respectively).

(i) *Human vs porcine insulin (Figure 4.20a)*. The hypoglycaemic response and incremental insulin levels were similar following human and porcine insulin at the lower dose level, except for one time point (240 min), when the glucose level was significantly lower following porcine insulin ($p < 0.05$). At 0.075 U/kg a faster rate of fall in plasma glucose was observed with both insulins reaching a similar nadir 90 min after injection. Thereafter, the plasma glucose remained significantly lower with human insulin between 150 and 180 min ($p < 0.05$). The incremental insulin profiles were similar for the two species of insulin, differing only at 210 min (porcine human: $p < 0.05$). At 0.15 U/kg a prompt and rapid fall in plasma glucose was observed with both insulins. Human insulin achieved a lower nadir at 90 to 120 min, although the difference between the insulins did not reach statistical significance until 180 min ($p < 0.05$). Subsequently, the trend was reversed with the glucose values lower on porcine insulin at 300 min ($p < 0.05$), due to a more rapid rate of recovery towards normoglycaemia following human insulin. This difference may be partly related to the lower glucose nadir achieved with human compared to porcine insulin, although the difference is more likely due to the higher incremental plasma insulin levels with human insulin during the first hour ($p < 0.05$ at 10, 40 min) and porcine insulin during the last two hours ($p < 0.05$ at 240 min).

(ii) *Human vs bovine insulin (Figure 4.20b)*. At both the low and high dose levels the initial hypoglycaemic response was similar for the two species of insulin. There was, however, a tendency towards a slower recovery with bovine insulin, the glucose levels being significantly lower than with human insulin at 270 min ($p < 0.05$–0.01). For the 0.05 and 0.15 U/kg dose levels the incremental insulin level was significantly higher ($p < 0.05$) with human than bovine insulin at 180 and 10 min, respectively.

The plasma glucose response to the two species of insulin at the 0.075 U/kg dose level showed a similar trend towards an earlier and shorter-lived

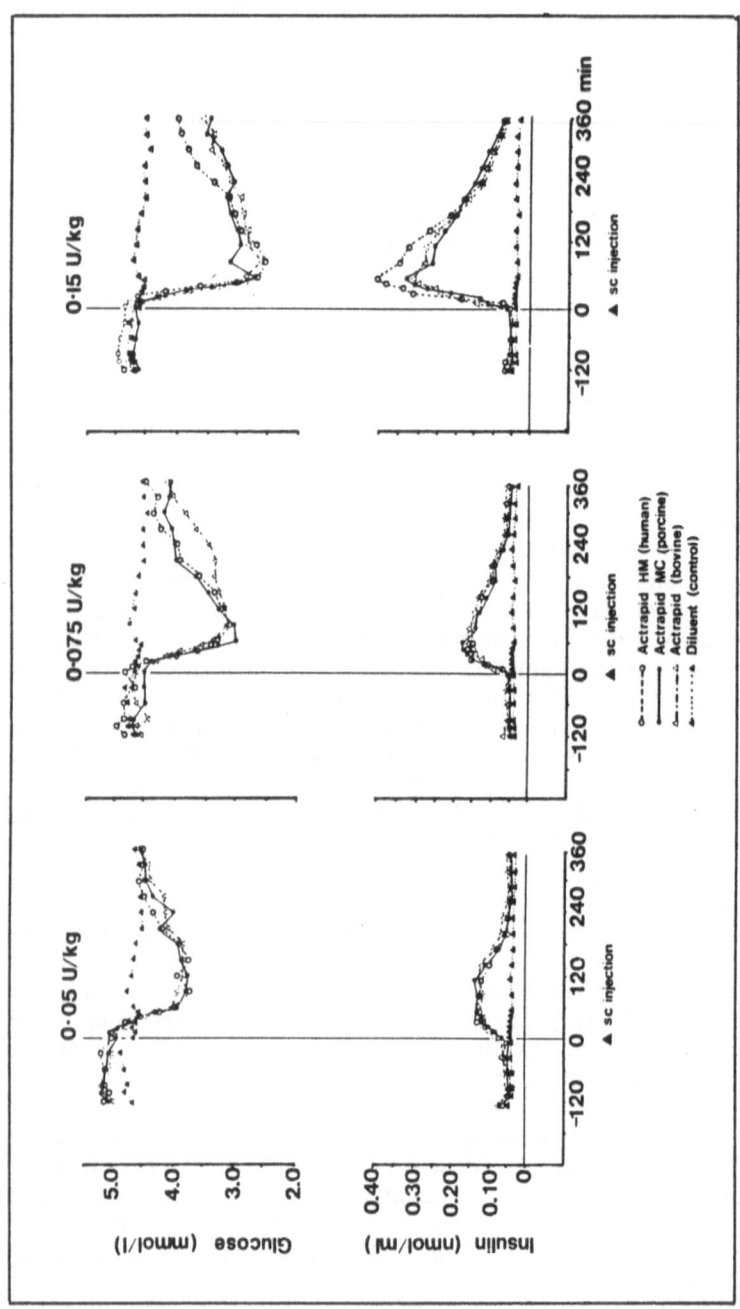

Figure 4.18 Effect of human, porcine and bovine insulins on plasma glucose and insulin (IRI) concentrations (means) in six subjects. Insulin (0.05, 0.075 and 0.15 U/kg) or diluent (control) given subcutaneously (sc) at time 0

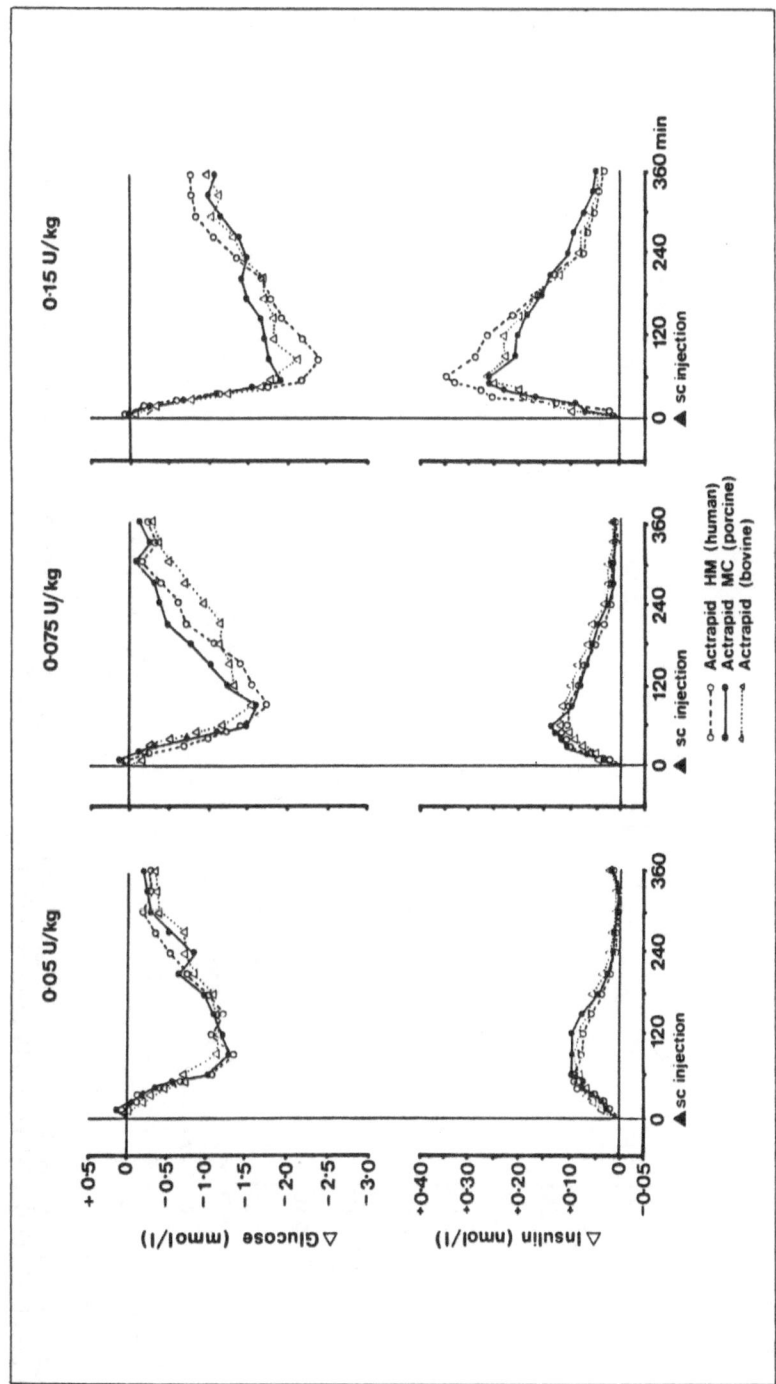

Figure 4.19a Effect of human, porcine and bovine insulins on plasma glucose and insulin (IRI) concentrations (means Δ values) in six subjects. Insulin (0.05, 0.075, 0.15 U/kg) given subcutaneously (sc) at time 0

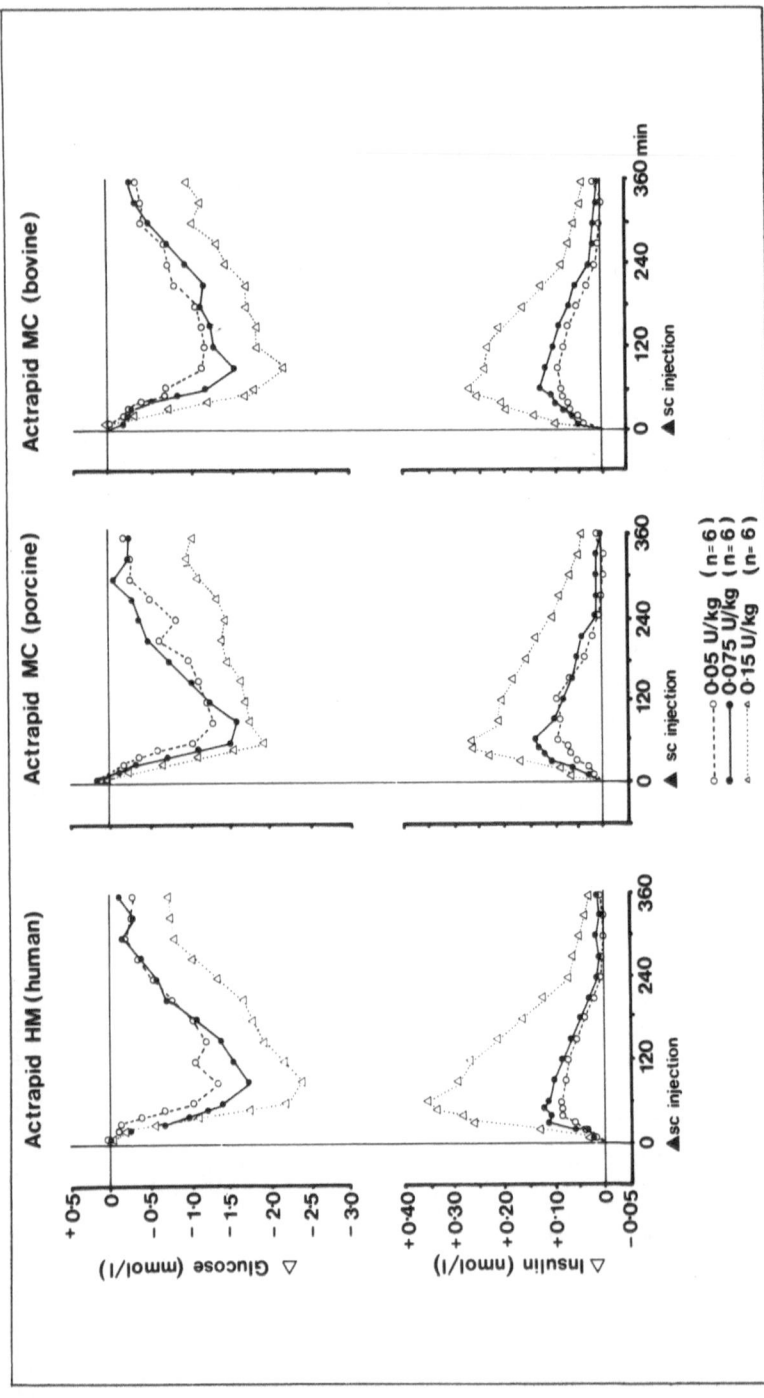

Figure 4.19b Effect of insulin dose on plasma glucose and insulin (IRI) concentrations (mean of Δ values) for human, porcine and bovine insulins in six subjects. Insulin (0.05, 0.075 and 0.15 U/kg) injected subcutaneously (sc) at time 0

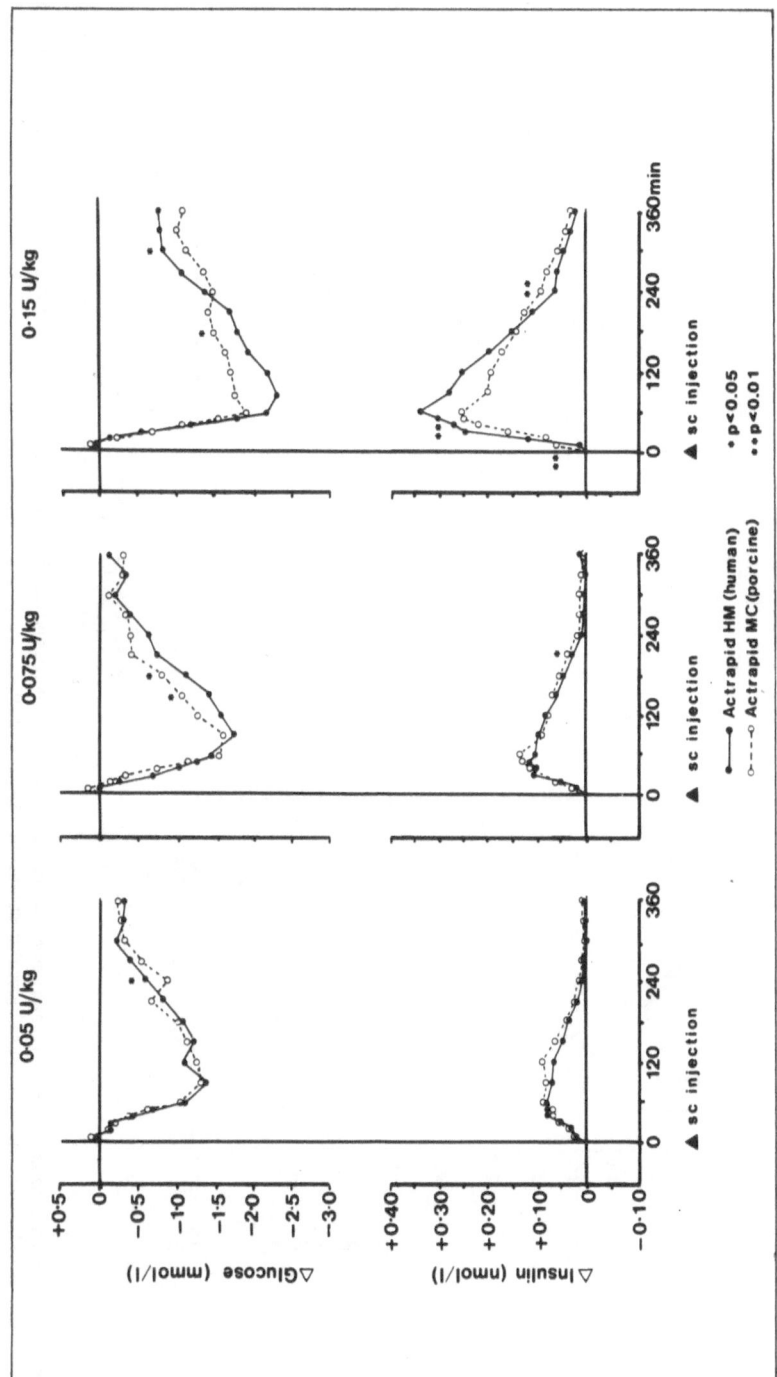

Figure 4.20a   Comparison of effect of human and porcine insulins on plasma glucose and insulin (IRI) concentrations (mean Δ values) in six subjects. Insulin (0.05, 0.075, 0.15 U/kg) or diluent (control) given subcutaneously (sc) at time 0

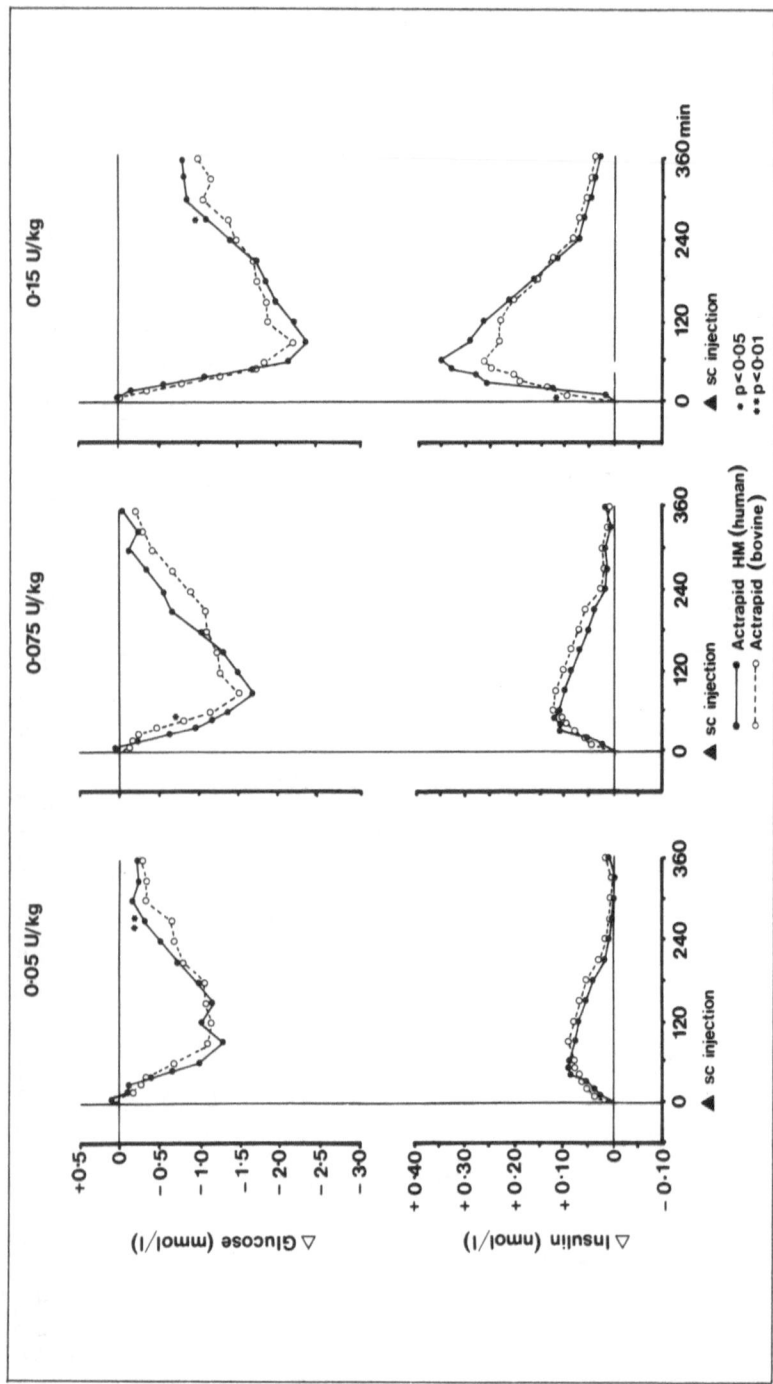

Figure 4.20b Comparison of effect of human and bovine insulins on plasma glucose and insulin (IRI) concentrations (mean of Δ values) in six subjects. Insulin (0.05, 0.075, 0.15 U/kg) or diluent (control) given subcutaneously (sc) at time 0

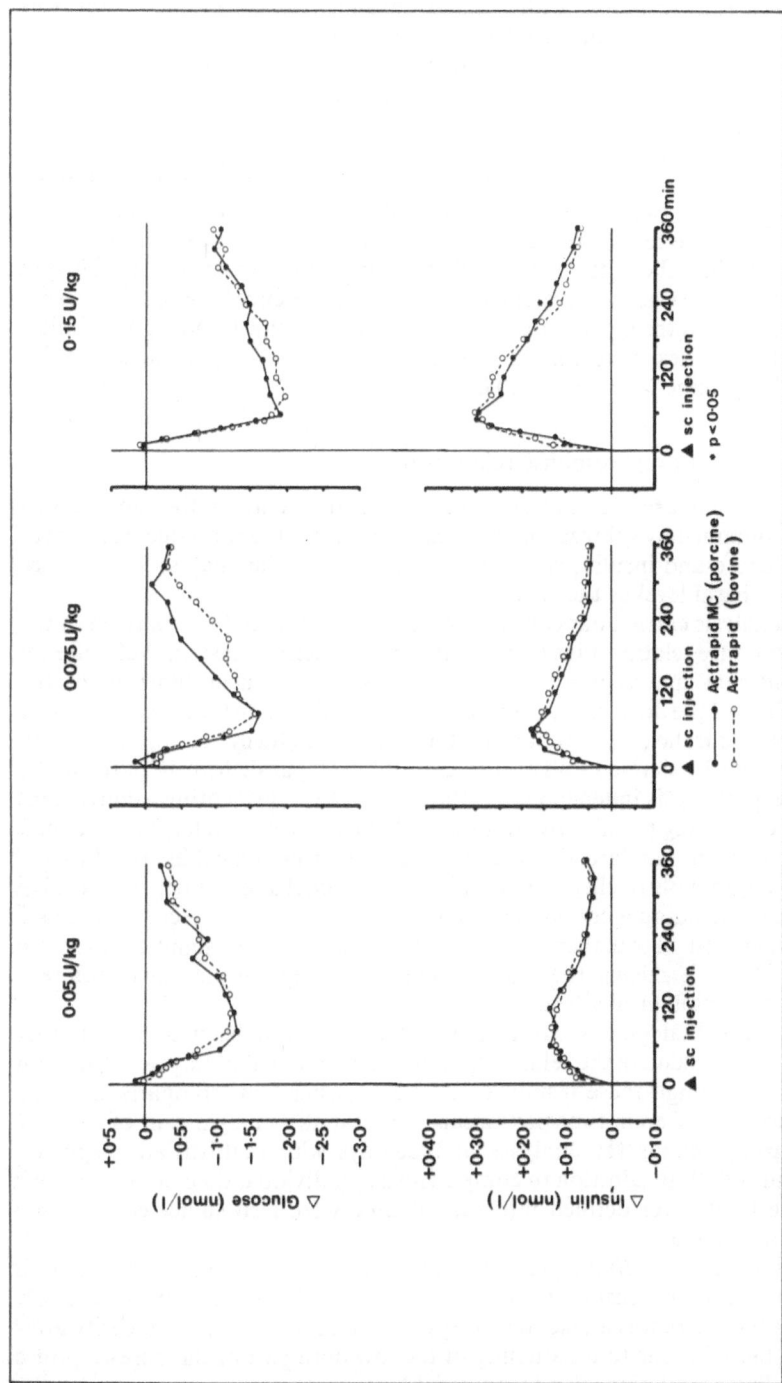

Figure 4.20c Comparison of effect of porcine and bovine insulins on plasma glucose and insulin (IRI) concentrations (mean of Δ values) in six subjects. Insulin (0.05, 0.075, 0.15 U/kg) or diluent (control) given subcutaneously (sc) at time 0

hypoglycaemic response with human insulin. The Δ glucose level was significantly lower with human than bovine insulin 50 min after administration ($p<0.05$). There was, however, no difference in the incremental plasma insulin concentrations between human and bovine insulin at this intermediate dose level.

(iii) *Porcine and bovine insulin (Figure 4.20c)*. The hypoglycaemic response and the incremental insulin profiles were identical for porcine and bovine insulin at the lowest dose level. At 0.075 U/kg, after a similar initial hypoglycaemic effect (0 to 120 min), a slower recovery was observed with bovine insulin, the difference reaching significance from 210 to 270 min ($p<0.05$). There was, however, no concomitant difference between the plasma insulin levels. At the highest dose level the hypoglycaemic response was similar for the two species of insulin, the insulin levels differing only at one time point (240 min, porcine $>$ bovine: $p<0.05$).

(b) Analysis of dose–response relationships

Preliminary covariance analysis confirmed that essentially the same results may be obtained by subtracting the mean basal from the subsequent levels for both glucose and insulin, rather than carrying out the analysis of variance using the basal level as the covariate.

The analysis carried out consisted of the estimation and comparison of the dose–response relationships between the three species of insulin. Very often it is found that the response can be described as a linear function of the logarithms of the dose. If the response versus log-dose line for the comparative insulins is parallel, an estimate of the relative 'potency' of one insulin to another can be derived. When the condition of parallelism is fulfilled the relative 'potency' is independent of the dose levels, representing a convenient way of expressing possible differential biological effects of related substances.

By means of standard methods for analysis of biological assays (Finney, 1978), it is possible to check the validity of the model and estimate the relative 'potency', including a confidence interval as a measure of precision and as a convenient test of whether the 'potency' estimate differs significantly from 100%. If so, it means that the comparative preparations have different quantitative biological effects.

The individual glucose or insulin values can also be used as separate responses to calculate the relative 'potency' and 'bioavailability' as a function of time. Although these responses are not independent, comparison of the 'potencies' at different time points can be accomplished by means of recently developed methods for analyses of bioassays with multivariate responses (Vølund, 1980). In addition to comparisons at individual time points, various average levels over defined intervals of time were also subjected to dose–response analysis.

(i) *Plasma glucose (biological 'potency'; Figure 4.21a)*. The conditions of linearity and parallelism referred to above could be met except for the low dose, where there was a tendency to systematic deviations from linearity after 120 to 180 min, due to a flattening of the low-dose part of the dose-response curve. The calculation of a meaningful 'potency' estimate also requires the

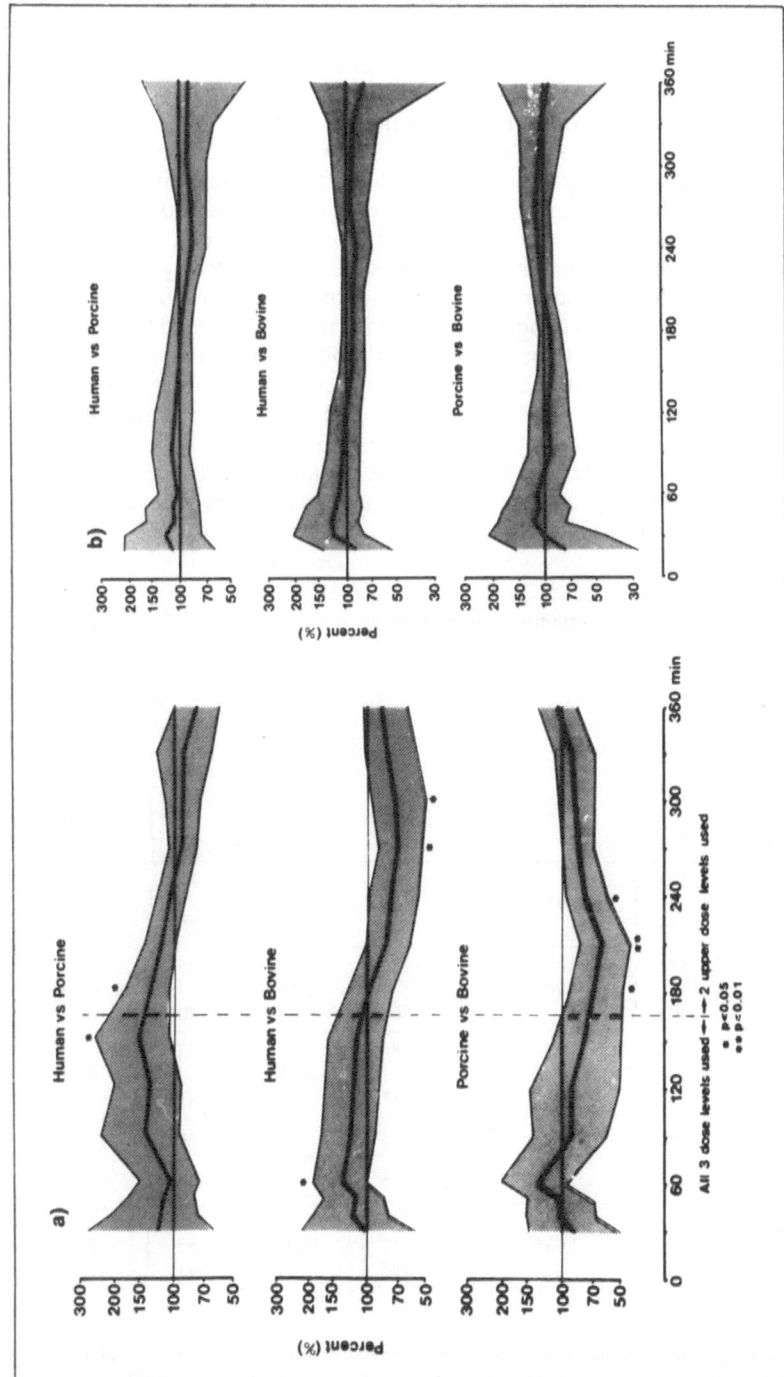

Figure 4.21 Estimates (with 95% confidence limits) of **(a)** relative hypoglycaemic 'potency' and **(b)** relative 'bioavailability' of human versus porcine; human versus bovine and porcine versus bovine insulin

slope to be significantly different from zero, which was not the case in the early responses at 10 and 20 min.

The estimated relative 'potency' with 95% confidence limits for human relative to both porcine and bovine insulin and porcine relative to bovine insulin is shown as a function of time in Figure 4.21a.

It appears that human insulin tended to be more potent than porcine insulin during the first hours after injection with the differences reaching statistical significance at 150 and 180 min ($p<0.05$). Human insulin was also more potent than bovine insulin over the first 180 min after administration, although the difference was barely significant at 60 min ($p<0.05$). Later, the hypoglycaemic response was greater with bovine than human insulin between 270 and 300 min ($p<0.05$). The comparison of porcine and bovine insulin indicated that porcine insulin, in general, tended to be less potent, although like human insulin there was a timing difference, porcine insulin being relatively more potent during the first 90 min after injection and less so subsequently. Between 180 and 240 min porcine insulin was significantly less potent ($p<0.05-0.01$) than bovine insulin (Figure 4.21a). These differences are brought out more clearly and compared more precisely when the average responses and time intervals are analysed simultaneously (Table 4.7).

Table 4.7 Multivariate dose–response analysis of average hypoglycaemic (Δ BG) responses over different time intervals

Time intervals (min)	Human vs porcine insulin		Human vs bovine insulin		Porcine vs bovine insulin	
	Rel. potency	χ^2	Rel. potency	χ^2	Rel. potency	χ^2
0–60	135		121		96	
		0.34		1.10		0.50
60–360	113		93		82*	
0–90	143		126		95	
		0.97		3.38		0.68
90–360	113		90		79*	
0–120	141		127		95	
		1.70		5.60*		0.76
120–360	109		86		80*	
0–150	144		128		93	
		3.64		8.78**		0.73
150–360	105		83*		81*	
0–180	143		121		86	
		6.05*		9.83**		0.18
180–360	101		79*		81*	
0–60	135		121		96	
60–180	144*	7.63*	121	11.31**	83	0.51
180–360	101		79*		81*	
0–360	115		95		83*	

*At the potency estimate mean that the associated (unvariate) 95% confidence interval does not contain the 100% value: * or ** at the χ^2 value means $p<0.05$ or $p<0.01$ respectively

There is statistically significant heterogeneity in the 'potency' of human relative to porcine or bovine insulin comparing the early and late hypoglycaemic responses. The differences between human and bovine insulin are larger and statistically more significant than those between human and porcine insulin. Whilst the differences between porcine and bovine insulin do not reach statistical significance, porcine insulin tends to be less potent overall than either bovine or human insulin.

After subcutaneous administration, human insulin has a stronger initial hypoglycaemic effect than either porcine or bovine insulin, whereas after 180 min bovine is more potent than human and porcine insulin. The insulins can therefore be ranked with respect to a high initial and a less delayed hypoglycaemic effect as follows: human>porcine>bovine.

(ii) *Plasma insulin ('bioavailability'; Figure 4.21b)*. The dose–response analysis was only carried out for the two higher dose levels for the same reasons given in the glucose dose–response analysis, i.e. flattening of the dose–response curve at the lower dose levels. The relative 'bioavailability' estimate as a function of time is shown in Figure 4.21b. Human insulin, relative to bovine insulin, shows the same time variation in 'bioavailability' as seen in hypoglycaemic 'potency', although the variation in 'bioavailability' over time is smaller than that of hypoglycaemic 'potency'. At no time point was there any difference between the insulin species.

Although analysis of the incremental insulin levels over the different time intervals (Table 4.8), shows no statistically significant difference between the species, the results are in the same direction as those observed between the hypoglycaemic potencies (Table 4.7). Differences in 'bioavailability' between

Table 4.8 Multivariate dose–response analysis of average (Δ IRI) responses over different time intervals

Time intervals (min)	Human vs porcine insulin		Human vs bovine insulin		Porcine vs bovine insulin	
	Rel. potency	χ^2	Rel. potency	χ^2	Rel. potency	χ^2
0–60	110		111		103	
		0.17		0.52		0.09
60–360	103		101		97	
0–120	113		111		98	
		1.30		1.53		0.00
120–360	98		95		98	
0–180	111		107		95	
		2.65		1.28		0.32
180–360	91		93		103	
0–60	110		111		103	
60–180	111	4.99	105	1.34	93	2.16
180 360	91		93		103	
0–360	105		103		98	

The 95% confidence intervals for all the individual estimates comprised 100%, i.e. no significant species differences the three species of insulin are relatively small, with the most pronounced difference between human and bovine insulin.

(iii) *Comparison of hypoglycaemic 'potency' and 'bioavailability'.* This was assessed by means of a direct comparison of the hypoglycaemic 'potency' and the 'bioavailability' by a multivariate bioassay using simultaneous glucose and insulin values. As it is a problem to select the most meaningful relationship between insulin and glucose levels, average Δ glucose values over defined periods have been compared with the corresponding insulin values and those relating to previous or subsequent periods (Table 4.9). Only one comparison of

Table 4.9 Multivariate dose–response analysis of Δ BG and Δ IRI levels

Time intervals (min)	Human vs porcine insulin Rel. potency			Human vs bovine insulin Rel. potency			Porcine vs bovine insulin Rel. potency		
	Δ BG	Δ IRI	χ^2	Δ BG	Δ IRI	χ^2	Δ BG	Δ IRI	χ^2
0–60	135	110	0.53	121	111	0.13	121	111	0.13
60–360	113	103	1.10	93	101	0.61	82*	97	3.11
0–120	141	113	1.24	127	111	0.65	95	98	0.03
120–360	109	98	1.59	86	95	1.21	86	95	1.21
0–180	143*	111	2.71	121	107	0.85	86	95	0.41
180–360	101	91	1.49	79*	93	2.34	81*	103	7.20*
60–180	144*	111	3.15	121	105	1.14	83	93	0.43
0–360	115	105	0.92	95	103	0.53	83*	98	2.58
0–60		110	} 1.48		111	} 0.99		103	} 3.11
60–360	113	103		93	101		82*	97	
0–60	135	110	} 0.53	121	111	} 1.41	96	103	} 1.02
60–360	113			93			82*		
0–120		113	} 2.67		111	} 3.09		98	} 5.11
120–360	109	98		86	95		80*	98	
0–120	141	113	} 1.86	127	111	} 6.42*	95	98	} 1.65
120–360	109			86			80		
0–180		111	} 3.22		107	} 5.52		95	} 7.25*
180–360	101	91		79*	93		81*	103	
0–180	143*	111	} 6.10*	121	107	} 11.00**	86	95	} 1.30
180–360	101			79*			81*		
0–180	143*	111	} 7.51	121	107	} 11.83**	86	95	} 7.42
180–360	101	91		79*	93		81*	103	

*At the potency estimate means that it deviates significantly from 100%
* or ** at the χ^2 value means that there is significant heterogeneity between the potencies (*$p < 0.05$ or **$p < 0.01$)

hypoglycaemic 'potency' and relative 'bioavailability' shows a statistically significant difference when comparing the hypoglycaemic effect and incremental insulin values between porcine and bovine insulin for the period 180 to 360 min. The hypoglycaemic 'potency' of porcine, relative to bovine insulin, was less than the relative 'bioavailability' in these comparisons except for the 0 to 60 min period.

When human is compared to porcine insulin, a higher hypoglycaemic 'potency' than relative 'bioavailability' is observed, especially during the first 180 min after injection (Table 4.9). The comparison between human and bovine insulin also showed a higher hypoglycaemic 'potency' than 'bioavailability' with the earlier responses, and vice-versa with the later effects.

The lower part of Table 4.9 shows comparisons of the early and late hypoglycaemic 'potency' relative to the early 'bioavailability', and the late hypoglycaemic 'potency' with the early and late relative 'bioavailability'. Compared to Table 4.7, the χ^2 values are essentially unchanged by the introduction of the early relative 'bioavailabilities', whereas relating the late hypoglycaemic 'potency' to the early and late 'bioavailability' increases the χ^2 value, indicating that the hypoglycaemic 'potencies' are more heterogeneous than the relative 'bioavailabilities'.

Discussion

Detailed analysis of the data has revealed significant time-dependent differences in the hypoglycaemic 'potency' of human, porcine and bovine Actrapid insulin following subcutaneous injection in man over a 360 min post-injection observation period. Human insulin possessed a stronger initial hypoglycaemic effect than either porcine or bovine insulin, whereas bovine insulin had a more prolonged action than either human or porcine insulin. In comparison, porcine insulin tended to be less potent in lowering plasma glucose than the other two species of insulin. Differences between the relative 'bioavailability' of the three species of insulin were in the same direction as the differences in hypoglycaemic 'potencies', although there were no significant differences. The clear differences in hypoglycaemic 'potency' and the relative absence of differences in 'bioavailability' imply that the species differ more in their biological effect than in their pharmacokinetic behaviour, suggesting that the insulins could still show differences in hypoglycaemic 'potency' with equivalent plasma levels.

Conflicting data prevail in the literature with regard to the relative 'bioavailability' and hypoglycaemic 'potency' of highly purified neutral, soluble porcine and human insulin (derived either from porcine insulin or employing DNA biotechnology) following bolus subcutaneous injection in normal man. Meaningful comparisons between the studies cannot be conducted due to differences in study design and procedures, insulin dosage, injection technique, site of administration, assay methodologies and details of 'potency' determinations with respect to the insulin preparations employed. The administration of 'semi-synthetic' human and porcine insulin by bolus subcutaneous injection into the anterior abdominal wall for the 0.05 and 0.075 U/kg dose levels results in similar plasma insulin profiles (Laube et al, 1981a, b;

Owens et al, 1981a, c; Owens et al, 1982; Ebihara et al, 1983). Comparison of the hypoglycaemic responses at a lower dose of 0.05 U/kg shows either a greater 'potency' with human insulin (Ebihara et al, 1983) or no difference, as seen in this study. Similarly, little or no difference exists between the two species at 0.075 U/kg (Owens et al, 1982). At the higher dose levels of 0.1 to 0.15 U/kg the results are more consistent in demonstrating the greater 'potency' of human relative to porcine insulin after subcutaneous injection in normal man. The differences in hypoglycaemic 'potency' may, or may not, reflect differences in insulin absorption or 'bioavailability' (Sundermann et al, 1981; Ebihara et al, 1983). Broadly similar results have been observed with 'biosynthetic' neutral, soluble human insulin. Equivalent hypoglycaemic responses to 'biosynthetic' human insulin and purified porcine insulin have been observed by the majority of investigators (Keen et al, 1980; Galloway et al, 1981b, 1982a; Weinges et al, 1981; Ebihara et al, 1982; Kemmer et al, 1982), with few exceptions (Federlin et al, 1981). At low dose levels, no difference in the resultant plasma insulin profiles has been observed (Ebihara et al, 1982; Pickup et al, 1982) whereas for doses of 0.1 U/kg and above, studies have shown that human insulin can achieve higher plasma insulin levels (Federlin et al, 1981; Galloway et al, 1982; Kemmer et al, 1982; Pickup et al, 1982).

This study demonstrates that at the low dose of 0.05 U/kg the subcutaneous administration of neutral, soluble human and porcine insulin results in similar insulin profiles and hypoglycaemic effects. With increasing doses, human insulin is more biologically potent than the equivalent formulation of porcine insulin, associated with a tendency towards better 'bioavailability' during the first hours after injection. Bovine insulin, prepared in an identical manner to the human and porcine insulin, has a weaker initial, but a more prolonged, hypoglycaemic effect than either human or porcine insulin. These differences are not inexplicable from the plasma insulin profiles. The data tentatively indicate that there are species differences in the timing of the hypoglycaemic response, which exceed those due to absorption or 'bioavailability' differences.

The results of this study, therefore, support earlier observations in both animals and man that a time-dependent variation in hypoglycaemic 'potency' exists between human, porcine and bovine insulin (Vølund et al, 1982; Owens et al, 1984a). The results also emphasise the need to use pure species insulin standards for the bioassay of the three species of insulin used clinically instead of the present mixed species (porcine/bovine) 4th International Standard (Bangham and Mussett, 1959).

4.1.6 Comparative study of intravenous and intramuscular administration of human insulin

Introduction

After the initial studies with subcutaneously administered neutral, soluble 'semi-synthetic' human and porcine insulin a further study, comparing intramuscular and intravenous bolus injections of human insulin, was conducted in normal male volunteer subjects for the purpose of comparing the three routes of administration. The route of administration is the main factor that influences the absorption of soluble insulin (Moore et al, 1959; Nora et al, 1964; Guerra and Kitabchi, 1976; Galloway et al, 1981a; Berger et al, 1982; Home et al, 1982b; Binder et al, 1984), being the only insulin preparation administered by the subcutaneous, intramuscular and intravenous route.

Subjects, materials and methods

The same six normal volunteer subjects who participated in the initial subcutaneous insulin study (cf. 4.1.1) were also entered into this study. Little or no changes had occurred in the subjects' weight since the original study which was conducted approximately 2 to 3 weeks previously.

The human insulin used in this study was 'semi-synthetic' human insulin. Diluting medium was used in the control studies and somatostatin was prepared for intravenous administration.

The dose of the insulin was 5 or 6 U administered by bolus injection. The insulin was given intramuscularly into the upper thigh or intravenously into an antecubital fossa vein. The protocol used in this study is summarised in the flow-diagram in Figure 4.22.

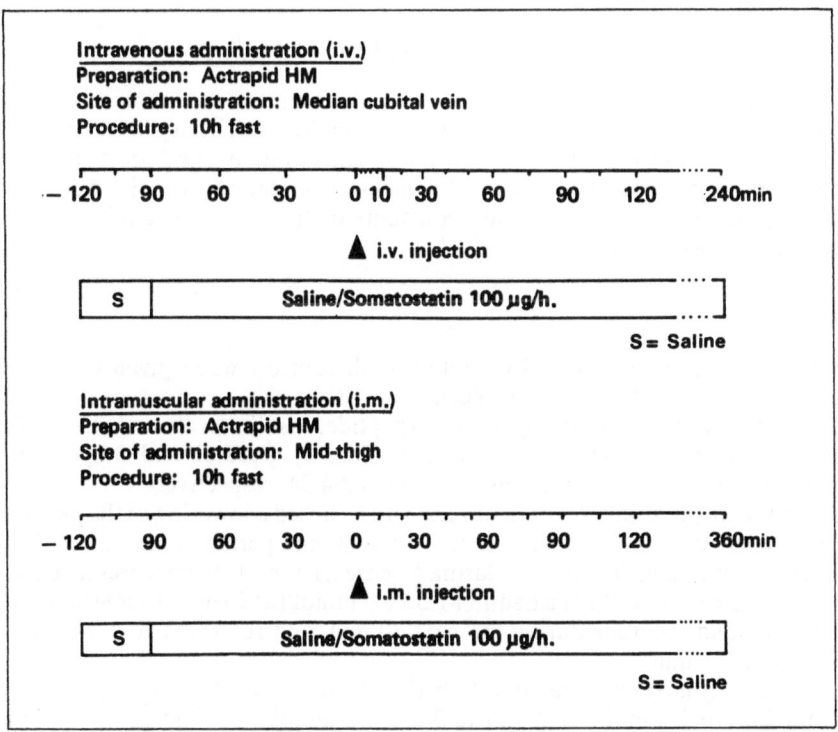

Figure 4.22

Somatostatin infusion was commenced after a 30 min basal period (–90 min), and continued for the remainder of both the intramuscular and intravenous studies. Human insulin was injected intramuscularly or intravenously at 0 min, i.e. 120 min from the start of the study and 90 min after the commencement of somatostatin. The blood sampling times after intravenous injection were 2, 4, 6, 8, 10, 15, 30, 40, 60, 75, 90, 105, 120, 150, 180, 210 and 360 min; and after intramuscular injection samples were taken at 10, 20, 30, 40, 50, 60, 75, 90, 105, 120 and every 30 min up to 360 min. The blood samples were taken into fluoride for plasma glucose (hexokinase), and into heparin for immunoreactive insulin (IRI) (Heding, 1972) and C-peptide (Heding, 1975) determinations. The concentrations of blood intermediary metabolites (lactate, alanine, glycerol and 3-hydroxybutyrate) were estimated in deproteinized blood (Lloyd et al, 1978).

Statistical methods

The results are expressed as means ± SE except where stated otherwise. The area under the insulin curve was estimated by the trapezoidal method. The analysis of the elimination kinetics of human insulin after intravenous bolus injection has been carried out by fitting a sum of two exponentials to the data from each of the six normal subjects, i.e.

$$c\ (t) = \alpha_0 + \alpha_1 \exp\ (-\beta_1 t) + \alpha_2 \exp\ (-\beta_2 t)$$

where $c(t)$ is the insulin concentration at time t after intravenous injection, and $\alpha_0, \alpha_2, \alpha_2, \beta_1$ and β_2 are constants derived from the data, i.e. α_0= basal insulin concentration just prior to intravenous injection; α_1 and α_2 = insulin concentration at time 0 determined by back-extrapolation from fitted curves, and β_1 and β_2 = elimination rate constants of the two exponential curves corresponding to α_1 and α_2.

Results

The human insulin was well tolerated in all subjects when given by bolus intravenous and intramuscular injection.

The means ± SE plasma glucose, C-peptide, insulin levels and the mean blood intermediary metabolite (lactate, alanine, glycerol and 3-hydroxy-butyrate) levels are shown in Figures 4.23 and 4.24, respectively.

Prior to insulin, somatostatin, as expected, caused a lowering of the plasma glucose by about 0.5 mmol/l over the initial 90 min period of infusion. After intravenous human insulin the plasma glucose fell rapidly from a pre-injection level of 4.5 ± 0.4 mmol/l to a nadir of 1.5 ± 0.2 mmol/l at 25 min, followed by an equally rapid recovery during the next 30 min, and returning to pre-insulin values at 210 min.

Following intramuscular injection the glucose levels fell more gradually from 4.4 ± 0.3 mmol/l at 0 min to 3.0 ± 0.2 mmol/l at 90 min, with a less dramatic recovery towards normoglycaemia, the plasma glucose reaching 4.4 ± 0.2 mmol/l at 360 min.

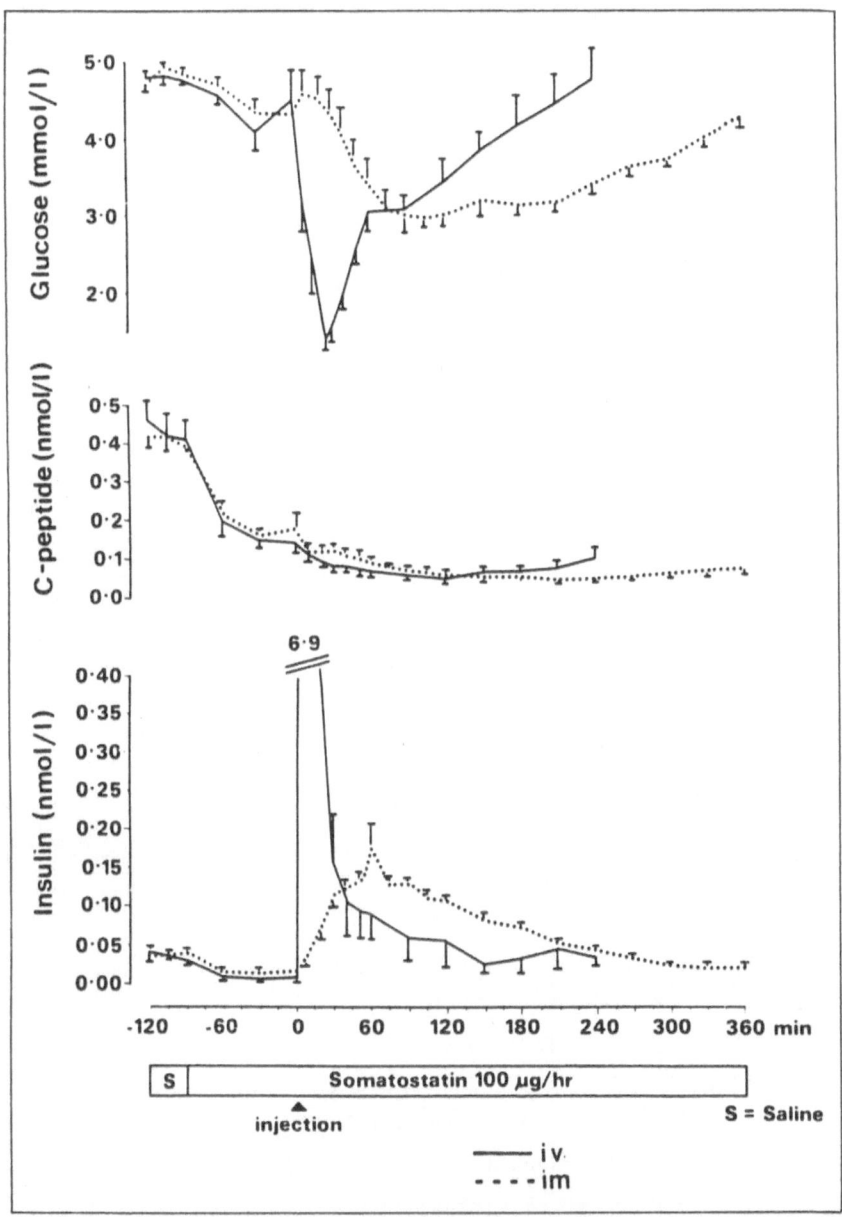

Figure 4.23 Effect of intravenous (iv) and intramuscular (im) bolus injections of human insulin on plasma glucose, C-peptide and insulin (IRI) concentrations (means ± SE) in six subjects. Somatostatin infused from –90 to 360 min. Insulin (~0.075 U/kg) given at time 0

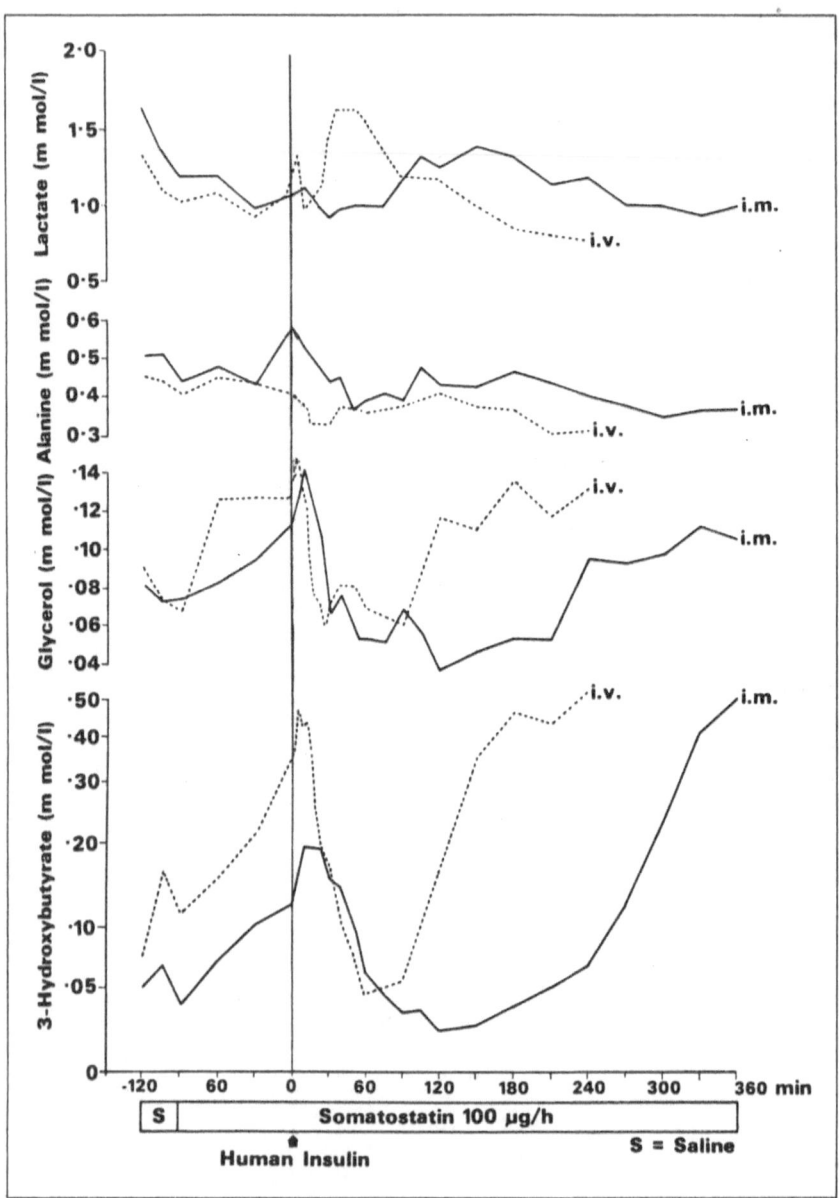

Figure 4.24 Effect of intravenous (iv) and intramuscular (im) bolus injections of human insulin on blood lactate, alanine, glycerol and 3-hydroxybutyrate concentrations (means) in six subjects. Somatostatin infused from –90 to 360 min. Insulin (~0.075 U/kg) given at time 0

During the basal (pre-insulin) periods of the intravenous and intramuscular studies, the somatostatin infusion lowered the plasma C-peptide level from 0.4 ± 0.07 to 0.14 ± 0.03 nmol/l, and from 0.4 ± 0.03 to 0.18 ± 0.5 nmol/l, respectively – a mean reduction of about 66% (Figure 4.23). Intravenous insulin resulted in a small additional suppression of C-peptide levels, reaching a nadir of 0.06 ± 0.01 nmol/l at 120 min. Following intramuscular administration the C-peptide levels fell from 0.18 ± 0.05 nmol/l to 0.05 ± 0.01 nmol/l at 120 min. At the end of the intravenous (240 min) and intramuscular (360 min) studies the C-peptide levels remained suppressed at 0.10 ± 0.03 and 0.07 ± 0.01 nmol/l, respectively. The basal plasma insulin level fell after 90 min of somatostatin infusion from 0.033 ± 0.007 and 0.04 ± 0.004 nmol/l to 0.011 ± 0.015 and 0.013 ± 0.003 nmol/l in the intravenous and intramuscular studies, respectively.

Intravenous insulin led to a steep rise in plasma insulin, reaching a peak level of 6.9 ± 0.73 nmol/l at 2 min. Thereafter, the plasma insulin level fell rapidly over the next 60 min returning to near fasting values at 150 min. In contrast, a more gradual increase in plasma insulin was observed following intramuscular injection, reaching a lower peak level of 0.18 ± 0.04 nmol/l at 60 min, returning to 0.02 ± 0.004 nmol/l by 360 min (Figure 4.23).

The blood levels of the intermediary metabolites, glycerol and 3-hydroxybutyrate increased with somatostatin prior to insulin administration, whereas lactate and alanine remained unchanged (Figure 4.24). Intravenous insulin produced a rapid increase in lactate levels during the first 90 min, with a lesser delayed response following intramuscular administration.

Intravenous insulin caused 3-hydroxybutyrate levels to fall rapidly after 10 min, when the mean value was 0.366 (0.025–0.690) mmol/l, reaching a nadir of 0.048 (0.010–0.090) mmol/l at 60 min (Figure 4.24). Intramuscular insulin produced a more gradual response, lowering the mean pre-injection 3-hydroxybutyrate of 0.198 (0.020–0.410) mmol/l, to 0.022 (0.010–0.035) mmol/l by 120 min. Thereafter there was a comparable post-hypoglycaemic rise occurring approximately 120 to 180 min earlier with the intravenous route of administration. Similar, but less dramatic, changes in blood glycerol concentrations were observed.

The mean plasma glucose, C-peptide, insulin and the glycerol and 3-hydroxybutyrate levels in response to human insulin administered either intravenously, intramuscularly or subcutaneously (cf. 4.1.1), are compared in Figures 4.25a and b, respectively. There was no statistically significant difference in the hypoglycaemic response to human insulin between the subcutaneous (anterior abdominal wall) and intramuscular (thigh) routes of administration. The plasma glucose level was, however, significantly lower with intravenous than intramuscular or subcutaneous injection between 10 and 50 min ($p < 0.05$–0.01), whereas from 120 min onwards the reverse was true. The plasma insulin profiles were similar during the first 120 min after subcutaneous and intramuscular injection, remaining higher after subcutaneous injection from 210 min onwards ($p < 0.01$–0.05). The insulin levels were significantly higher with intravenous than either intramuscular or subcutaneous insulin during the first 20 min after administration; the reverse being the case from 150 min onwards.

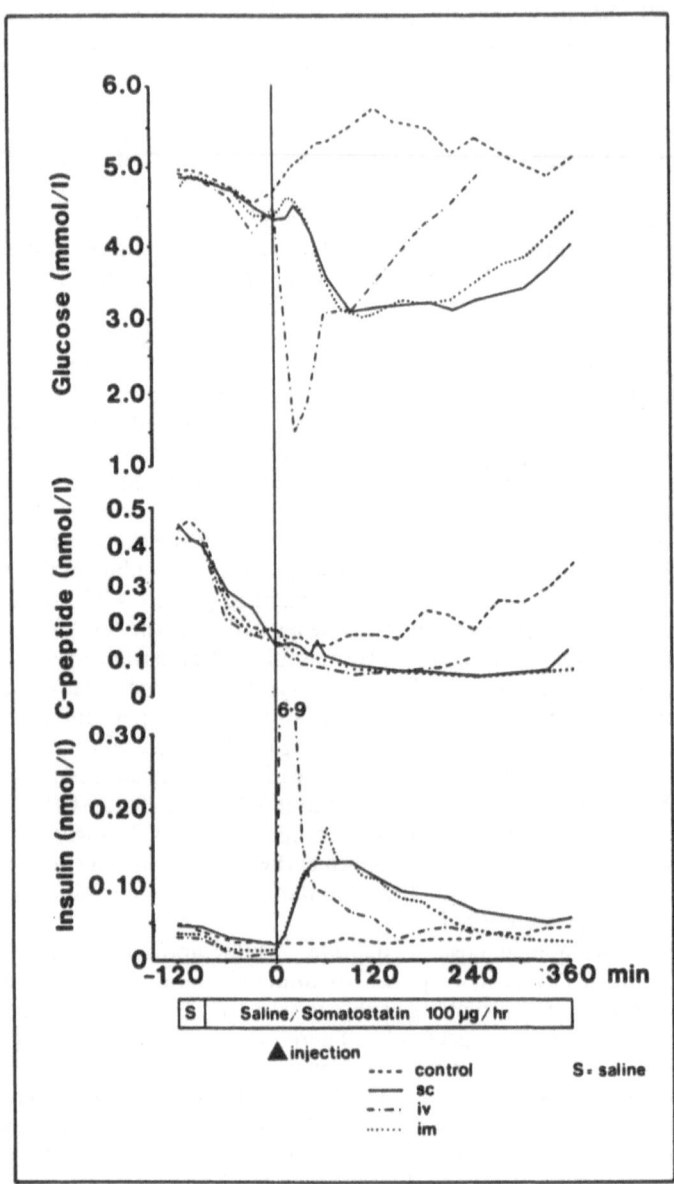

Figure 4.25a Effect of subcutaneous (sc), intravenous (iv) and intramuscular (im) bolus injections of human insulin on plasma glucose, C-peptide and insulin (IRI) concentrations (means) in six subjects. Somatostatin infused from –90 to 360 min. Insulin (~0.075 U/kg) or sc diluent (control) given at time 0

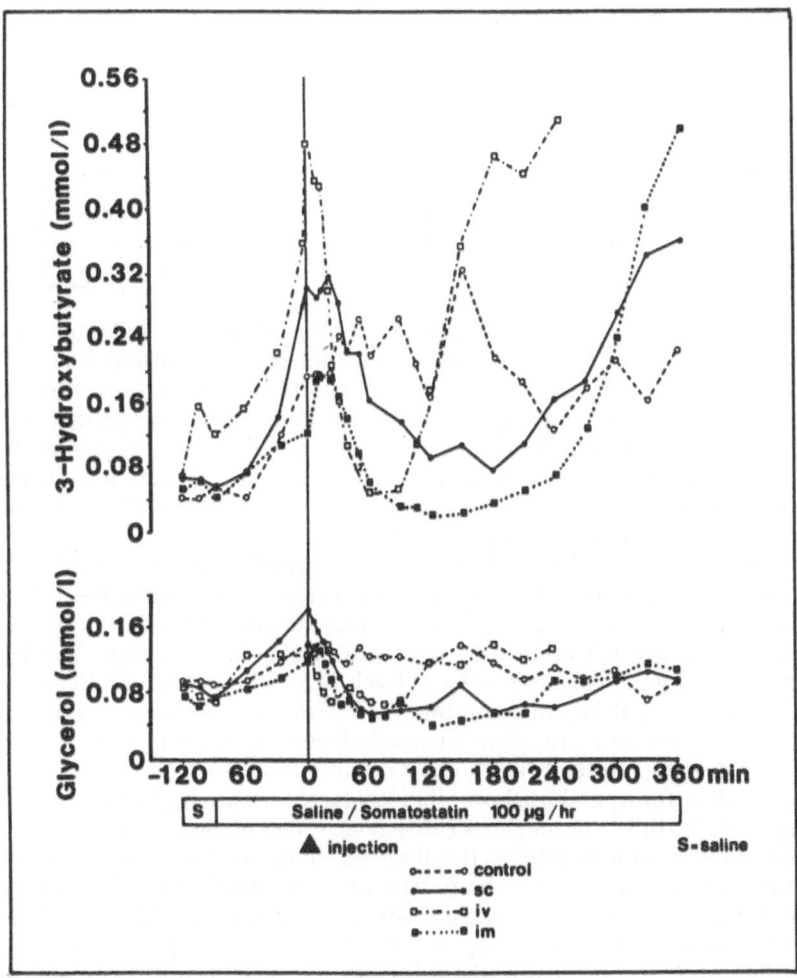

Figure 4.25b Effect of subcutaneous (sc), intravenous (iv) and intramuscular (im) bolus injections of human insulin on blood 3-hydroxybutyrate and glycerol concentrations (means) in six subjects. Somatostatin infused from –90 to 360 min. Insulin (~0.075 U/kg) or sc diluent (control) given at time 0

Insulin kinetics

The areas under the plasma insulin curves (AUC) for human insulin given by the three routes of administration are included in Table 4.10.

As the comparison of the areas calculated in this way is only meaningful when the times of measurement are the same, the intravenous data cannot be compared to that of intramuscular or subcutaneous administration. However, assuming that the few differences in measurement times between the intramuscular and subcutaneous studies are probably unimportant, there are apparently no differences between these two routes of administration.

Table 4.10 Pharmacokinetic analyses

Route of administration	Time interval (min)	Insulin AUC (nmol/1/min)						
		Subjects						
		1	2	3	4	5	6	$\overline{X}$
Intravenous	0–240	37.4	96.2	62.2	48.2	36.3	34.5	52.5
Intramuscular	0–360	18.4	28.5	36.4	19.7	24.2	24.4	25.3
Subcutaneous	0–360	28.1	26.2	21.4	32.4	31.5	30.6	28.4

The elimination kinetics of human insulin after intravenous bolus injection has been analysed by fitting the sum of two exponentials to the data from each of the six normal volunteers. The 2 and 4 min insulin values were not included, since insulin may not be homogeneously distributed in the plasma that early after injection. The computer-fitted values of α and β are two expressions for the goodness of fit, i.e. the absolute residual standard deviation (SD) and coefficient of variation (CV), expressed as a percentage of the insulin concentration, are included in Table 4.11.

In one case the best fit was obtained with $\alpha_0 = 0$ indicating total inhibition of insulin secretion by somatostatin. Three other cases had α_0 values close to zero (<0.006 nmol/l), demonstrating that somatostatin infusion had depressed the basal insulin concentration to a level that was practically zero. The two remaining subjects had elevated basal levels of 0.023 nmol/l and 0.15 nmol/l. The sum of α_1 and α_2, representing the insulin concentration at time zero determined by back-extrapolation from the fitted curve, is rather similar in all but one subject (subject 4 value almost double; Table 4.11).

The values for α_1 and α_2 show relatively large variations (Table 4.11). The magnitude for this variation is reflected in the values of the SD and CV, which describe the deviations between the observed values and the fitted curves. The coefficients of variation, which are relevant in the high concentration range and for judgement of the semilogarithmic plot, are between 2.5 and 10.5%.

With a dose of ~ 0.075 U/kg, i.e. ~ 0.5 nmol/kg, the apparent volume of distribution (dose/$\alpha_1 + \alpha_2$) is about 0.1 l/kg (range 0.06–0.11 l/kg), and the plasma clearance rate is approximately 1.0 l/min (range 0.6–1.3 l/min).

The values of β_1 are fairly close together and correpond to an initial rapid elimination component with a $T_{\frac{1}{2}}$ in the range of 3.3 to 5.1 min (Table 4.12).

Table 4.11

Subject no.	nmol/l			min^{-1}		SD (nmol/l)	CV (%)
	α_0	α_1	α_2	β_1	β_2		
1	0.0227	5.673	0.053	0.162	0.019	0.023	4.6
2	0.	4.911	0.195	0.158	0.012	0.031	6.2
3	0.1535	5.571	0.315	0.135	0.020	0.052	10.5
4	0.0230	9.201	1.134	0.212	0.066	0.013	2.5
5	0.0042	5.044	0.118	0.164	0.0218	0.018	3.5
6	0.0029	4.362	0.107	0.180	0.0491	0.031	6.1

Table 4.12

Subject no.	β_1 (min^{-1})	$T_{1/2}$ (min)	β_2 (min^{-1})	$T_{1/2}$ (min)
1	0.162	4.3	0.019	36.5
2	0.158	4.4	0.012	57.8
3	0.135	5.1	0.020	34.7
4	0.212	3.3	0.0661	10.5
5	0.164	4.2	0.0219	31.8
6	0.180	3.9	0.0491	14.1
$\bar{x}$	0.169	4.2	0.0778	30.9

$T_{1/2}$ = half time of disappearance (min)
β_1, β_2 = elimination rate constants of the two exponential curves corresponding to α_1 and α_2

The disappearance half-time for the slower elimination component was 31 min (range 11 to 58 min; Table 4.12).

Discussion

The human insulin was well tolerated in all subjects after both intravenous and intramuscular administration.

The hypoglycaemic response to a bolus intravenous injection of human insulin was rapid, reaching a nadir at 25 min followed by recovery to pre-insulin levels within 210 min, similar to that seen with other soluble insulins (Greenwood and Landon, 1966). Peak insulin levels were achieved between 2 and 4 min after administration, which is also in agreement with previous data (Stimmler et al, 1972; Ginsberg et al, 1973; Guerra and Kitabchi, 1976; Galloway et al, 1981a). This was followed by an initial rapid elimination with a half-time of disappearance ($T_{1/2}$) in the range of 3 to 5 min. Previous findings with porcine, bovine and human pancreatic soluble insulin in normal man are similar, although the values vary from study to study within the range of 3 to 15 minutes (Ørskov and Christensen, 1966; Stimmler, 1966; Martin et al, 1967; Sönksen et al, 1973; Burt and Davidson, 1974; Bellmann and Hartmann, 1975; Lind et al, 1977). The estimation of insulin kinetics after a single-pulse intravenous injection is limited since insulin disappearance curves are multi-exponential, dependent on insulin dose and timing of samples, contributing to the varying estimates quoted above (Sherwin et al, 1974; Navalesi et al, 1978). There are also considerable difficulties in the interpretation of *in vivo* studies using unlabelled insulin, due to the presence of endogenous insulin secretion (Frost et al, 1973; Tranberg and Dencker, 1978). In this study we have used somatostatin to inhibit insulin secretion, so that the plasma insulin concentrations reflect more precisely the kinetics of the exogenous insulin. There are, however, inherent problems in the use of somatostatin, due to its known inhibitory effect on splanchnic blood flow (Felig and Wahren, 1976). The estimated apparent volume of distribution (AVD) and plasma clearance rates (PCR) are similar to that found by Tranberg and Dencker (1978), i.e. AVD approximately 0.1 l/kg body weight and PCR approximately 14ml/kg/min. The presence of insulin antibodies in insulin-dependent diabetics will result in a much longer $T_{1/2}$ for insulin of up to 54 min (Berson et al, 1956; Kruse, 1981).

In comparison to intravenous insulin, the intramuscular route of administration resulted in a less dramatic hypoglycaemic response, reflecting the differences observed in the plasma insulin levels. The hypoglycaemic response to intramuscular insulin in the thigh region was similar to that seen previously with subcutaneous injection into the anterior abdominal wall, although tending to be of shorter duration after intramuscular injection. Similar mean plasma insulin peak concentrations were achieved at approximately the same time (60 to 90 min) for both im and sc routes of administration, followed by a slightly more rapid clearance after intramuscular injection.

The blood glycerol and 3-hydroxybutyrate levels rose during somatostatin infusion and fell after insulin, the response being more rapid in onset and shorter in duration with intravenous relative to intramuscular and subcutaneously injected insulin.

The studies demonstrated that the new neutral, soluble 'semi-synthetic' human insulin was well tolerated when given as a single bolus intravenous, intramuscular or subcutaneous injection at a dose level of 0.075 U/kg body weight to normal man (Owens et al, 1981d).

4.1.7 A study of intravenous (human, porcine, bovine) and intramuscular (human) insulin in normal man

Introduction

The previous study, involving the intravenous and intramuscular administration of insulin during an intravenous infusion of somatostatin to suppress endogenous insulin secretion, was repeated in fasting subjects without the concomitant use of somatostatin.

The purpose of this study was to follow the insulin kinetics and metabolic responses in normal subjects following:

(1) bolus intravenous (iv) injection of human, porcine and bovine insulin and diluting medium (control),
(2) intramuscular injection of human insulin and diluting medium (control).

Subjects, materials and methods

Six healthy normal male volunteer subjects were entered into the study, all of

Table 4.13

	Actrapid HM (human)	Actrapid MC (porcine)	Actrapid MC (bovine)	Actrapid diluent
Nitrogen (mg/ml)	0.216	0.215	0.215	—
Potency[a] (IU/ml)	39.9	39.8	39.8	—

[a]Theoretical potency 185 IU/mgN

whom were within 10% of ideal body weight. Five subjects were involved in the intravenous part of the study and six in the intramuscular section. The preparations used in the study are shown in Table 4.13. The insulin dose for both routes of administration was ~0.075 U/kg, i.e. 6 U, with an equivalent volume of diluting medium for the control studies. There was a separate control day for both the intravenous and intramuscular part of the study.

The basic protocol was the same as that used for the earlier study (cf. 4.1.6) of intravenous and intramuscular human insulin, but omitting the somatostatin infusion. All the subjects (except one) underwent both parts of the study involving a total of six separate study days, i.e. 4 days for the intravenous and 2 days for the intramuscular section. The treatments for each part of the study were randomised, with the intramuscular study started only after the completion of the intravenous section. Frequent blood samples were taken throughout both studies and subsequently assayed for glucose (hexokinase), insulin (IRI) (Heding, 1972) and intermediary metabolites (lactate, alanine, glycerol and 3-hydroxybutyrate) (Lloyd et al, 1978).

Statistical methods

The results are expressed as means ± SE except where stated otherwise. The concentrations of 3-hydroxybutyrate were log transformed to normalise distribution (Foster et al, 1978). The individual pairs of treatments were compared using the Student's t-test. The paired comparisons were carried out on both the absolute and the Δ values (derived by subtracting the mean basal level (–120 to 0 min) from all subsequent levels on each study day).

The insulin (IRI) data have also been analysed by means of standard pharmacokinetic methods. Although the previous study indicated that a two-compartment model is more appropriate to analyse the insulin data following bolus intravenous injection, the simple one-compartment model was used in view of the relatively infrequent sampling during the first hour. Therefore, the kinetic parameters should be regarded more as approximate measures, thus the use of the word 'apparent'. The parameters calculated included the individual estimated values of the constants α_0, α_1, β_1 (α_0 = basal insulin concentrations prior to intravenous injection; α_1 = insulin concentration at time zero by back-extrapolation from fitted curve; β_1 = plasma clearance rate constant of the exponential curve corresponding to α_1; the coefficient of variation (CV); areas under curve (AUC) estimated from the fitted exponential (0–120 min = 0–infinity), the area estimated by the trapezoidal method 0–240 min, half-time of disappearance ($T_{1/2}$) = $0.693/\beta_1$; apparent volume of distribution (AVD) = dose/α_1; and plasma clearance = $\beta_1 \times$ AVD.

Results

(i) Intravenous study

The mean Δ plasma glucose and insulin values after bolus intravenous injection of diluting medium (control), human, porcine and bovine insulin are

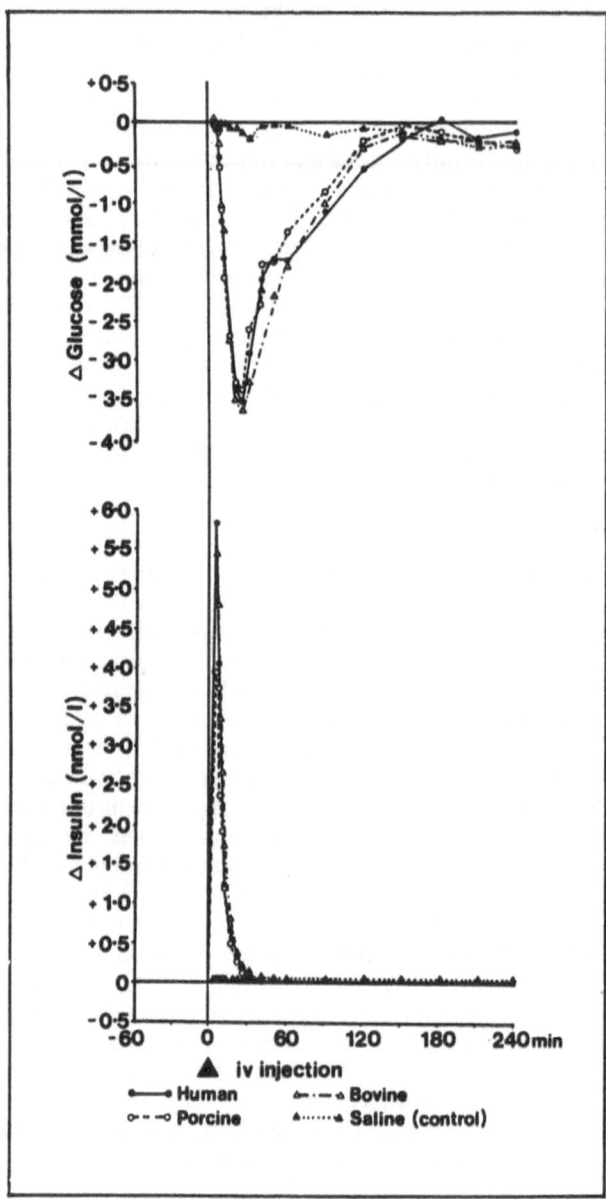

Figure 4.26a Effect of human, porcine and bovine insulins on plasma glucose and insulin (IRI) concentrations (means) in five subjects. Insulin (~0.075 U/kg) or saline (control) given intravenously (iv) at time 0. Results shown as mean of Δ values

illustrated in Figure 4.26a. During the control day the plasma glucose gradually fell from 4.7 ± 0.2 mmol/l at –120 min to 4.3 ± 0.2 mmol/l at 240 min.

Similarly, the fasting plasma insulin fell during the control study from 0.062 ± 0.01 to 0.04 ± 0.01 nmol/l. After the intravenous administration of human, porcine and bovine insulin, the plasma glucose levels fell rapidly from pre-injection levels of 4.5 ± 0.2, 4.8 ± 0.2 and 5.0 ± 0.1 mmol/l to nadirs of 1.0 ± 0.1, 1.5 ± 0.1 and 1.4 ± 0.2 mmol/l, respectively at 25 min after injection. Thereafter, the plasma glucose rapidly recovered reaching pre-insulin levels between 120 and 180 min. There was no difference in the hypoglycaemic response between the three species of insulin.

Table 4.14 Pharmacokinetic analyses

(a) Human insulin

Subject no.	Dose (U)	α_0	α_1	β_1	CV (%)	AUC(nmol/l/min)		$T_{1/2}$ (min)	AVD (litre)	Clearance (litre/min)
						0–120	0–240			
1	6	0.0685	6.3177	0.1423	19.73	52.60	58.08	4.9	5.98	0.84
2	6	0.0330	5.8480	0.1266	23.41	50.16	50.26	5.5	6.36	0.61
3	6	0.324	7.2586	0.2647	17.22	50.81	49.03	4.5	5.13	0.79
4	6	0.0674	5.2439	0.1261	17.84	49.69	53.88	5.4	7.09	0.89
5	6	0.0637	6.8954	0.1524	17.54	52.88	54.57	4.5	5.39	0.82

(b) Porcine insulin

Subject no.	Dose (U)	α_0	α_1	β_1	CV (%)	AUC(nmol/l/min)		$T_{1/2}$ (min)	AVD (litre)	Clearance (litre/min)
						0–120	0–240			
1	6	0.0371	6.2141	0.1397	26.79	48.95	49.60	5.0	5.98	0.84
2	6	0.0247	6.8417	0.1558	23.16	46.87	44.08	4.4	5.44	0.85
3	6	0.0295	5.7466	0.1627	35.01	38.86	39.68	4.3	6.5	1.05
4	6	0.0361	4.7901	0.1361	23.02	39.54	39.09	5.1	7.77	1.06
5	6	0.0587	4.0953	0.1320	20.59	38.07	39.64	5.3	9.08	1.20

(c) Bovine insulin

Subject no.	Dose (U)	α_0	α_1	β_1	CV (%)	AUC(nmol/l/min)		$T_{1/2}$ (min)	AVD (litre)	Clearance (litre/min)
						0–120	0–240			
1	6	0.0467	8.2153	0.1424	14.03	63.30	60.33	4.9	4.5	0.65
2	6	0.0330	9.4921	0.1605	24.96	63.12	67.18	4.3	3.9	0.63
3	6	0.0294	7.355	0.1500	17.58	52.58	50.03	4.6	5.1	0.76
4	6	0.0371	6.105	0.1465	20.87	46.13	44.87	4.7	6.1	0.89
5	6	0.0757	6.969	0.1236	22.43	56.40	66.40	5.6	5.3	0.66

α_0	= basal insulin concentration prior to iv injection
α_1	= insulin concentration at time 0 determined by back extrapolation from fitted curve
β_1	= plasma clearance rate constant of the exponential curve corresponding to α_1
CV	= coefficient of variation
AUC	= area under insulin curve estimated by the trapezoidal method
$T_{1/2}$	= $0.693/\beta_1$
Clearance	= $\beta_1.AVD$
AVD	= apparent volume of distribution: Dose/α_1.

The mean pre-injection plasma insulin level was similar for the comparative groups at about 0.05 nmol/l. The levels increased dramatically after the intravenous injection of each of the three preparations, reaching peak levels at 2 min of 5.9 ± 0.77, 4.0 ± 0.62 and 5.5 ± 0.5 nmol/l following human, porcine and bovine insulin, respectively. The insulin profiles were similar for the three species of neutral, soluble insulin.

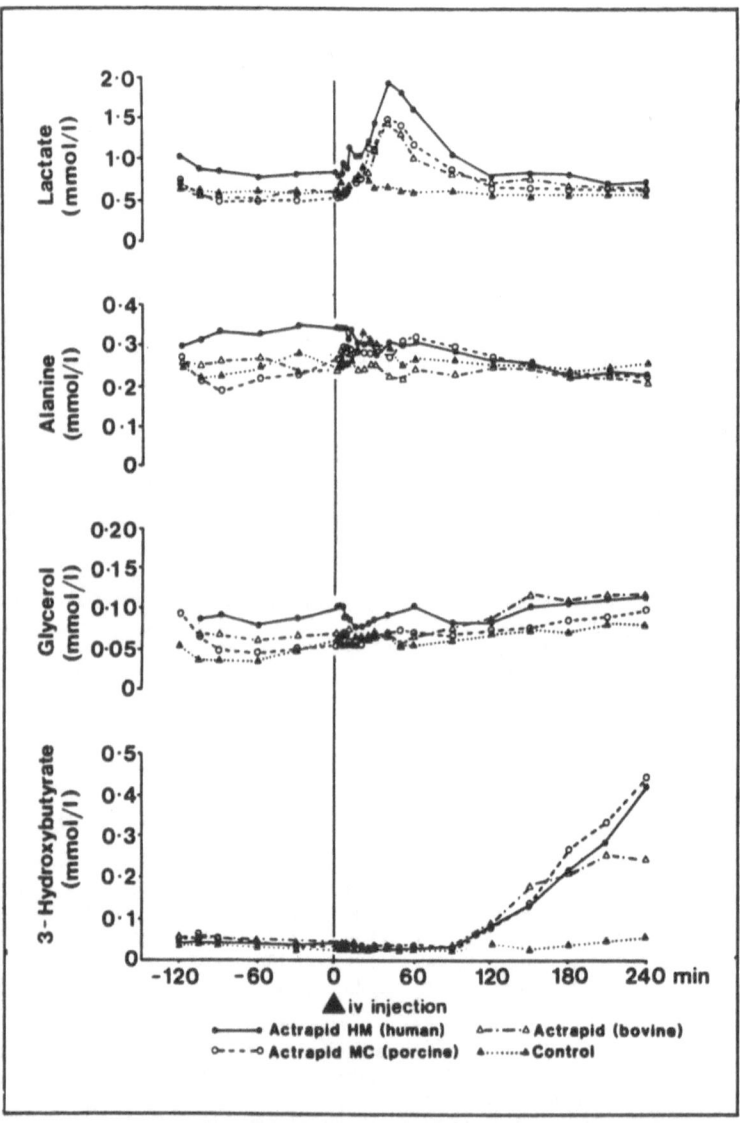

Figure 4.26b Effect of human, porcine and bovine insulins on blood lactate, alanine, glycerol and 3-hydroxybutyrate concentrations (means) in five subjects. Insulin (~0.075 U/kg) or saline (control) given intravenously (iv) at time 0

Relatively crude analysis of the insulin kinetics was carried out using a simple one-compartment model. The individual estimated values for human, porcine and bovine insulin are given in Tables 4.14a, 4.14b and 4.14c, respectively. The apparent $T_{1/2}$ (mean range) for human, porcine and bovine insulin was 5(4.5–5.5), 4.8(4.3–5.3) and 4.8(4.3–5.6) min, respectively, with an apparent volume of distribution (AVD) of 6(5.1–7.1), 6.9(5.4–9.1) and 5(3.9–6.1) litres, respectively, i.e. approximately 0.1 l/kg. The plasma clearance rates were 0.83(0.79–0.89), 1.0(0.84–1.20) and 0.7(0.63–0.89) l/min for human, porcine and bovine insulin, respectively (i.e. approximately 13 ml/kg/min). There was a tendency to higher AUC (0–240) with human than porcine insulin ($p<0.01$). Also, bovine insulin gave higher AUCs than porcine insulin ($p<0.05$), associated with a slower plasma clearance rate ($p<0.05$) and a smaller apparent volume of distribution ($p<0.05$). Similarly, the clearance and, to some extent, the volume of distribution were less ($p<0.05$) with bovine relative to human insulin. These analyses indicate that, whilst the direct comparison of the insulin (IRI) levels did not show any statistically significant differences, this does not preclude any pharmacokinetic differences.

The blood intermediary metabolite levels are shown in Figure 4.26b. After intravenous insulin administration there was an early rise in lactate levels reaching a peak at 40 min post-injection, returning to basal levels within 120 min. There was no significant difference in the lactate response between the three species of insulin. The blood alanine and glycerol levels remained essentially unchanged throughout the total 8 hour study period. In contrast there was a marked post-hypoglycaemic rise in 3-hydroxybutyrate levels from 120 min onwards which was similar with all three insulins (Figure 4.26b).

(ii) Intramuscular study

The mean Δ plasma glucose and insulin levels during the control and human insulin study days are illustrated in Figure 4.27a. The plasma glucose fell slowly during the control study, whereas after intramuscular insulin there was a relatively rapid fall from 4.8 ± 0.1 mmol/l at 0 min to 3.4 ± 0.3 mmol/l at 105 min. The plasma glucose then gradually increased, reaching near control levels at 360 min. At the beginning and end of the control day the plasma insulin levels were 0.058 ± 0.01 nmol/l and 0.04 ± 0.01 nmol/l, respectively. Following intramuscular injection, the plasma insulin level increased reaching a peak of 0.14 ± 0.05 nmol/l at 50 min. This was followed by a slow decline to fasting levels over the remaining three hours.

There was no change in the blood lactate, alanine and glycerol levels following the intramuscular injection of human insulin (Figure 4.27b). There was, however, a small rise in 3-hydroxybutyrate levels from 180 min onwards.

(iii) Comparison of intravenous and intramuscular insulin

The comparison between the responses to intravenous and intramuscular human insulin can be seen in Figures 4.28a and 4.28b. Whereas a very rapid fall in plasma glucose values, reaching a nadir at 25 min with an almost equally rapid recovery, was observed following intravenous administration, a much

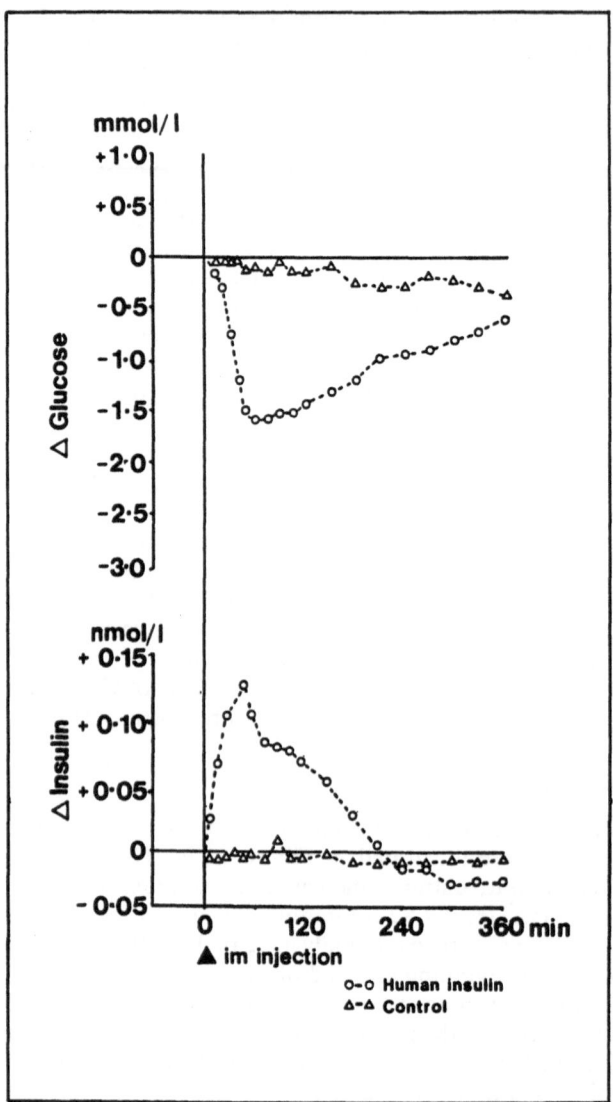

Figure 4.27a Effect of bolus intramuscular (im) injection of human insulin on plasma glucose and insulin (IRI) concentrations (means) in six subjects. Insulin (~0.075 U/kg) or im saline (control) given at time 0. Results shown as mean of Δ values

slower fall in plasma glucose was observed with intramuscular injection, reaching a nadir much later, between 90 and 120 min, followed by a slow recovery to near basal levels at 360 min (Figure 4.28a). The maximum reduction in plasma glucose was approximately 3.5 mmol/l and 1.5 mmol/l following intravenous and intramuscular human insulin, respectively.

Peak plasma insulin levels were reached within 2 min after intravenous

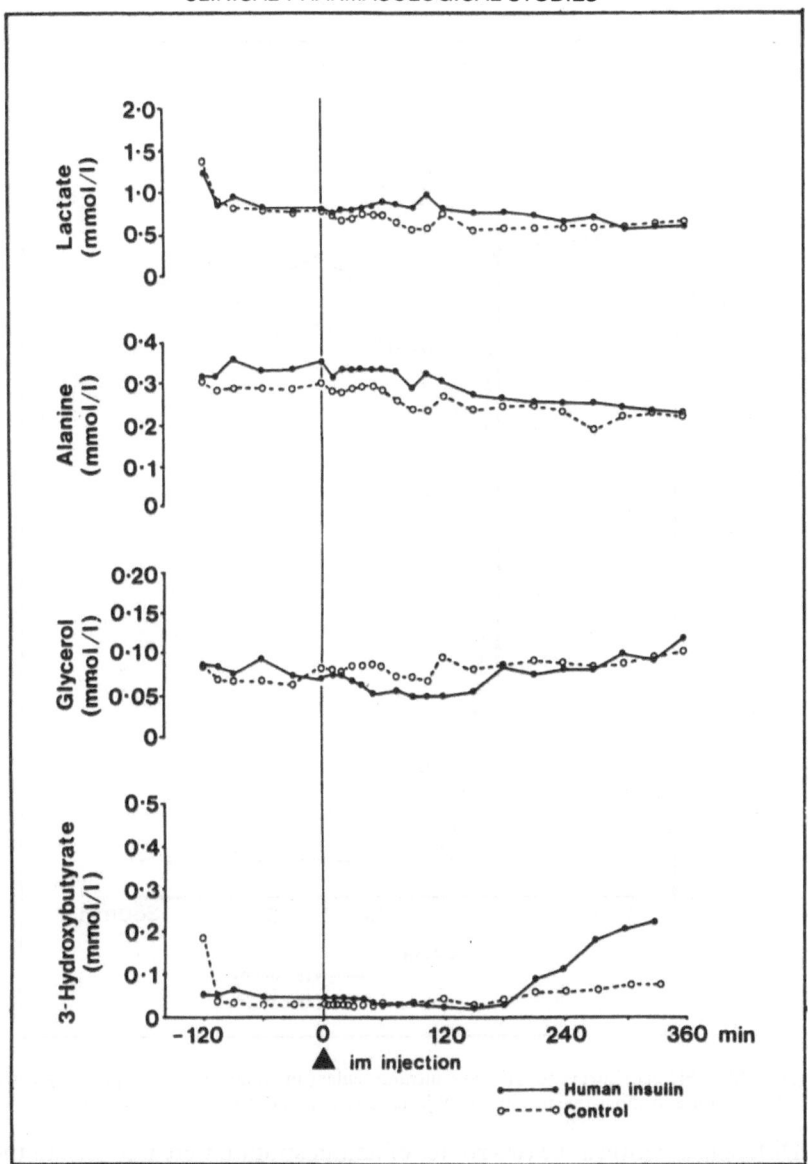

Figure 4.27b Effect of bolus intramuscular (im) injection of human insulin on blood lactate, alanine, glycerol and 3-hydroxybutyrate concentrations (means) in six subjects. Insulin (~0.075 U/kg) or im saline (control) given at time 0

compared to 60 min after intramuscular injection, with the peak levels approximately thirty-fold higher following intravenous administration. The mean area under the insulin curve, following intravenous injection (AUC_{0-240}) was 53.2 compared to 24.2 and 45.4 nmol/min/l for the 0 to 240 and 0 to 360 min periods, respectively, after intramuscular administration.

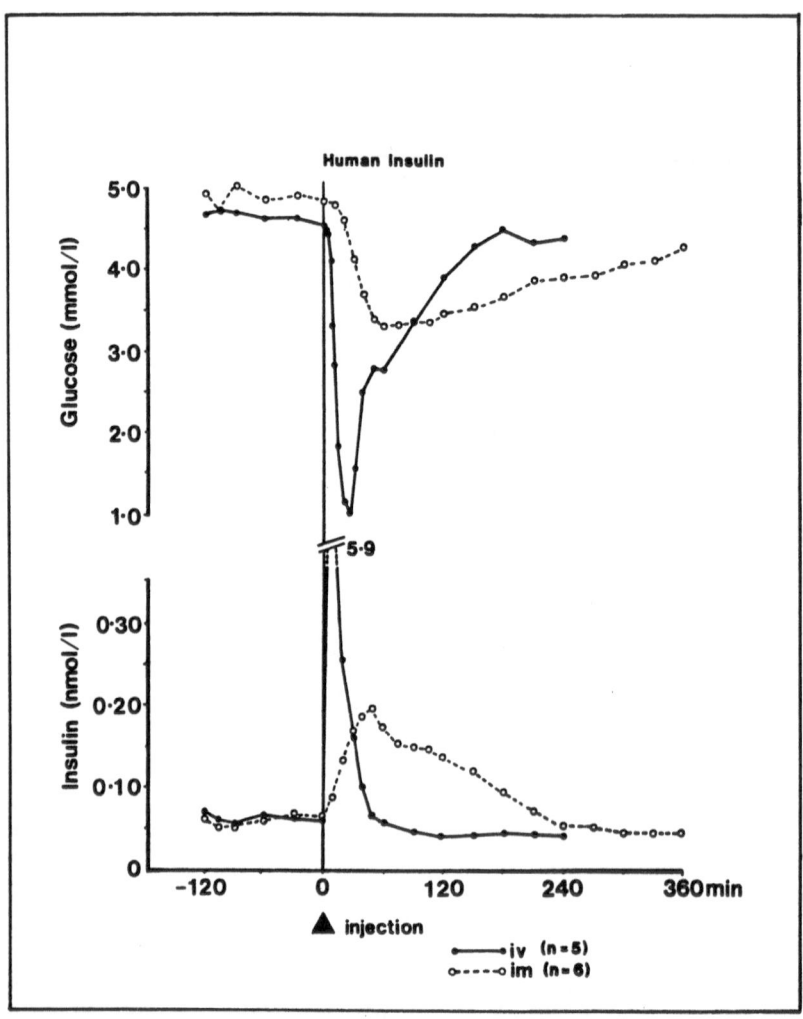

Figure 4.28a Effect of intravenous (iv) and intramuscular (im) human insulin on plasma glucose and insulin concentrations (means) in six subjects. Insulin (~0.075 U/kg) given at time 0

Differences between the two routes of administration were also seen in the lactate and 3-hydroxybutyrate responses. Whereas there was little change in lactate levels with intramuscular insulin, a sharp, short-lived increase followed intravenous administration. In addition, a much earlier post-hypoglycaemic rise in 3-hydroxybutyrate levels was seen with intravenous than with intramuscular insulin (Figure 4.28b).

Discussion

The results are in agreement with those of other investigators, demonstrating

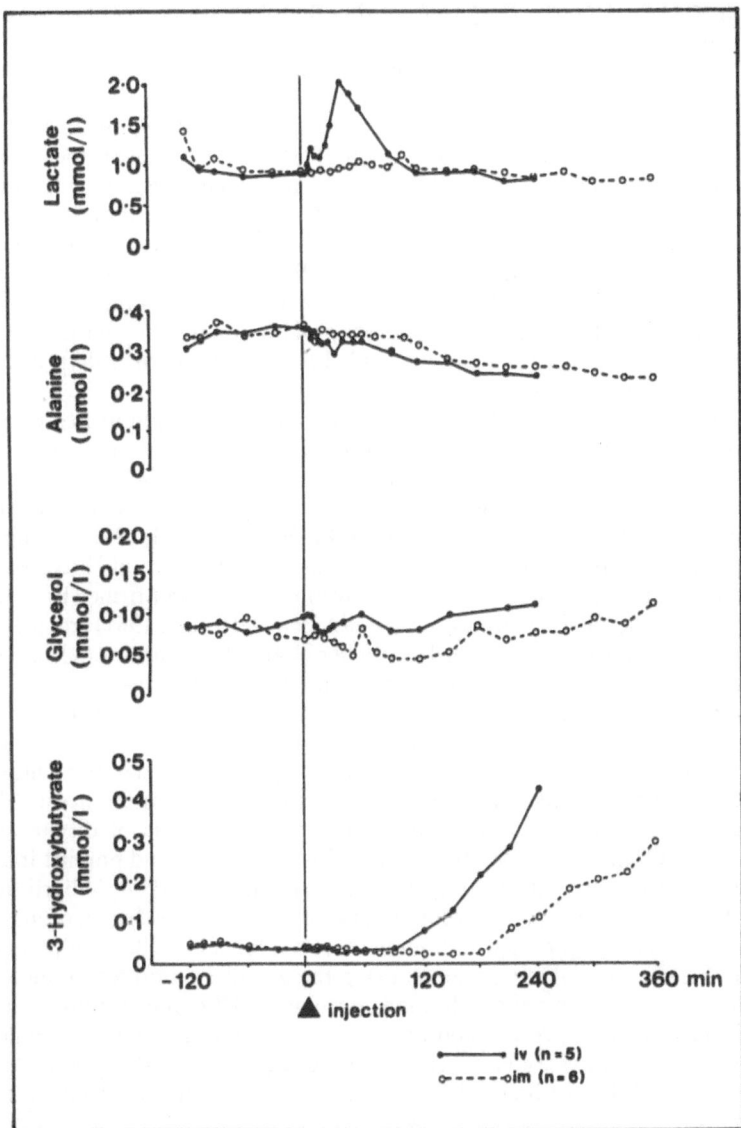

Figure 4.28b Effect of intravenous (iv) and intramuscular (im) human insulin on blood lactate, alanine, glycerol and 3-hydroxybutyrate concentrations (means) in six subjects. Insulin (~0.075 U/kg) given at time 0

an equivalent hypoglycaemic response and plasma insulin profiles with neutral, soluble 'semi-synthetic' human and porcine insulins when administered by bolus intravenous injection to normal man (Laube et al, 1981a, b, 1982; Ebihara et al, 1983; Arias et al, 1984). The crude analysis of the intravenous kinetics of the three species of insulin indicates that there may be some species differences. However, further analyses are required to validate these results.

Using a priming-dose constant-infusion technique, the metabolic clearance rate, half-disappearance time ($T_{1/2}$) and apparent distribution space are similar for 'semi-synthetic' human and porcine insulin (Gerlis et al, 1982; Adeniyi-Jones et al, 1983). Home and co-workers (1982a, 1983), using the glucose clamp technique, demonstrated that human and porcine insulin, when given intravenously by constant infusion, are identical with respect to glucose requirements and blood intermediary metabolite responses. Confirmatory findings have been obtained in similar studies involving diabetic patients (Charles et al, 1983; Home et al, 1983; Mirouze et al, 1983; Staten et al, 1984). Using a similar technique, a higher 'potency' of human insulin on the liver has however been suggested (Chisholm et al, 1983; Müller et al, 1984), but not conclusively demonstrated.

Intravenous injections of 'biosynthetic' human insulin and purified porcine insulin in normal man also achieve comparable hypoglycaemic responses (Ebihara et al, 1982; Federlin et al, 1981; Galloway et al, 1981b; Raptis et al, 1981; Weinges et al, 1981) and similar plasma insulin profiles (Federlin et al, 1981; Schlüter et al, 1981; Ebihara et al, 1982; Brogard et al, 1983). Using the euglycaemic clamp technique the equivalent 'potency' of intravenous 'biosynthetic' human insulin and porcine insulin has been confirmed by several investigators both in normal subjects (Massi-Benedetti et al, 1981) and insulin-dependent diabetics (Beyer et al, 1981; Klier et al, 1981; Raptis et al, 1981).

Therefore, all studies agree that the hypoglycaemic response to a bolus intravenous injection of human ('semi-synthetic' and 'biosynthetic') and purified porcine insulin are similar. However, Brogard et al (1984), whilst finding no difference in the hypoglycaemic response between 'biosynthetic' human and porcine insulin, suggested that there was a difference in their biological half-life, elimination rate and apparent volume of distribution. Also, when administered by intravenous infusion, human and porcine insulin possess identical hypoglycaemic 'potencies' (Keen et al, 1980; Viberti et al, 1981; Pickup et al, 1982). Occasionally, however, a greater degree of glucose disposal has been observed with human insulin (Doi et al, 1983; Schlüter et al, 1983a). Studies in diabetic patients, using the glucose clamp technique, also demonstrate that intravenous human, porcine and bovine insulins achieve identical free insulin profiles and have equivalent hypoglycaemic 'potencies' (Home et al, 1983; Gray et al, 1984). The absence of a difference in direct comparisons of the insulin levels does not, however, exclude pharmacokinetic differences.

Despite similar hypoglycaemic responses to intravenous human and porcine insulin, inconsistent differences in the hormonal counterregulatory responses to the two species of insulin have been recorded (Rosak et al, 1982; Schlüter et al, 1982, 1983a, b; Brogard et al, 1984), which need further exploration.

This study clearly demonstrates the difference in the plasma insulin concentrations and subsequent metabolic responses between intravenous and intramuscular human insulin. In contrast to the very early and profound fall in plasma glucose with intravenous insulin, a more gradual reduction occurs with intramuscular injection, reaching a nadir approximately 30 to 90 min later, approximately 40% less than that observed with the intravenous route. After intravenous injection the maximum insulin levels were seen at 2 min, in contrast to 50 min after intramuscular administration. Differences between the two routes of administration were also reflected in the blood lactate and 3-hydroxybutyrate responses. A marked increase in blood lactate and an earlier post-hypoglycaemic rise in 3-hydroxybutyrate levels were observed with intravenous compared to intramuscular insulin.

4.1.8 A study of the hormonal counterregulatory responses to subcutaneous and intravenous human ('semi-synthetic', 'biosynthetic') and porcine insulins

Introduction

The increasingly convincing evidence that poor metabolic control is associated with microvascular complications (Tchobroutsky, 1978; Pirart, 1977; Skyler, 1979; Raskin et al, 1983; Camerini-Davalos et al, 1983; Siperstein, 1983), commits the diabetologist to strive for the best possible glycaemic control, whilst avoiding the dangers of hypoglycaemia (Unger, 1982). The increasing use of intensified conventional insulin regimens (Skyler et al, 1982; Schade et al, 1983) and insulin by continuous subcutaneous infusion (Pickup et al, 1979) underlines the critical importance of the glucose counterregulatory systems in the insulin-treated diabetic patient (Cryer and Gerich, 1983). Impairment in glucose counterregulation is not an uncommon finding in insulin-dependent diabetics (Gerich et al, 1973; Cryer and Gerich, 1983), due either to deficiencies in counterregulatory hormone release (Hilsted et al, 1981; Hoeldtke et al, 1982; Boden et al, 1981; Polonsky et al, 1982; Rudman et al, 1981), concomitant therapy with beta-adrenergic blocking agents (Popp et al, 1982), or unknown factors (Polonsky et al, 1982).

The recently introduced neutral, soluble formulations of 'semi-synthetic' and 'biosynthetic' human insulin (Chance et al, 1981a, b; Markussen et al, 1981, 1982), have similar hypoglycaemic actions to their porcine counterparts when administered intravenously (Federlin et al, 1981; Galloway et al, 1981b; Owens et al, 1981d; Home et al, 1982a). In comparison, when using the subcutaneous route of administration, the hypoglycaemia is either the same with the two species of insulin (Galloway et al, 1981b; Owens et al, 1981a, 1982), or sometimes greater with human insulin (Federlin et al, 1981; Sundermann et al, 1981; Kemmer et al, 1982). Despite similar hypoglycaemic effects, differences in the hormonal counterregulatory responses have been recorded between human and porcine insulin (Schlüter et al, 1981, 1982, 1983a, b; Petersen et al, 1982; Rosak et al, 1982; Owens et al, 1983a). The earlier studies (cf. 4.1.4) also suggest a lesser glucagon and growth hormone response with human insulin when compared to its porcine counterpart.

Schlüter and co-workers observed, following bolus intravenous injection of 'biosynthetic' human insulin and porcine insulin, an identical hypoglycaemic response but a less pronounced increase in serum cortisol and growth hormone levels with human insulin (Schlüter et al, 1981, 1982). Even under euglycaemic conditions, porcine insulin has been shown to cause a small but significant increase in both serum growth hormone and cortisol concentrations, which was not observed after 'biosynthetic' human insulin (Schlüter et al, 1983a, b). Others have failed to demonstrate any difference in the glucagon, catecholamine, cortisol and growth hormone response following 'biosynthetic' human and porcine insulin when given by bolus intravenous injection resulting in identical hypoglycaemic effects (Ebihara et al, 1983; Landgraf-Leurs et al, 1984). The observation of a greater prolactin response with porcine insulin (Rosak et al, 1982; Landgraf-Leurs et al, 1984), together with the anecdotal observations that hypoglycaemic symptoms seem less severe with human insulin, implies a different pattern of hormonal responses with the two species of insulin (Schlüter et al, 1981). The existence of a lower hormonal response to human insulin may, therefore, offer theoretical advantages to the insulin-treated diabetic (Lundbaek et al, 1971). There is, however, no consistent difference in the glucagon and growth hormone response between human and porcine insulin in normal and diabetic patients (Schlüter et al, 1981, 1982; Rosak et al, 1982; Christensen et al, 1984; Landgraf-Leurs et al, 1984).

Therefore, in view of the initial findings of a difference in the hormonal counterregulatory responses between porcine and 'semi-synthetic' human insulin, when given subcutaneously (cf. 4.1.4), and the possible implications of such an observation, the study was repeated in a new group of volunteer subjects (study 4.1.8.1). In addition, a second study was conducted to compare the counterregulatory response to bolus intravenous injections of porcine insulin, 'semi-synthetic' and 'biosynthetic' human insulins in a separate group of normal subjects (study 4.1.8.2).

The subcutaneous (study 4.1.8.1) and intravenous (study 4.1.8.2) studies are presented separately.

4.1.8.1 Subcutaneous study

The purpose of this study was to compare the growth hormone, glucagon and cortisol responses following subcutaneously administered porcine and 'semi-synthetic' human insulin at a dose level of 0.075 U/kg body weight in normal subjects observed over a 330 min post-injection period.

Subjects, materials and methods

Six normal male volunteer subjects were recruited with each subject involved in two study days conducted 1–3 weeks apart. Details of the insulins used are shown in Table 4.15.

Table 4.15

	Actrapid HM (human)	Actrapid MC (porcine)
Nitrogen (mg/ml)	0.218	0.213
Potency[a] (IU/ml)	40.3	39.4

[a]Theoretical potency: 185 IU/mgN

Methods

The procedure was as described for studies 4.1.3 and 4.1.5. The dose of the comparative insulin preparations was 0.075 U/kg, administered into the anterior abdominal wall. The study consisted of a 1 h basal period, followed by a 330 min post-injection period.

Venous blood samples were taken for the determinations of plasma glucose (hexokinase method), insulin (Heding, 1972), C-peptide (Heding, 1975), cortisol (Baum et al, 1974), glucagon (Heding, 1971) and growth hormone (Boden and Soeldner, 1976).

Statistical methods

The results are expressed as means ± SE except where stated otherwise. The Student's t-test was used for paired comparisons of both the absolute and Δ values (derived by subtracting the mean basal value (–60 to 0 min) from all subsequent readings on each study day).

Variation in the hypoglycaemic response may bias the comparison of the hormonal counterregulatory responses to subcutaneously administered human and porcine insulins. Therefore an analysis of covariance was carried out to see whether the responses to the comparative insulin preparations differed after adjustment was made for differences in hypoglycaemia. The covariables used to characterise the hypoglycaemic response were:

1. rate of decrease between 10 and 60 min,
2. average level, 0 to 330 min (area),
3. average decrease from initial level,
4. minimum level.

These covariables were used in connection with analysis of the growth hormone, glucagon and cortisol responses expressed as:

(a) average (area under curve) level, 0 to 330 min;
(b) average increment for growth hormone and glucagon (average minus mean level (–60 to 0 min)); for cortisol, maximum level after 50 min minus the 50 min level;
(c) maximum value (after 50 min in the case of cortisol).

Results

The mean absolute and Δ plasma glucose, C-peptide, insulin, glucagon, growth hormone and cortisol levels during the 'semi-synthetic' human and porcine insulin studies are represented in Figure 4.29.

Following the subcutaneous injection of human and porcine insulin, the plasma glucose fell rapidly from a mean pre-injection level of 5.1 mmol/l, to a nadir of 3.3 ± 0.3 and 3.4 ± 0.3 mmol/l at 90 and 60 min, respectively. Thereafter, a similar recovery towards normoglycaemia was observed with the plasma glucose levels reaching 4.5 mmol/l at 330 min. The mean plasma

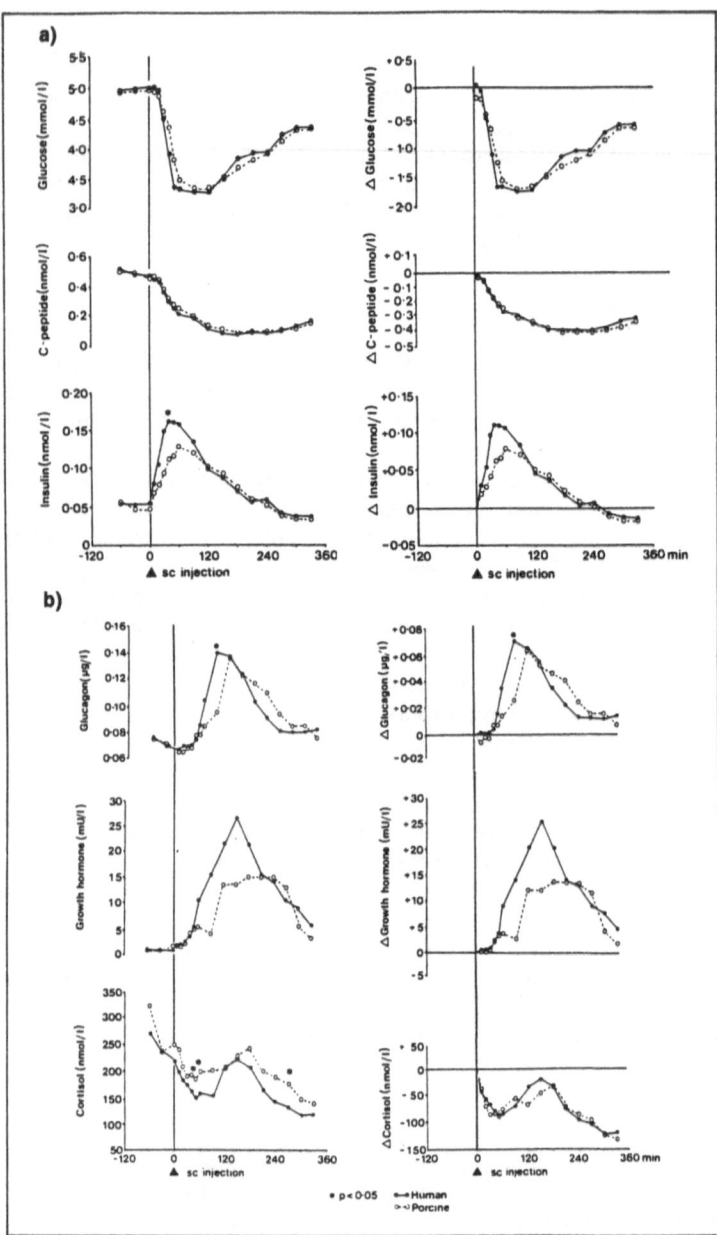

Figure 4.29 Effect of human and porcine insulins on (**a**) plasma glucose, C-peptide and insulin (IRI) concentrations, (**b**) plasma glucagon, growth hormone and cortisol concentrations in six subjects. Insulin (~0.075 U/kg) given subcutaneously (sc) at time 0. Results shown as means and mean Δ values

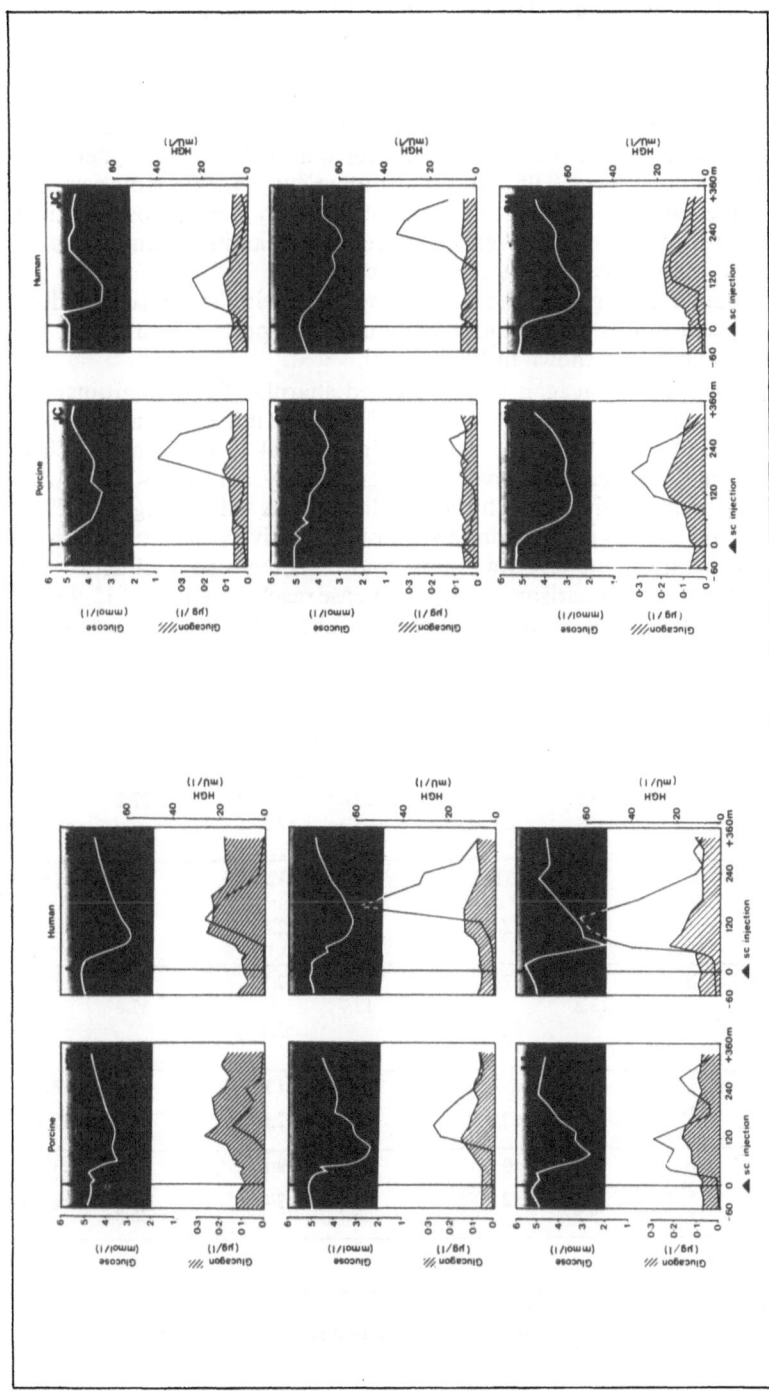

Figure 4.30 Effect of human and porcine insulins on the plasma glucose, glucagon and growth hormone concentrations in each of the six subjects. Insulin (~0.075 U/kg) given subcutaneously (sc) at time 0

C-peptide levels were identical throughout the two comparative study periods.

After administration of human insulin the plasma insulin levels increased, reaching a peak mean concentration of 0.17 ± 0.03 nmol/l at 40 min. In comparison, following porcine insulin, a more gradual increase in plasma insulin levels was observed, with a lower peak level of 0.14 ± 0.02 nmol/l achieved at 60 min. The plasma insulin level was significantly higher with human insulin 40 min ($p<0.05$) after injection (Figure 4.29a). However, the subsequent levels from 120 min to the end of the study were almost identical with the two insulins. The difference between the mean incremental plasma insulin levels did not reach statistical significance.

The glucagon and growth hormone responses with the corresponding glucose concentrations before and after human and porcine insulin, for the individual subjects, are shown in Figure 4.30.

The mean plasma glucagon level increased sharply after human insulin, from a pre-injection value of 0.07 ± 0.01 μg/l at time 0 min to a peak of 0.14 ± 0.03 μg/l at 90 min. With porcine insulin a similar peak level was not reached until 120 min. The glucagon level was significantly higher ($p<0.05$) with human insulin at 90 min for both the absolute and Δ values (Figure 4.29b). One hour after human insulin administration, a relatively steep rise in mean plasma growth hormone levels was observed reaching a peak of 27.3 ± 9.5 mU/l at 150 min. In comparison, a slower increase reaching a peak of 15.9 ± 4.6 mU/l at 180 min was observed with porcine insulin. There was no significant

Table 4.16 Analysis of covariance of growth hormone response to hypoglycaemia

		AUC^1 0–330 min		$Incr.^2$		Max^3 0–330 min	
Direct	Human	13.9		12.8		37.2	
estimates			±2.4		±2.5		±6.5
	Porcine	10.1		8.8		26.2	
Adjusted: PG	b	364	±314	401	±321	1276	±761
rate of	Human	15.7		14.8		43.3	
decrease			±2.8		±2.8		±6.7
	Porcine	8.3		6.8		20.0	
Adjusted: PG	b	−1.08	±7.01	−0.99	±7.32	3.7	±19.0
area	Human	13.8		12.7		37.6	
(0–330 min)			±2.8		±2.9		±7.6
	Porcine	10.2		8.9		25.7	
Adjusted: PG	b	−9.5	±13.5	−11.9	±13.7	−17.8	±37.7
decrease	Human	13.8		12.8		37.1	±7.1
	Porcine	10.2	±2.8	8.9	±2.6	26.3	
Adjusted: PG	b	11.3	±9.2	10.9	±9.8	22.4	±37.0
minimum	Human	14.1	±2.3	13.0	±2.4	37.5	±6.7
	Porcine	9.9		8.7		25.8	

PG = Plasma glucose
b   = Regression coefficient (between response and co-variate)
[1]   Average (area under curve) level 0–330 min
[2]   Increment, average minus initial mean level (−60 to 0 min)
[3]   Maximal value

Table 4.17   Analysis of covariance of glucagon response to hypoglycaemia

		AUC^1 0–330 min		$Incr.^2$		$Max.^3$ 0–330 min	
Direct	Human	0.102		0.031		0.158	
estimates			±0.004		±0.003		±0.008
	Porcine	0.101		0.029		0.148	
Adjusted: PG	b	0.115	±0.321	−0.135	±0.397	−1.10	±1.08
rate of	Human	0.103	±0.003	0.031	±0.007	0.153	±0.010
decrease	Porcine	0.100		0.029		0.153	
Adjusted: PG	b	0.0025	±0.0062	−0.0018	±0.0078	−0.037	±0.015
area	Human	0.103		0.031		0.154	
(0–330 min)			±0.002		±0.003		±0.006
	Porcine	0.100		0.029		0.152	
Adjusted: PG	b	0.0056	±0.0125	−0.0118	±0.0147	−0.054	±0.03
decrease	Human	0.102		0.031		0.158	
			±0.002		±0.003		±0.007
	Porcine	0.101		0.029		0.148	
Adjusted: PG	b	−0.0053	±0.0093	0.0036	±0.0118	0.060*	±0.020
minimum	Human	0.102		0.031		0.159	
			±0.002		±0.003		±0.005
	Porcine	0.101		0.029		0.147	

PG = Plasma glucose
b = Regression coefficient (between response and co-variate)
[1] Average (area under curve) level 0–330 min
[2] Increment, average minus initial mean level (−60 to 0 min)
[3] Maximal value
* $p < 0.05$

difference between the growth hormone responses to human and porcine insulin.

The fasting plasma cortisol levels continued to fall during the pre-injection period, and for the first hour after insulin administration. Subsequently, the levels increased reaching a peak at 150 and 180 min with human and porcine insulin, respectively. The values observed with porcine insulin were significantly higher at 50, 60 and 270 min ($p < 0.05$; Figure 4.29b). There was, however, no statistically significant difference in the Δ values between human and porcine insulin.

The results of the analysis of covariance for the three response variables for growth hormone, glucagon and cortisol are contained in Tables 4.16, 4.17 and 4.18, respectively. None of the analyses showed any statistically significant difference in the hormonal counterregulatory responses to human and porcine insulin. It is noted, however, that the rate of fall of glucose, when used to adjust the growth hormone responses, increased the difference between the estimated mean for human and porcine insulin, in contrast to the other covariables (Table 4.17). Interestingly, there was a significant correlation ($p < 0.05$) between the maximum glucagon response and the minimum glucose level for the two insulins (Table 4.18).

Table 4.18 Analysis of covariance of cortisol response to hypoglycaemia

		AUC^1 0–330 min		$Incr.^2$		$Max.^3$ 0–330 min	
Direct estimates	Human	169		250		97	
			±11		±25		±28
	Porcine	200		272		86	
Adjusted: PG rate of decrease	b	459	±1710	2901	±3517	3093	±3939
	Human	172		264		112	
			±15		±31		±35
	Porcine	198		258		71	
Adjusted: PG area (0–330 min)	b	8.5	±33.2	91	±58	115	±58.6
	Human	171		262		112	
			±13		±23		±24
	Porcine	199	.	261		71	
Adjusted: PG decrease	b	-15.2	±67.6	124	±136	178	±141
	Human	169		251		98	
			±13		±26		±26
	Porcine	200		272		85	
Adjusted: PG minimum	b	5.85	±51.2	-117	±97	-160	±97
	Human	170		249		95	
			±13		±24		±24
	Porcine	200		274		88	

PG = Plasma glucose
b = Regression coefficient (between response and co-variate)
1 Average (area under curve) level 0–330 min
2 Increment, average minus 50 min level
3 Maximal value after 50 min

Discussion

The results demonstrate that subcutaneous neutral, soluble porcine and 'semi-synthetic' human insulin, at a dose level of approximately 0.075 U/kg body weight, resulted in a similar hypoglycaemic response and suppression of C-peptide levels in normal man. There was, however, a trend towards higher plasma insulin levels with human compared to porcine insulin. Comparison of the glucagon response to human and porcine insulin revealed a higher incremental level with human insulin 90 min after injection. There were no differences in the growth hormone and cortisol responses between the two insulins. Analysis of covariance did not show any statistically significant differences in the counterregulatory responses between the two species of insulin. Apart from a significant correlation ($p<0.05$) between the maximum glucagon response and the minimum glucose level, no other correlation could be established between the hypoglycaemic effects and the hormonal counterregulatory responses.

In view of the small size of the study, no firm conclusions can be drawn regarding the difference between human and porcine insulin, or the relationship between the hormonal and hypoglycaemic responses. A larger study would therefore be necessary to explore the possibility that the growth hormone response is best correlated to the rate of fall of glucose, whereas with glucagon the minimum glucose level is the most important covariate.

The results are in contrast to the previous studies (cf. 4.1.3, 4.1.5) which showed a greater glucagon and growth hormone response with porcine compared to human insulin, despite an equivalent hypoglycaemic response. The discrepancy between the studies is difficult to explain on the available results.

It has to be concluded that the study has limited power to detect differences in the hormonal counterregulatory responses between human and porcine insulin; therefore further studies are necessary. The relationship between the hormonal response, hypoglycaemia (Gerich et al, 1973; Palmer and Ensinck 1975) and the prevailing insulin level (Weir et al, 1976) also requires further investigation.

4.1.8.2 Intravenous study

The purpose of this study was to compare in normal subjects the glucagon, adrenaline, cortisol and growth hormone responses to intravenous injections of porcine insulin (Actrapid MC), 'semi-synthetic' (Actrapid HM) and 'bio-synthetic' (Humulin S) human insulins, using saline as control.

Subjects, materials and methods

Six normal male subjects, aged between 21 and 30 years, were entered into the study. Each subject was involved in four separate study days 1 to 3 weeks apart, during which they received, in random order, porcine insulin, 'semi-synthetic' and 'biosynthetic' human insulin at a dose level of 0.1 U/kg body weight and an equivalent volume of saline during a control day. After a 40 min basal period the test materials were administered by bolus intravenous injection, after which samples were taken every 10 min during the first hour and then at 75, 90, 120, 150, 180, 210 and 240 min for plasma glucose (hexokinase), immunoreactive insulin (Heding, 1972), C-peptide (Heding, 1975), glucagon (Heding, 1971), adrenaline (Da Prada and Zürcher, 1976), cortisol (Baum et al, 1974) and growth hormone (Boden and Soeldner, 1976) determinations.

The blood samples were aliquoted into EDTA for glucose estimation, lithium heparin bottles containing either freeze-dried reduced glutathione for adrenaline, or aprotinin (Trasylol: Bayer A/G) for the remaining assays. Details of the insulin preparations used are included in Table 4.19.

Table 4.19

	Actrapid MC (porcine: Novo A/S)	Actrapid HM (human: Novo A/S)	Humulin S (human: Eli Lilly)
Nitrogen (mg/ml)	0.213	0.218	—
Potency (IU/ml)	39.4[a]	40.3[a]	40.5[b]

[a]Theoretical potency 185 IU/mgN
[b]Potency determination performed by a quantitative HPLC method

Statistical methods

The statistical analysis of the differences between the three insulin preparations was carried out as three sets of paired comparisons (Student's t-test) of the values defined as the differences between the mean basal value (–40, –20 and 0 min) and all subsequent values on each study day. The results are expressed as means ± SE unless stated otherwise. For the pharmacokinetic analysis the standard one- and two-compartment models were fitted to the individual insulin curves. Further analyses were conducted to estimate the elimination rate, area under curve, clearance and apparent volume of distribution for the three insulin preparations.

Results

The mean absolute and Δ plasma glucose, C-peptide, insulin, adrenaline, glucagon, cortisol and growth hormone are shown in Figures 4.31 and 4.32, respectively.

(i) Control day. During the control day the plasma glucose fell gradually from 4.9 ± 0.1 mmol/l to 4.7 ± 0.1 mmol/l over the 4 h study period. There was a fall in C-peptide levels from 0.38 ± 0.10 to 0.25 ± 0.03 nmol/l and insulin levels from 0.023 ± 0.004 to 0.019 ± 0.004 nmol/l during the control study.

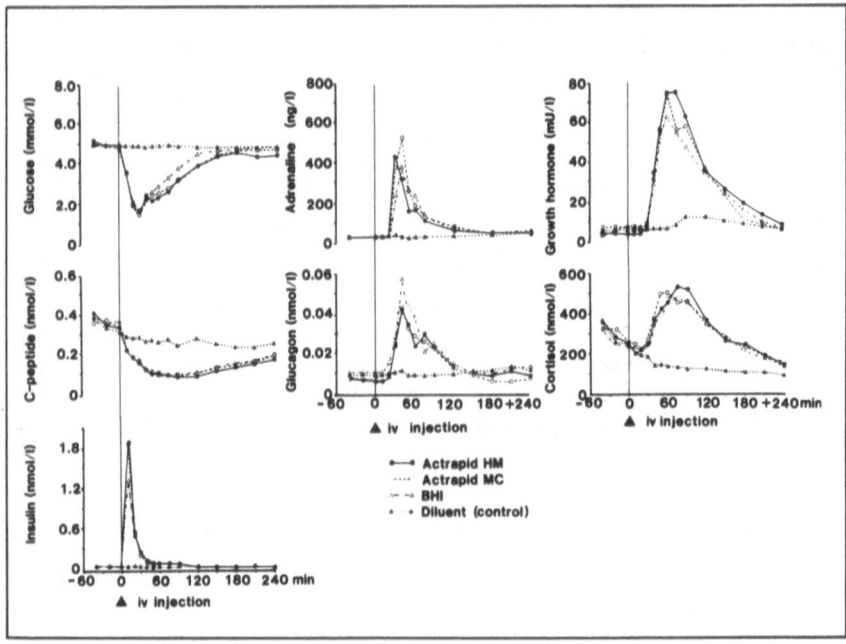

Figure 4.31 Effect of 'semi-synthetic' (Actrapid HM), 'biosynthetic' (BHI) human and porcine (Actrapid MC) insulins on plasma glucose, C-peptide and insulin (IRI) concentrations (means) in six subjects. Insulin (0.1 U/kg) or diluent (control) given intravenously (iv) at time 0

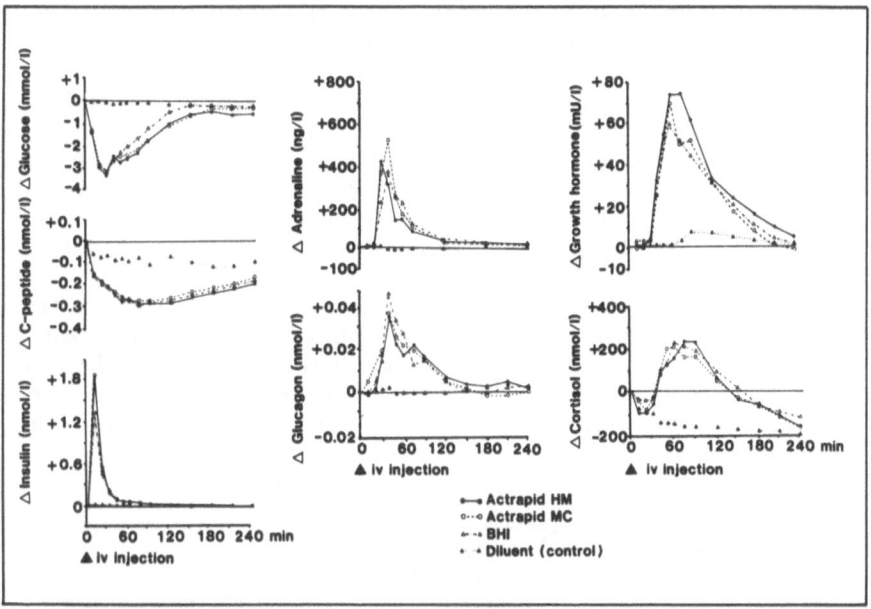

Figure 4.32 Effect of 'semi-synthetic' (Actrapid HM), 'biosynthetic' (BHI) human and porcine (Actrapid MC) insulins on plasma glucose, C-peptide and insulin (IRI) concentrations in six subjects. Insulin (0.1 U/kg) or diluent (control) given intravenously (iv) at time 0. Results shown as means of Δ values

There was no change in the plasma glucagon level which remained at approximately 0.3 nmol/l or the plasma adrenaline concentration at about 30 ng/l during the control day. In contrast, the plasma cortisol level fell from 365 ± 21 nmol/l at −40 min to 90 ± 12 nmol/l at 240 min.

(ii) Insulin study days

Glucose.   A similar and rapid fall was observed reaching nadir values at 30 min of 1.4 ± 0.2, 1.5 ± 0.2 and 1.6 ± 0.2 mmol/l after intravenous injection of porcine, 'semi-synthetic' and 'biosynthetic' human insulins, respectively (Figure 4.31). Subsequently, a faster recovery was observed with 'biosynthetic' human insulin, with the hypoglycaemic effect significantly less than porcine insulin between 90 and 150 min ($p < 0.05$) and human insulin from 60 to 150 min and at 240 min ($p < 0.05$). There was no difference in the hypoglycaemic response between porcine and 'semi-synthetic' human insulin.

C-peptide.   An identical reduction in plasma C-peptide levels was observed with the three species of insulin, with the concentration reaching a nadir 75 min after insulin administration. This was followed by a gradual increase to about 50% of basal values by the end of the study.

Insulin.   The peak insulin levels for the three insulins were observed at 10 min, the first sample time-point after injection. The levels reached were 1.92 ± 0.22, 1.90 ± 0.28 and 1.38 ± 0.15 nmol/l for porcine, 'semi-synthetic' and 'biosynthetic' human insulin, respectively (Figure 4.31). The insulin levels were lower after 'biosynthetic' human insulin than after the other two insulins during the first 20 min after administration, although the differences are not statistically significant due to a large variation in the observed insulin levels during this period. Later, however, when the insulin concentrations had returned to near-fasting values, the levels were significantly higher with porcine and 'semi-synthetic' human insulin than 'biosynthetic' human insulin at 60 min ($p<0.01$) and between 90 and 120 min ($p<0.05$), respectively.

The results of the pharmacokinetic analyses are shown in Table 4.20. The two-compartment open model could only be fitted to the insulin measurements (10 to 120 min) for 5 out of the 18 study days, although the first model could be fitted consistently. This was probably due to the relatively infrequent sampling during the first hour after injection. In order to give an impression of the ability of the models to fit the data, Figure 4.33 shows the

Table 4.20 Pharmacokinetic analysis (one- or two-compartment open models were fitted to the insulin (IRI) data after intravenous injection)

Subject	Insulin	Model	α_0 (nmol/l)	α_1 (nmol/l)	α_2 (nmol/l)	β_1 (min^{-1})	β_2 (min^{-1})	CV(%)	AUC (nmol/l/min)	PCR (ml kg.min)	AVD V_1 (l/kg)	AVD V_2 (l/kg)
1	PI	1	0.016	2.27	–	0.080	–	5	34.3	17	0.022	–
	SSHI	1	0.041	6.46	–	0.149	–	8	43.3	14	0.09	–
	SSHI	1	0.031	2.90	–	0.095	–	8	30.5	20	0.21	–
	BHI	2	0.017	45.60	1.01	0.428	0.054	2	125.4	5	0.01	0.01
2	PI	1	0.043	4.59	–	0.100	–	10	45.9	13	0.13	–
	SSHI	1	0.044	5.84	–	0.141	–	11	41.5	14	0.10	–
	BHI	1	0.033	4.40	–	0.093	–	3	47.0	13	0.14	–
3	PI	1	0.051	10.25	–	0.138	–	6	74.0	8	0.06	–
	PI	2	0.041	16.66	1.65	0.217	0.075	3	98.7	6	0.03	0.01
	SSHI	1	0.054	10.13	–	0.115	–	4	88.0	7	0.06	–
	BHI	1	0.015	4.03	–	0.093	–	6	43.2	14	0.15	–
4	PI	1	0.018	5.55	–	0.127	–	4	43.8	14	0.11	–
	PI	2	0.007	6.68	0.223	0.153	0.036	2	50.0	12	0.09	0.02
	SSHI	1	0.027	5.94	–	0.117	–	6	50.7	12	0.10	–
	BHI	1	0.031	7.41	–	0.154	–	8	48.0	12	0.08	–
5	PI	1	0.019	8.74	–	0.137	–	8	63.6	9	0.07	–
	PI	2	0.000	16.01	0.734	0.212	0.049	2	90.0	7	0.04	0.01
	SSHI	1	0.017	5.97	–	0.131	–	6	45.7	13	0.10	–
	BHI	1	0.032	1.73	–	0.063	–	7	27.5	22	0.34	–
6	PI	1	0.030	5.21	–	0.118	–	7	44.2	13	0.11	–
	SSHI	1	0.024	4.47	–	0.110	–	7	40.6	15	0.13	–
	BHI	1	0.027	2.99	–	0.107	–	6	27.9	21	0.20	–
	BHI	2	0.011	3.95	0.234	0.148	0.029	4	34.6	17	0.14	0.08

PI = Porcine Novo insulin
SSHI = Human Novo insulin
BHI = Human Lilly insulin
AUC = Area under the plasma insulin curve
AVD = Apparent volume of distribution
PCR = Elimination rate

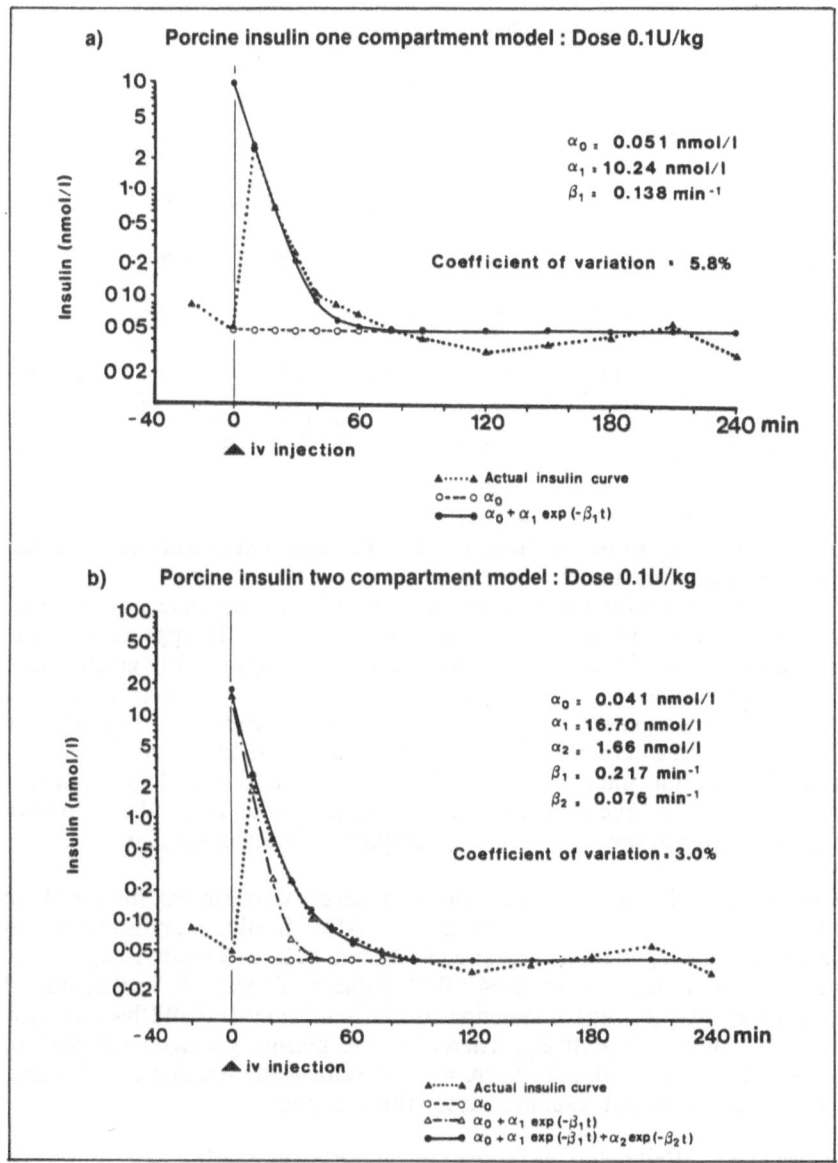

Figure 4.33 Pharmacokinetic analysis: comparison of the (a) one- and (b) two-compartment model fitted to the plasma insulin concentrations from 10 to 240 min following the intravenous (iv) administration of porcine insulin in one subject. Insulin (0.1 U/kg) given at time 0

results for one subject with porcine insulin which gave an intermediate coefficient of variation (6%) according to a one-compartment model. With the two-compartment model the coefficient of variation decreased to 3%. Similar tendencies were observed in other cases, indicating that the two-compartment

Table 4.21   Two-way analysis of variance

Kinetic parameters	Neutral, soluble insulin preparations			Common SE	F(2,10) insulins	F(5,10) subjects
	Porcine	SSHI	BHI			
Elimination rate (min⁻¹)	0.117	0.127	0.101	0.011	0.49	0.35
AUC (nmol/l/min)	51.0	51.6	37.4	4.5	3.26	3.38*
Clearance ml(kg.min)	12.3	12.5	17.0	1.2	4.71*	2.41
AVD l/kg	0.117	0.097	0.187	0.025	3.47	1.00

PI   = Porcine Novo insulin   AUC = Area under the plasma insulin curve
SSHI = Human Novo insulin   AVD = Apparent volume of distribution
BHI   = Human Lilly insulin   * $p < 0.05$

model is more appropriate. However, for the reasons stated above it was not possible to use this model.

The comparison of the various pharmacokinetic parameters of the one-compartment model are summarised in Table 4.21. It appears that the clearance of the 'biosynthetic' human insulin was significantly greater than that of the other two insulins, whereas the other parameters showed no significant heterogeneity. The increased clearance appears to be due to a larger apparent volume of distribution, rather than due to an increased elimination rate. The analysis indicates that the differences between the hypoglycaemic responses may be due to an increased clearance of the 'biosynthetic' human insulin relative to the porcine and 'semi-synthetic' human insulins.

Glucagon.   The fasting plasma glucagon levels were similar for the three treatment groups at about 0.03 nmol/l. After insulin administration an increase in glucagon levels was already evident at 20 to 30 min. Peak plasma glucagon concentrations of 0.064 ± 0.01, 0.063 ± 0.01 and 0.078 ± 0.01 nmol/l were observed at 40 min with porcine insulin, 'semi-synthetic' and 'biosynthetic' human insulins, respectively. Thereafter the plasma glucagon returned to pre-insulin levels at 150 min. There were no statistically significant differences between the glucagon responses to the three insulins.

Adrenaline.   Following the intravenous injection of porcine, 'semi-synthetic' and 'biosynthetic' human insulin there was a rapid increase from similar basal values of 23.3 ± 4.7, 24.5 ± 5.2 and 26.8 ± 3.7 ng/l to peak levels of 523 ± 101, 424 ± 62 and 379 ± 76 ng/l at 20, 30 and 40 min, respectively. The increment in plasma adrenaline was significantly greater following 'semi-synthetic' than 'biosynthetic' human insulin at 50 min ($p < 0.05$). The adrenaline concentration returned to fasting levels at 180 min after insulin administration.

Cortisol.   There was a fall in the plasma cortisol levels from about 350 nmol/l to 250 nmol/l during the 40 min basal period. Following porcine and 'biosynthetic' human insulin administration, the levels continued to fall for the first 10 to 20 min, before increasing to peak levels of 507 ± 42, and 492 ± 59 nmol/l at 60 min. A similar peak level of 539 ± 65 nmol/l was reached half an hour later with 'semi-synthetic' human insulin. There were no differences between the three test insulins.

Growth hormone. Thirty minutes after insulin administration, the plasma growth hormone levels started to increase reaching peak levels of 76 ± 10, 76 ± 5, and 64 ± 15 mU/l at 60 min, with 'semi-synthetic' human, porcine and 'biosynthetic' human insulin, respectively. The levels returned to the pre-injection basal range by 240 min. There was no significant difference in the growth hormone responses between the three insulin preparations.

Discussion

This study demonstrates essentially similar hormonal counterregulatory responses to hypoglycaemia induced by intravenous bolus injections of neutral, soluble porcine, 'semi-synthetic' and 'biosynthetic' human insulins in normal fasting subjects. Other investigators, using a similar protocol in healthy volunteers, have observed a more prominent response in both the primary (adrenaline and glucagon) and secondary (growth hormone and cortisol) glucose counterregulatory hormones (Schlüter et al, 1981; Rosak et al, 1982) with porcine compared to human insulin.

In this study the bolus intravenous administration of equivalent formu-lations of porcine and 'semi-synthetic' human insulin resulted in identical plasma insulin levels, hypoglycaemia and consequent increases in the levels of the counterregulatory hormones adrenaline, glucagon, cortisol and growth hormone. In comparison it appears that the glucose response to 'biosynthetic' human insulin was significantly less than to the other two insulins, which may account for the lower adrenaline levels following 'biosynthetic' relative to 'semi-synthetic' human insulin. The shorter hypoglycaemic effect of 'bio-synthetic' human insulin may be due to an increased clearance compared to the other insulins. In view of the inherent weakness of the methods of analysis it is not possible to draw firm conclusions about the pharmacokinetic differences between the three insulins compared.

Less subjective symptoms of hypoglycaemia, associated with a significantly lower prolactin release, have been observed with human compared to animal species insulin, at a dose level of 0.075 U/kg body weight, suggesting a different direct or indirect effect at hypothalamic level (Rosak et al, 1982; Schlüter and Kerp, 1983b; Landgraf-Leurs et al, 1984). This difference is not evident, however, at higher dose levels (Landgraf-Leurs et al, 1984), confirming the validity of using human insulin in hypothalamic pituitary function tests.

In conclusion, these results do not support the suggestion of a differential hormonal glucose counterregulatory response with human compared to porcine insulin when administered by bolus intravenous injection to normal subjects.

With the advent of intensified conventional insulin regimens, differences in subcutaneous absorption, antigenicity of porcine and human insulins and the ensuing hypoglycaemic effect are more likely to influence the pattern of the hormonal counterregulatory response than any direct influence of insulin species alone.

4.2 INSULIN PREPARATIONS WITH PROLONGED EFFECT

Introduction

Following the discovery of insulin and its introduction for the treatment of diabetes (Banting and Best, 1922a, b; Banting et al, 1922b), the only preparation available up to 1936 was an acid solution of a very impure unmodified insulin. The necessity for multiple daily injections of this 'short-acting' insulin prompted numerous attempts to prolong the subcutaneous absorption of insulin, thereby extending its hypoglycaemic effect. Early attempts involved mixing insulin with gum arabic solutions (Burgess et al, 1923), oil suspensions (Leyton, 1929), lecithin emulsions (Suranyi and Szalai, 1930) and vasoconstrictor substances (Wermer and Monguio, 1933; Clausen, 1934). Little success attended these early efforts to prolong the action of insulin (reviewed by Best, 1937; Dörzbach and Müller, 1971). Soon afterwards the addition of certain metal ions to the insulin solutions was seen to extend insulin action (Maxwell and Bischoff, 1935; Scott and Fisher, 1935). Also the use of strongly basic proteins (protamines) combined with neutral suspensions of insulin delayed absorption (Beecher and Krogh, 1936). During 1936 Hagedorn and co-workers made available the first clinically useful protracted insulin, protamine insulin (Hagedorn et al, 1936). The neutral suspension of protamine insulin was unstable, although the problem was solved by using excess protamine and adding a small amount of zinc (Scott and Fisher, 1936). The resulting preparation, protamine zinc insulin (PZI), had a very prolonged hypoglycaemic effect (Colwell, 1947), requiring the addition of soluble insulin to achieve an intermediate timing of action (Campbell et al, 1936; Lawrence and Archer, 1937; Colwell et al, 1942). Such a mixture, however, was also shown later to be very unstable (Peck and Schechter, 1944).

The need to have a more 'intermediate-acting' insulin, better able to deal with post-prandial glucose excursions, was quickly appreciated. In 1939 Globin insulin was developed, having an 'intermediate' duration of effect (Bauman, 1939; Reiner et al, 1939). Surfen, a synthetically produced urea derivative, was also developed as a possible substitute for protamine (Umber et al, 1938). In 1946, Hagedorn and co-workers introduced a stable PZI modification, the crystalline NPH insulin (Neutral Protamine Hagedorn) with a stoichiometric ratio between insulin and protamine (Krayenbühl and Rosenberg, 1946). NPH insulin is prepared by combining the insulin and protamine in 'isophane' proportions (no excess of insulin or protamine) at neutral pH, in the presence of a small amount of zinc and phenol and/or phenol derivatives to form an amorphous precipitate which is gradually transformed into tetragonal oblong crystals. This insulin preparation quickly became, and has remained, popular as a once- or twice-daily insulin used alone, or admixed with soluble insulin as required (Hagedorn, 1946; Oakley et al, 1966).

Following the demonstration that added zinc ions prolonged the action of insulin (Scott and Fisher, 1935; Bischoff and Jemtegaard, 1937; Blatherwick et al, 1938) protracted insulin preparations, without added foreign proteins or synthetic compounds, became available in 1951 (Hallas-Møller et al, 1951, 1952, 1954; Hallas-Møller, 1956). The Lente trilogy of insulins, comprising Semilente, Lente and Ultralente, were developed by Hallas-Møller and co-workers by complexing neutral suspensions of insulin with small amounts of zinc ions and utilising the influence of physical state and size of the suspended zinc insulin particles on duration of action. With substitution of the small amorphous insulin particles of Semilente by crystals, as in Ultralente, the duration of action resembles PZI. Lente insulin contains a 3:7 mixture of amorphous and crystalline particles, thereby having an intermediate timing of action similar to NPH (isophane) insulin (Whitehouse et al, 1961; Bressler and Galloway, 1978). The original Lente insulin consisted of amorphous porcine insulin and a bovine crystalline fraction, whereas in Monotard, a preparation of the Lente type, the suspended insulin particles (amorphous and crystalline) are porcine in origin. Further exploitation of the difference in the solubility of porcine and bovine insulin at neutral pH resulted in the introduction of Rapitard insulin, consisting of approximately 25% porcine insulin in solution and 75% bovine insulin crystals in suspension (Schlichtkrull, 1959; Schlichtkrull et al, 1961, 1965).

Recently, human insulin prepared from porcine insulin by an enzymatic process (Markussen, 1980) has been formulated as *NPH*: Human Protaphane (Protaphane HM); *Lente*: human Monotard (Monotard HM) and *Ultralente*: human Ultralente (Ultratard HM) insulin preparations.

A series of studies have been carried out to describe the pharmacokinetics and pharmacodynamic responses to the new 'intermediate-' and 'long-acting' human 'semi-synthetic' insulin preparations following subcutaneous injection in normal subjects. The insulin preparations and dosage levels used in these studies are summarised in Figure 4.34.

4.2.1 'Intermediate-acting' insulin preparations

4.2.1.1 *A study of human ('semi-synthetic') and porcine Lente (Monotard) insulins (U-40)*

The widespread use of twice a day mixtures of soluble and Lente porcine insulin preparations underlines the importance of ascertaining any difference in the pharmacokinetics and pharmacodynamic responses between the new human and the well-established porcine Monotard insulin. In contrast to the extensive clinico-pharmacological studies comparing the two species of insulin formulated as neutral, soluble 'short-acting' insulins, only a very limited amount of data is available for the 'intermediate-acting' human and porcine insulin zinc suspensions. The results so far obtained are inconsistent, demonstrating either an earlier and more profound hypoglycaemic response

Study	Dose levels U/kg	Human Insulin 'Semi-synthetic' Lente (Monotard HM) U40	U100	Ultralente (Ultratard HM) U100	NPH (Protaphane HM) U40	U100	Human Insulin Biosynthetic NPH (Humulin I) U40	U100	Porcine Insulin Lente (Monotard MC) U40	U100	Ultralente (Ultratard MC) U100	NPH (Protaphane MC) U40	U100	Bovine Insulin Ultralente U100
A	0.10	x							x					
A	0.15	x							x					
A	0.30	x							x					
B	0.15				x		x		x			x		
B	0.30				x	x			x			x		
C	0.15	x			x							x		
C	0.30	x	x		x							x		
D	0.30			x							x			x

Figure 4.34 Schematic summary of studies involving 'intermediate-acting' and 'long-acting' insulin preparations

with human insulin (Vander Hoogen et al, 1982) or, more usually, similar hypoglycaemic effects and plasma insulin profiles following the subcutaneous administration of porcine and human Monotard insulin (Galloway et al, 1982a; Sestoft et al, 1982; Sonnenberg et al, 1983).

The purpose of this study was to compare the hypoglycaemic response ('potency') and insulin profiles ('bioavailability') following the bolus subcutaneous injection of human and porcine Monotard at three dose levels (0.1, 0.15 and 0.3 U/kg body weight) in normal fasting subjects.

Subjects, materials and methods

Six normal male volunteers aged between 28 and 38 years of age were included into the study, all of whom were within 20% of their ideal body weight (Metropolitan Life Insurance Company, 1960). Details of the insulin preparations used in the study are shown in Table 4.22. Each subject underwent

Table 4.22

	Porcine Monotard MC	Human Monotard HM	Diluting medium
Nitrogen (mg/ml)	0.210	0.217	—
Potency[a] (IU/ml)	38.9	40.1	—

[a]Theoretical potency based on 185 IU/mgN

seven study days which included a control day and six additional study days on human and porcine Monotard at the three dose levels: 0.1, 0.15 and 0.3 U/kg. On each of the study days, following a 1 hour basal period, a bolus subcutaneous injection of the test preparation was given into the anterior abdominal wall using a Plastipak SFP 1 ml syringe (Becton–Dickinson). Thereafter, $\frac{1}{2}$-hourly samples were taken for the first 3 hours, and hourly during the remainder of the 11 hour post-injection period.

Blood was taken into fluoride for glucose estimation (glucose analyser: Yellow Springs, Ohio, USA) and heparin for immunoreactive insulin (IRI) (modification of Heding, 1972) and C-peptide (modification of Heding, 1975) determinations.

Statistical methods

The results are expressed as means ± SE except where stated otherwise. The initial analysis comparing individual pairs of data was carried out using the Student's t-test. This method was chosen as it does not require assumptions about variance homogeneity. The analysis was conducted on both the observed and adjusted values (Δ values) defined as the observed minus the corresponding control day value from which is subtracted the mean basal (pre-injection) level on each study day for each of the response variables (glucose, C-peptide, insulin).

137

(i) *Estimation of exogenous insulin.* Estimates of the plasma exogenous insulin (IRI_{EXOG}) concentration were derived using two separate methods, both based on the assumption that the insulin radioimmunoassay measures exogenous and endogenous insulin in an additive manner and utilising the C-peptide level as an index of endogenous insulin secretion (Eaton et al, 1980). The use of insulin:C-peptide ratios, as a reflection of the relationship of the two beta-cell secretory peptides at any one time, is limited due to the marked differences in their plasma half-lives and the paucity of information on the kinetics and metabolism of insulin and C-peptide under different conditions (Polonsky and Rubenstein, 1984). Therefore, the calculation of the peripheral endogenous insulin level (IRI_{END}), based on a factor (F) which is the ratio between insulin and C-peptide concentrations and the prevailing C-peptide ($C\text{-peptide}_{OBS}$) level, i.e. $IRI_{END} = F \times C\text{-peptide}_{OBS}$, can only be expected to be approximate provided that the observed insulin (IRI) and C-peptide do not change too rapidly. Based on certain assumptions about constancy (in time) of insulin and C-peptide kinetics, including endogenous secretion in constant ratio, the use of the ratios (F) to derive an approximate estimate of the exogenous insulin has been evaluated according to the equation:

$$IRI_{EXOG} = IRI_{OBS} - F \times C\text{-peptide}_{OBS}$$

The accuracy of this approximation will improve when the endogenous component is small relative to the observed insulin (IRI_{OBS}).

Different sets of data have been used to calculate the ratio factors:

(a) IRI and C-peptide levels during a control day from which serial IRI: C-peptide ratios are derived for each individual subject, referred to as the 'control day method', and

(b) insulin and C-peptide levels during the initial basal (pre-insulin) period for all study days for each subject to derive the individual mean insulin: C-peptide ratio, i.e. the 'initial ratio method'.

Partial validation of the two methods was undertaken to see if the 'control day method' gave zero 'exogenous' insulin levels for the basal samples on other study days, and whether the 'initial ratio method', when applied to the control day, also gave zero values. In addition, a direct comparison of the estimates of exogenous insulin using both methods was made. Data from a former study (cf. 4.1.3) and the present study were used for this methodological analysis.

Study 4.1.3 involved six subjects given human and porcine neutral, soluble insulin and diluting medium (control) in random order on three separate days. With the 'control day method', the mean ratio was calculated for each serial time-point ($n = 22$) to estimate the IRI_{EXOG} both before and after insulin administration. In the 'initial ratio method' the mean ratio for each subject was derived from the six basal (pre-insulin) samples on each of the three study days ($n = 18$) which were then used to estimate the IRI_{EXOG} in all samples after time 0 min on the control day. Thereafter, the estimated mean exogenous insulin levels after insulin administration according to both methods were compared. The same procedures were also adopted for the present study.

(ii) *Insulin 'potency' and 'bioavailability' estimations*   Further analyses were conducted to examine the dose–response relationships for the two insulins, from which the relative 'potency' and 'bioavailability' of human and porcine insulins were estimated using the parallel line model (Finney, 1978).

Results

The mean ± SE absolute and Δ plasma glucose, C-peptide and insulin levels are shown in Figures 4.35a and 4.35b, respectively. The results are presented as follows:

(a) control day,
(b) comparison of response variables at each dose level,
(c) estimation of exogenous insulin,
(d) dose–response analysis and potency estimations.

(a) *Control day (Figure 4.35a)*.   During the control day there was a gradual fall in the plasma glucose level from 5.3 ± 0.1 at -2 h to 4.7 ± 0.2 mmol/l at 11 h. This was accompanied by a fall in C-peptide levels from 0.42 ± 0.1 to 0.23 ± 0.1 nmol/l and insulin concentrations from 0.063 ± 0.015 to 0.027 ± 0.004 nmol/l.

(b) *Comparison of response variables at each dose level (Figures 4.35a, 4.35b)*

(i) Dose: 0.10 U/kg body weight.   Following porcine Monotard the plasma glucose fell from 5.1 ± 0.1 to a nadir of 4.3 ± 0.2 mmol/l at 6 h, and remained at this level to the end of the study with only minor fluctuations in between (Figure 4.35a). Human Monotard resulted in an identical fall in plasma glucose over the first 3 h but the level continued to fall reaching a lower nadir of 4.1 ± 0.3 mmol/l between 4 and 6 h after injection. Thereafter, as for porcine insulin, the level remained essentially unchanged for the remainder of the study period. The glucose values were significantly lower with human than porcine insulin at 5 and 8 h after injection ($p < 0.05$).

A similar reduction in plasma C-peptide was observed with human and porcine insulin, the concentrations falling from pre-insulin levels of 0.35 ± 0.04 and 0.33 ± 0.03 nmol/l to nadir values of $0.09 + 0.04$ and $0.08 + 0.02$ nmol/l at 5 and 6 h, respectively (i.e. a reduction of 75%). There were no subsequent changes in the C-peptide levels during the remainder of the study period.

After the injection of human insulin there was a gradual increase in plasma insulin levels from 0.04 ± 0.01 nmol/l at time 0 h to a peak level of 0.08 ± 0.07 nmol/l at 3 h, returning to basal levels by about 9 h after administration. In comparison a more gradual rise was observed with porcine insulin, reaching a lower peak level of 0.064 ± 0.07 nmol/l at 5 h. The mean plasma insulin level was higher after human insulin between 2 and 4 h after injection, although the difference did not reach statistical significance.

Comparing the Δ values for the two species indicated that the hypoglycaemic effect of human insulin was greater than that of its porcine counterpart at 5 h and 8 h ($p < 0.05$) associated with higher incremental plasma

139

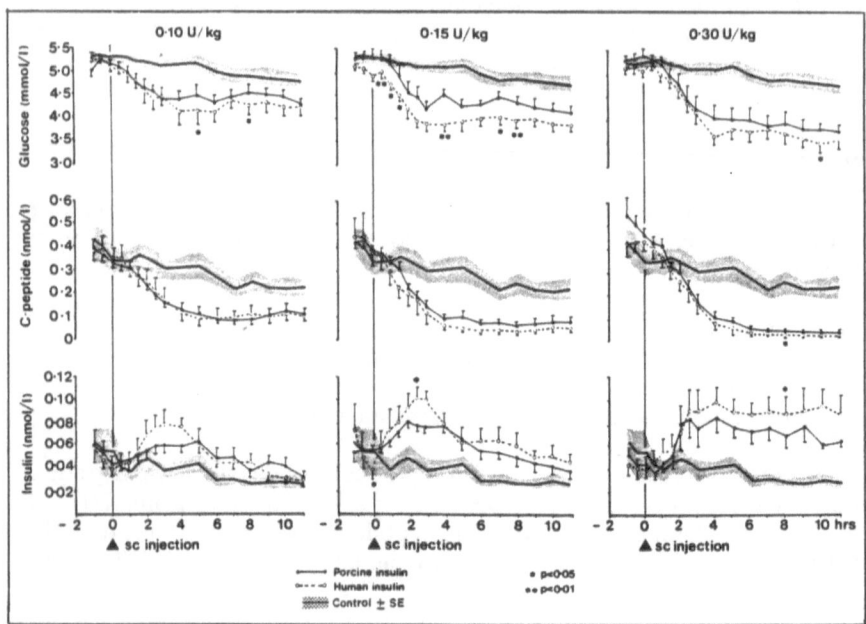

Figure 4.35a Comparison of effect of human and porcine Monotard insulins on plasma glucose, C-peptide and insulin (IRI) concentrations (means ± SE), in six subjects. Insulin (0.10, 0.15 and 0.30 U/kg) or diluent (control) injected subcutaneously (sc) at time 0

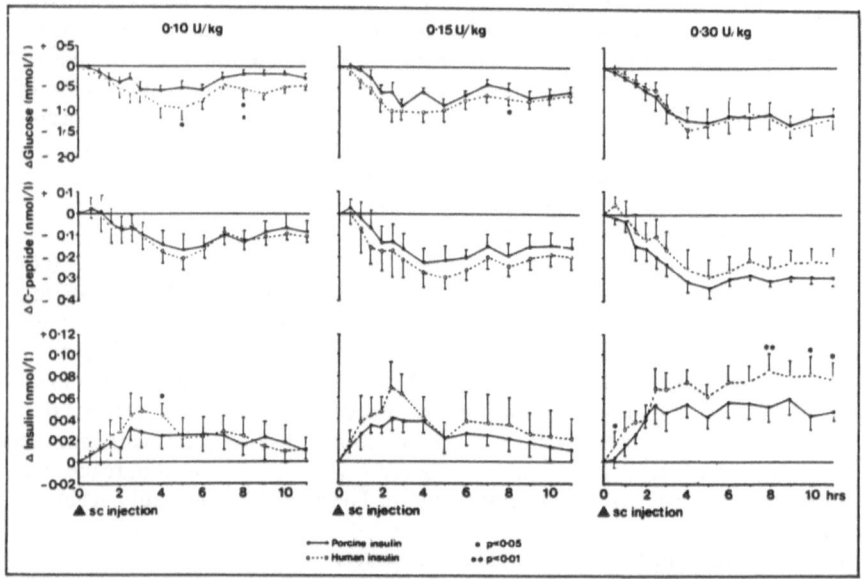

Figure 4.35b Comparison of effect of human and porcine Monotard insulins on plasma glucose, C-peptide and insulin (IRI) concentrations in six subjects. Insulin (0.10, 0.15 and 0.30 U/kg) injected subcutaneously (sc) at time 0. Results shown as means ± SE of Δ values

140

insulin concentrations during the first 4 h after injection, the difference reaching significance at 4 h ($p<0.05$).

(ii) Dose: 0.15 U/kg body weight.   The plasma glucose level immediately before insulin injection on the human and porcine insulin study days was 4.9 ± 0.1 and 5.3 ± 0.1 mmol/l, respectively. Both human and porcine insulins resulted in a relatively steeper fall than that observed with the lower dose level (Figure 4.39). Nadir glucose levels of 3.9 ± 0.1 and 4.2 ± 0.2 mmol/l were achieved at 4 and 3 h following human and porcine insulin, respectively. The glucose levels were significantly lower on human insulin at 0.5 to 1.5, 4, 7 and 8 h ($p<0.05$–0.01). However, when the values were adjusted to take account of the difference observed between the pre-insulin periods, the hypoglycaemic effect differed only at 8 h ($p<0.05$).

There were similar reductions in plasma C-peptide levels with the two insulins, the levels reaching approximately 11% and 18% of basal values by 6 h with human and porcine insulin, respectively.

The mean plasma insulin levels increased after human insulin from 0.04 ± 0.01 nmol/l at time 0 h to a peak of 0.1 ± 0.01 nmol/l at 2.5 h, followed by a gradual fall, returning to 0.046 ± 0.01 nmol/l at the end of the study. In comparison a lower peak level of 0.08 ± 0.01 nmol/l was reached at 2 h with porcine insulin. The plasma insulin level was significantly higher with human insulin at 2.5 h ($p<0.05$). From 4 h onwards the plasma insulin profiles were similar for the two species of insulin. There was no difference in the incremental insulin levels between human and porcine insulin.

(iii) Dose: 0.30 U/kg body weight.   After the injection of human insulin the plasma glucose level fell from a mean level of 5.1 ± 0.1 to 3.6 ± 0.1 mmol/l within 4 h and remained at this level for the last 7 h. The hypoglycaemic response was similar following human and porcine insulin at this dose level except that at 10 h the level was significantly lower ($p<0.05$) after human insulin. The Δ glucose values were identical for the two insulins.

A similar fall in fasting C-peptide levels from 0.43 ± 0.01 and 0.46 ± 0.04 nmol/l to a nadir of 0.02 ± 0.01 and 0.03 ± 0.01 nmol/l at 8 and 9 h was observed after human and porcine insulin, respectively.

The plasma insulin levels increased relatively quickly during the first 2.5 h after injection of human and porcine insulin, reaching peak levels of 0.09 ± 0.02 and 0.08 ± 0.02 nmol/l at 4 h, respectively. With human insulin the plasma levels remained unchanged for the remainder of the study, compared to a very gradual fall on the porcine insulin, the difference reaching significance at 8 h ($p<0.05$).

The difference between the insulins was more apparent for the incremental values (Δ values), which were significantly higher with human compared to porcine insulin at 0.5, 8, 10 and 11 h ($p<0.05$–0.01).

(c) *Estimation of exogenous insulin (Figures 4.36–4.38)*. For the 'short-acting' insulin study (cf. 4.1.3), the results show that the 'control day method' did not estimate any apparent exogenous insulin during the pre-insulin period, although there was a tendency to deviations from zero which did not reach

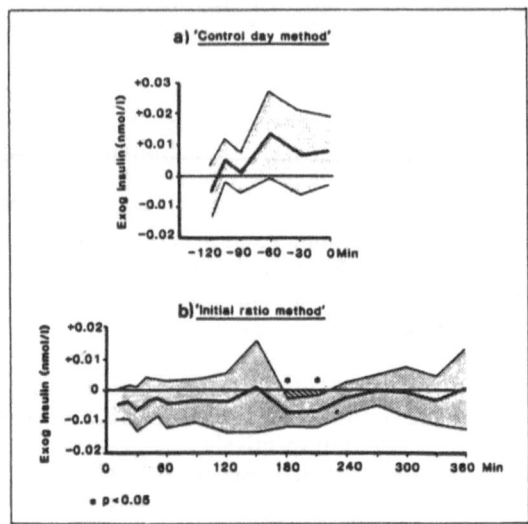

Figure 4.36a, b Plasma exogenous insulin estimates (with 95% confidence limits) using (**a**) the 'control day method' and (**b**) the 'initial ratio method'. Data derived from previous 'short-acting' insulin study (cf. 4.1.3)

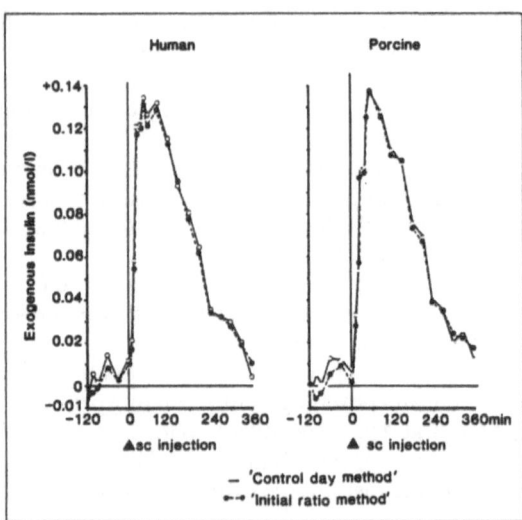

Figure 4.36c Comparison of exogenous insulin estimated according to the 'control day method' and 'initial ratio method' following the administration of human and porcine neutral, soluble insulin to six subjects. Insulin (0.075 U/kg) given subcutaneously (sc) at time 0

statistical significance (Figure 4.36a). When utilising the 'initial ratio method' for the time points after 0 min on the control day, the estimated mean exogenous insulin levels tended to be below zero, reaching significance at 180 and 210 min (Figure 4.36b). The analyses indicate that with both methods,

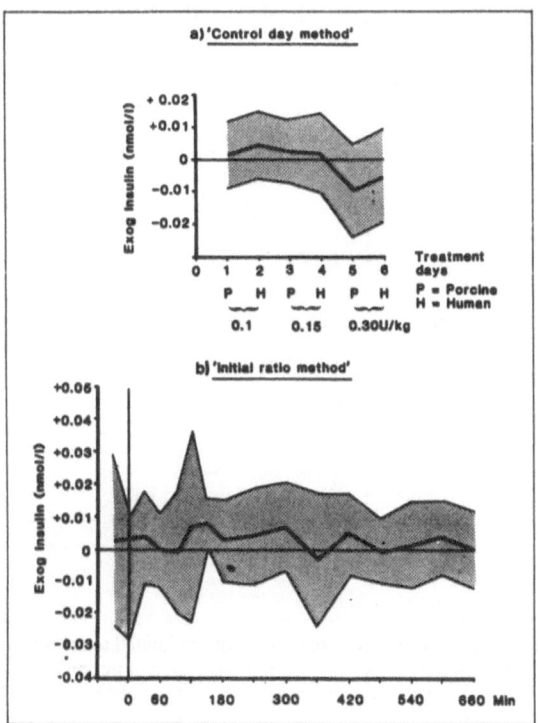

Figure 4.37a, b Plasma exogenous insulin estimates (with 95% confidence limits) using (**a**) the 'control day method' and (**b**) the 'initial ratio method'

none, or only very little, apparent exogenous insulin is estimated during periods when no insulin has been administered. Comparison of the two methods following the administration of insulin demonstrates that nearly the same results are obtained, with a correlation coefficient (r) of 0.992 ($n = 183$). There was a tendency to slightly lower values with the initial compared to the control day ratio method (Figure 4.36c).

In the present study the control day insulin:C-peptide ratios are more variable than those obtained in the previous study, but the estimated means (IRI$_{EXOG}$) for the three initial basal samples on each of the six insulin (treatment) days do not differ much from the expected zero (Figure 4.37a). Similarly with the 'initial ratio method' no apparent exogenous insulin was estimated during the 11h control day (Figure 4.37b). There is also good agreement between the two methods after insulin administration (Figure 4.37c). Despite the more gradual changes in insulin and C-peptide levels in this study, the general agreement is not as good as seen in study 4.1.3, which is reflected in the slightly decreased correlation coefficient between the estimated exogenous insulin values ($r = 0.953$; $n = 488$).

The mean plasma insulin (IRI$_{OBS}$), the estimated endogenous (IRI$_{END}$) and exogenous (IRI$_{EXOG}$) insulin levels using the 'control day method' for human

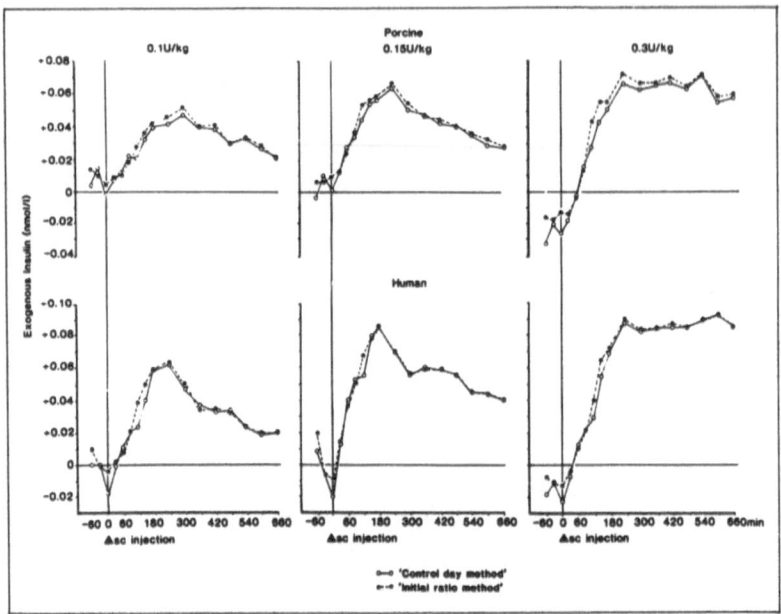

Figure 4.37c Comparison of plasma exogenous insulin estimated according to the 'control day method' and 'initial ratio method' following the administration of porcine and human Monotard insulin (0.10, 0.15 and 0.30 U/kg) to six subjects. Insulin given subcutaneously at time 0

and porcine insulin at the three dose levels are shown in Figure 4.38a. Whereas the estimated exogenous insulin level tended to be higher on human insulin, the difference did not reach statistical significance (Figure 4.38b).

(d) *Dose–response analysis and 'potency' estimations (Figures 4.39, 4.40).* The mean Δ plasma glucose, C-peptide and insulin values for the three dose levels of human and porcine Monotard insulin are shown in Figure 4.39. The results of the dose-response analysis for porcine and human insulin using the analysis of covariance with time 0h as covariate are summarised in Figures 4.40a and 4.40b, respectively.

There was no significant difference in the hypoglycaemic response between the two lower doses of porcine insulin, whereas with the human insulin the effect was greater with 0.15 U/kg at 1.5, 7 and 11h ($p<0.05$). There was also a dose-related glucose-lowering effect for human insulin between the 0.15 and 0.30 U/kg dose levels occurring at 1.5h, 2h ($p<0.01$) and 2.5h ($p<0.05$) after injection. For both porcine and human insulin there was a dose-related hypoglycaemic effect between the low and the high doses from 8 to 11h ($p<0.05$–0.01) and at 3, 5, 7 to 10h ($p<0.05$–0.01), respectively as reflected in the C-peptide results (Figures 4.40a and 4.40b).

There were no dose-related increments in plasma insulin levels with porcine insulin comparing the low and intermediate dose levels in contrast to human insulin where there were differences at 2.5 and 6h ($p<0.05$). No dose-related

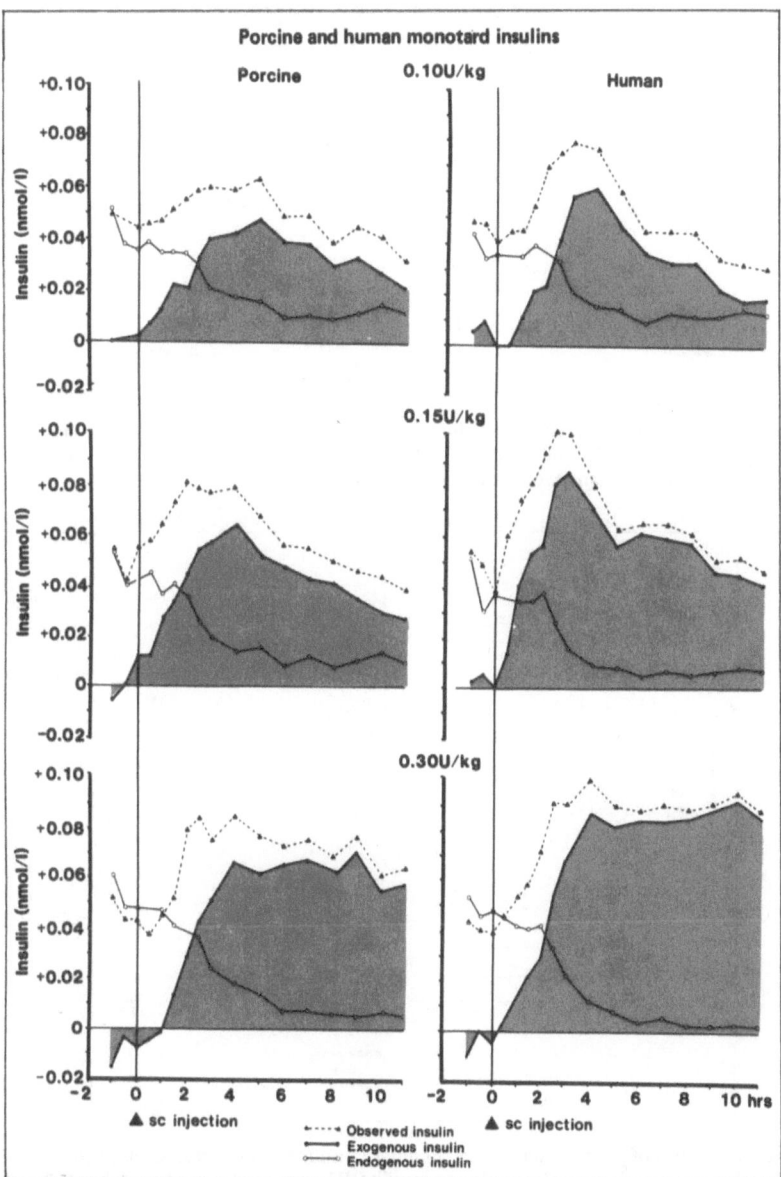

Figure 4.38a Effect of porcine and human Monotard insulins on plasma insulin (observed) and the estimated endogenous and exogenous ('control day method') insulin concentrations (means) in six subjects. Insulin (0.10, 0.15 and 0.30 U/kg) given subcutaneously (sc) at time 0

increments in plasma insulin with either species occurred between the 0.15 and 0.30 U/kg dose levels, whereas comparing the low and high dose levels, there was a significant ($p<0.05$–0.01) dose effect from 9 h onwards for human insulin and at 8, 9 and 11 h with porcine insulin.

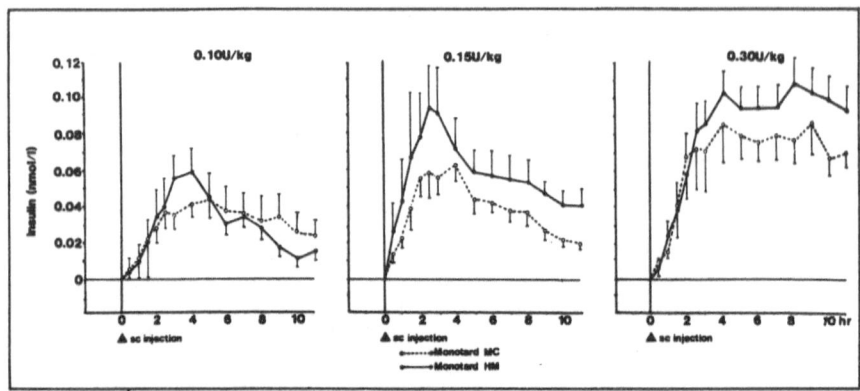

Figure 4.38b Comparison of the estimated plasma exogenous ('control day method') concentrations (means SE) following the subcutaneous (sc) injection at time 0 of porcine (Monotard MC) and human (Monotard HM) insulin

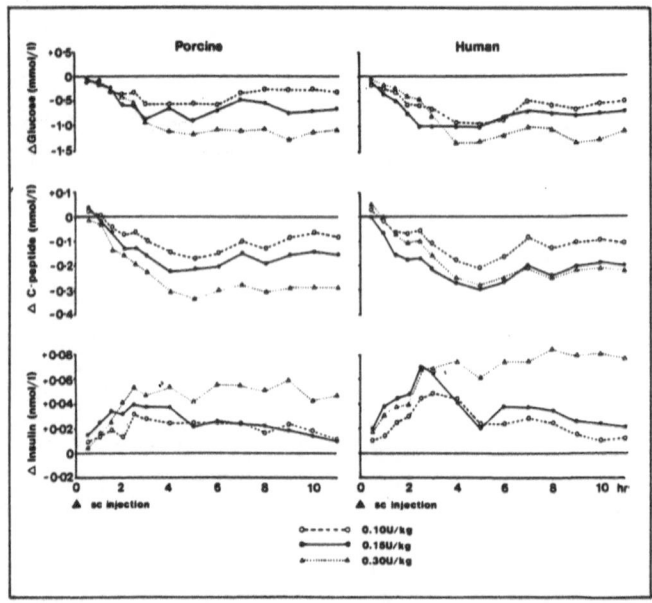

Figure 4.39 Effect of porcine and human Monotard insulins at three dose levels (0.10, 0.15 and 0.30 U/kg) on plasma glucose, C-peptide and insulin (IRI) concentrations in six subjects. Insulin given subcutaneously (sc) at time 0. Results shown as means of Δ values

Subsequent to the above, further dose–response analyses were conducted for the mean responses computed for the periods 0 to 3, 3 to 7 and 7 to 11 h. The 'potency' estimates of human relative to porcine insulin using the parallel line model for each parameter are represented in Table 4.23 and Figure 4.41. The analysis of the glucose values demonstrates a greater 'potency' of human

a) Porcine Monotard

Time h	Glucose 0.1 vs 0.15	Glucose 0.15 vs 0.30	Glucose 0.10 vs 0.30	C-peptide 0.1 vs 0.15	C-peptide 0.15 vs 0.30	C-peptide 0.10 vs 0.30	Insulin 0.1 vs 0.15	Insulin 0.15 vs 0.30	Insulin 0.10 vs 0.30
0.5			$p < 0.05$						
1									
1.5	$p < 0.05$	$p < 0.01$							
2		$p < 0.01$							
2.5		$p < 0.05$					$p < 0.05$		
3									
4									
5									
6							$p < 0.05$		$p < 0.05$
7	$p < 0.05$								
8			$p < 0.05$						
9			$p < 0.01$	$p < 0.05$					$p < 0.05$
10			$p < 0.01$	$p < 0.001$		$p < 0.05$			$p < 0.01$
11	$p < 0.05$		$p < 0.05$	$p < 0.01$		$p < 0.05$			$p < 0.05$

b) Human Monotard

Time h	Glucose 0.1 vs 0.15	Glucose 0.15 vs 0.30	Glucose 0.10 vs 0.30	C-peptide 0.1 vs 0.15	C-peptide 0.15 vs 0.30	C-peptide 0.10 vs 0.30	Insulin 0.1 vs 0.15	Insulin 0.15 vs 0.30	Insulin 0.10 vs 0.30
0.5			$p < 0.05$						
1									
1.5	$p < 0.05$	$p < 0.01$							
2		$p < 0.01$							
2.5		$p < 0.05$					$p < 0.05$		
3									
4									
5									
6							$p < 0.05$		$p < 0.05$
7	$p < 0.05$								
8			$p < 0.05$						
9			$p < 0.01$	$p < 0.05$					$p < 0.05$
10			$p < 0.01$	$p < 0.001$		$p < 0.05$			$p < 0.01$
11	$p < 0.05$		$p < 0.05$	$p < 0.01$		$p < 0.05$			$p < 0.05$

Figure 4.40 Dose–response analysis using analysis of covariance (with time 0 as covariate) for (a) porcine and (b) human Monotard. Insulins given subcutaneously at the three dose levels 0.10, 0.15 and 0.30 U/kg body weight

relative to porcine insulin for the 3 to 7, 7 to 11 and 0 to 11 h periods. It is of interest to note that similar trends are seen for the Δ glucose values, which is in agreement with the trend towards higher plasma insulin levels with human insulin, although the differences do not reach statistical significance.

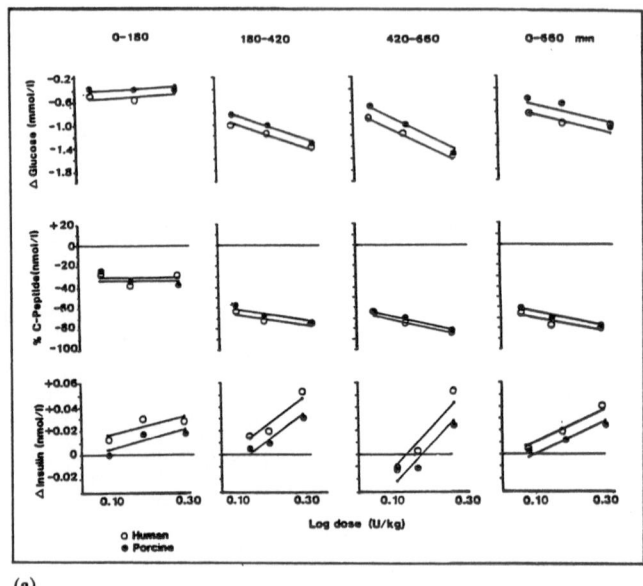

(a)

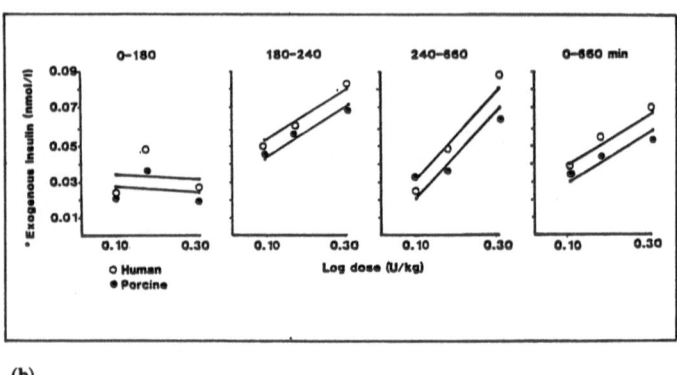

(b)

Figure 4.41a, b   Dose-response analysis of effect of human and porcine Monotard insulins on plasma glucose, C-peptide and insulin (IRI) concentrations in six subjects. Insulin (0.10, 0.15 and 0.30 U/kg) given subcutaneously (sc) at time 0. Results shown as means of (**a**) Δ glucose, % C-peptide, Δ insulin and (**b**) estimated exogenous insulin ('control day method') values for the periods 0–180, 180–420, 420–660 and 0–660 min

Discussion

The Lente trilogy of insulins (Semilente, Lente and Ultralente) were produced in the early 1950s (Hallas-Møller, 1956) and Monotard, a purely porcine Lente insulin, was introduced into clinical practice in 1975. The majority of the early clinical–pharmacological studies with Lente insulin have used radiolabelled

Table 4.23 Dose–response analysis and 'potency' estimates (with 95% confidence limits) of human relative to porcine Monotard insulin determined using the parallel line model (Finney, 1978)

	Periods (area means)			
Response	0–3 h	3–7 h	7–11 h	0–11 h
Glucose	—	219 (111–2750)*	151 (108–238)*	214 (118–1139)*
Δ Glucose	—	150 (89–372)	123 (94–167)	140 (93–247)
C-peptide	—	—	122 (73–241)	—
Δ C-peptide	—	103 (43–268)	99 (57–169)	99 (45–212)
% C-peptide	—	168 (62–∞)	124 (83–205)	143 (66–884)
IRI	—	147 (84–411)	127 (88–201)	143 (87–308)
Δ IRI	—	154 (94–362)	135 (95–214)	147 (97–279)
Exog IRI (1)	—	163 (88–700)	130 (91–203)	155 (92–399)
Exog IRI (2)	—	148 (85–403)	125 (91–186)	144 (89–307)

Exog IRI (1): Exogenous insulin estimated by the 'control day method'
Exog IRI (2): Exogenous insulin estimated by the 'initial ratio method'
* The relative potencies are significantly different at the 5% level when the 95% interval does not contain the 100% value
– No estimates are given when the dose-response relationship was not significant at the 5% level

insulin (Binder, 1969; Faber et al, 1975; Schlichtkrull, 1977), as almost all insulin-treated diabetics had, to varying degrees, circulating insulin antibodies which invalidated the measurement of insulin in the plasma (Berson and Yalow, 1964). Despite the fact that the 'intermediate-acting' insulins account for over 80% of all insulins used, there is still a paucity of meaningful pharmacological studies in man with the Lente insulin preparations (Griffin et al, 1980; Galloway et al, 1981a; Fukomoto et al, 1982). Therefore with the advent of human insulin (Chance et al, 1981a, b; Markussen et al, 1982) there have been attempts to describe the pharmacokinetics and pharmacodynamic responses of both the old and the new Lente insulins in normal man (Galloway et al, 1982a; Vander Hoogen et al, 1982) and diabetic patients (Sestoft et al, 1982; Colagiuri et al, 1983; Greene et al, 1983; Mann et al, 1983; Home et al, 1984).

In this study an attempt has been made to evaluate the plasma glucose, C-peptide and insulin responses to bolus subcutaneous injection of human and porcine Monotard insulin at the three dose levels of 0.1, 0.15 and 0.3 U/kg body weight in a small number of normal subjects.

The results demonstrate that with both human and porcine Monotard insulin the plasma glucose level fell gradually at the rate of about 0.25 mmol/l per hour over the initial 4 h post-injection period. Thereafter the glucose level remained unchanged for the two higher dose levels, whereas there was a gradual recovery towards fasting values from 5 to 6 h onwards with the low dose. The study period was too short, however, to determine the total duration of the hypoglycaemic response in the normal subjects.

Comparison of the plasma glucose levels for each time point during the human and porcine insulin study days, revealed a trend towards lower levels on human insulin, although the difference reached significance at only a few time points for the unadjusted data and fewer for the adjusted data. There was little or no difference between the C-peptide response to the two insulins. There was, however, a tendency for the plasma insulin levels to be higher on human insulin between 2.5 and 4 h for the low and intermediate dose levels and from 3 h onwards for the 0.3 U/kg dose level. As for the glucose response, the study period was too short to indicate the subsequent course of the plasma insulin profile, especially for the 'intermediate' and high dose levels.

When the responses were combined over arbitarily defined periods of time after injection and using the parallel line method to determine the relative hypoglycaemic 'potencies' and 'bioavailabilities', the results indicate that the hypoglycaemic effect of human insulin was greater than porcine insulin between 3 to 7 and 7 to 11 h associated with a tendency to higher insulin levels.

Two methods were used to estimate exogenous insulin levels. Whereas the methods were in good agreement, this does not mean that either is capable of estimating the exogenous insulin correctly. However, based on certain assumptions about constancy of insulin and C-peptide kinetics, provided that the observed insulin and C-peptide levels do not change too rapidly, $IRI_{EXOG} = IRI_{OBS} - F \times C\text{-peptide}_{OBS}$ with good approximation, the ratio factor (F) having been derived either from a control day or the basal (fasting) samples. The 'control day method' should be able to adjust for possible individual changes in the ratio during prolonged study periods, as well as for variation from subject to subject. The usefulness of the 'initial ratio method' was assessed, as many similar studies do not employ a control day. Attempts to estimate the exogenous insulin levels were made in view of the relatively low incremental insulin levels observed with the 'intermediate-acting' insulins, which were exaggerated by the suppression of endogenous insulin secretion accompanying the hypoglycaemia. Additional studies and analytical methods are necessary to estimate further the validity and usefulness of these crude methods.

In conclusion, the results demonstrate that both human and porcine Lente (Monotard) insulin, following subcutaneous administration in normal man at 0.1, 0.15 and 0.3 U/kg dose level, achieved maximal or near-maximal hypoglycaemic responses within 4 h of administration. Over the following 6 h there was little or no further reduction with either the 'intermediate' or high dose levels, only a moderate recovery towards normoglycaemia occuring at the low dose level for both preparations. At the two lower dose levels, peak insulin concentrations were observed between 2.5 and 5 h after injection, followed by a gradual fall over the remaining period. At the high dose level, the plasma insulin level increased relatively quickly over the first 2 to 3 h, reaching a lower plateau on porcine compared to human insulin. From 8 to 10 h after injection the insulin levels started to fall.

There was a trend towards lower glucose and higher insulin levels with human compared to porcine Lente (Monotard) insulin following sub-cutaneous injection in healthy normal subjects. The study protocol with its small number of subjects demands conservative interpretation of the comparisons between human and porcine insulin. Further studies involving a more prolonged observation period and more subjects are necessary to explore any potential clinically relevant difference between human and porcine Lente (Monotard) insulin.

Any difference that may be present between the two preparations in this study does not appear to prejudice the safety of the diabetic patient transferred from porcine to human insulin used as admixtures of soluble and insulin zinc suspensions administered once or twice a day (Greene et al, 1983; Mann et al, 1983; Birtwell et al, 1984; Home et al, 1984). The data also re-emphasises that small dosage changes of the 'intermediate-acting' insulins are unlikely to have any clinical relevance in the majority of patients (Lauritzen et al, 1982; Hildebrandt et al, 1984a).

4.2.1.2   A study of human ('semi-synthetic' and 'biosynthetic') and porcine NPH ('isophane') insulins (U-40)

Prior to the 1980s NPH insulin consisted of bovine, porcine or a mixture of bovine and porcine insulin. Human insulin derived either from porcine insulin by enzymatic conversion (Markussen, 1982a, b) or by employing recombinant DNA technology (Chance et al, 1981a, b) has resulted in the recent availability of human NPH insulins for clinical use.

The purpose of this study was to compare the plasma glucose and C-peptide responses and insulin levels following the subcutaneous administration of three highly purified NPH insulin preparations, i.e. porcine, 'semi-synthetic' and 'biosynthetic' human NPH insulins at two dose levels (0.15 and 0.30 U/kg body weight) in normal man.

Subjects, materials and methods

Six healthy normal male subjects aged 24–38 years and weighing 66–80 kg were entered into the study. Details of the three NPH insulin preparations used in the study are included in Table 4.24.

Table 4.24

	Human NPH insulin		Porcine NPH
	'Semi-synthetic'	'Biosynthetic'	insulin
Potency[a] (IU/ml)	40.9	40.5	39.6
Protamine sulphate (mg)	0.142	0.144	0.145
Glycerol (mg)	16	16	16
m-Cresol (mg)	1.5	1.6	1.5
Phenol (mg)	0.65	0.72	0.65
Sodium phosphate (mg)	2.4	—	2.4

[a]Determined by quantitative HPLC gel permeation chromatography method with monocomponent porcine insulin as standard

All the subjects participated on six separate study days, 1–4 weeks apart. Following a basal period of 1 h, the comparative insulin preparations or diluting medium (control) were administered by subcutaneous injection into the anterior abdominal wall. The porcine and 'semi-synthetic' human insulin were administered at the two dose levels: 0.15 and 0.30 U/kg body weight, and the 'biosynthetic' human insulin at the low dose level only (0.15 U/kg body weight). Blood samples were taken ½-hourly during the basal period and for the first 3 h after injection, then hourly up to 11 h. The blood was aliquoted into fluoride for plasma glucose (hexokinase), heparin for immunoreactive insulin (modification of Heding, 1972) and C-peptide (modification of Heding, 1975) determinations.

Statistical methods

The results are expressed as means ± SE unless stated otherwise. The individual pairs of treatments were compared using the Student's *t*-test as this method does not require assumptions about variance homogeneity. The analyses were conducted on the absolute values and on the data after adjusting for the corresponding control values and pre-injection (basal) concentrations, i.e. Δ values.

An approximate estimate of the exogenous plasma insulin levels was calculated using the 'control day method' described in study 4.2.1.1.

In addition, dose–response analyses were carried out and the hypoglycaemic 'potency' and 'bioavailability' of 'semi-synthetic' human relative to porcine and

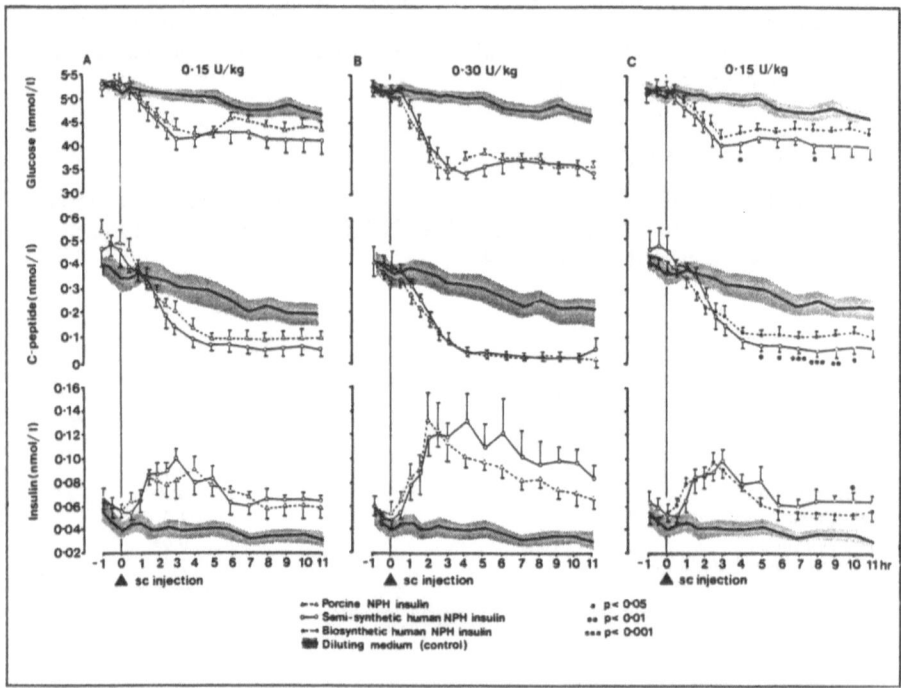

Figure 4.42 Comparison of effect of porcine, 'semi-synthetic' and 'biosynthetic' human NPH insulins on plasma glucose, C-peptide and insulin (IRI) concentrations (means ± SE) in six subjects. Porcine, 'semi-synthetic' human (0.15 and 0.30 U/kg) and 'biosynthetic' human (0.15 U/kg) NPH insulins or diluent (control) injected subcutaneously (sc) at time 0

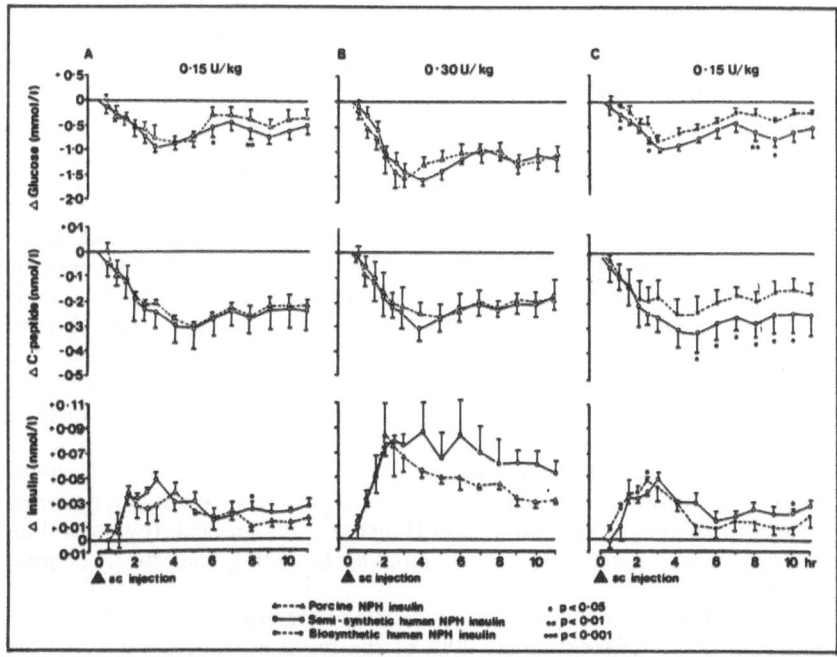

Figure 4.43 Comparison of effect of porcine, 'semi-synthetic' and 'biosynthetic' human NPH insulins on plasma glucose, C-peptide and insulin (IRI) concentrations in six subjects. Porcine, 'semi-synthetic' human (0.15 and 0.30 U/kg) and 'biosynthetic' human (0.15 U/kg) NPH insulins or diluent (control) injected subcutaneously (sc) at time 0. Results shown as means ± SE of Δ values

'biosynthetic' human insulin were determined according to the parallel line model (Finney, 1978). The relative estimates were calculated for the 0 to 3, 3 to 7, 7 to 11 and 0 to 11 h time intervals for the variables; plasma glucose, C-peptide and insulin.

Results

The mean ± SE plasma glucose, C-peptide and insulin levels following subcutaneous porcine and 'semi-synthetic' human NPH insulin at 0.15 and 0.30 U/kg body weight and 'biosynthetic' human insulin at 0.15 U/kg body weight are shown in Figure 4.42. The corresponding values adjusted for the control and basal levels, i.e. Δ values, are represented in Figure 4.43. The results are presented as follows:

  (i) control day,
 (ii) comparisons between the insulin preparations at each dose level,
(iii) exogenous insulin estimations,
(iv) dose–response analysis and 'potency' estimations.

(i) *Control day (Figure 4.42).* During the control day the plasma glucose concentration fell from 5.3 ± 0.1 mmol/l at -1 h to 4.6 ± 0.1 mmol/l at 11 h. Similarly, the endogenous pancreatic beta-cell secretion was reduced over the 12 h study period as depicted by a lowering in plasma C-peptide levels from 0.42 ± 0.05 to 0.21 ± 0.05 nmol/l and insulin levels from 0.055 ± 0.007 to 0.028 ± 0.003 nmol/l.

(ii) *Comparisons between insulin preparations (Figures 4.42 and 4.43)*

Dose: 0.15 U/kg.   After the subcutaneous injection of porcine and 'semi-synthetic' human NPH insulin at the low dose level of 0.15 U/kg body weight, the plasma glucose fell from a pre-injection level of 5.4 ± 0.1 mmol/l to a nadir of 4.3 ± 0.1 mmol/l at 4 h and 4.1 ± 0.2 mmol/l at 3 h, respectively (Figure 4.42A). There followed a short-lived recovery in plasma glucose (0.2–0.3 mmol/l) over the ensuing 2 to 4 h period, with the subsequent levels falling again to 4.4 ± 0.2 and 4.1 ± 0.2 mmol/l for porcine and human insulin, respectively. There was no significant difference in the observed glucose levels during the porcine and 'semi-synthetic' human NPH insulin study days. Comparison of the Δ values did, however, indicate that the hypoglycaemic response to 'semi-synthetic' human NPH insulin was significantly greater than its porcine counterpart at 6 h ($p<0.05$) and 8 h ($p<0.01$), respectively (Figure 4.43A).

Both insulins resulted in a similar reduction in the mean plasma C-peptide concentration to approximately 20% of the basal level between 5 and 8 h post-injection and remained essentially unchanged up to the end of the study period.

The plasma insulin concentration increased with porcine insulin from 0.057 ± 0.01 nmol/l to a peak of 0.091 ± 0.01 nmol/l at 4 h. In comparison, following the administration of 'semi-synthetic' human NPH insulin the level increased from 0.055 ± 0.01 nmol/l at time 0 h to an earlier and higher peak level of 0.099 ± 0.01 nmol/l at 3 h (Figure 4.42A). Comparison of the absolute values revealed no difference between these insulins, although the incremental plasma insulin level was significantly higher with human insulin at 8 h only ($p<0.05$; Figure 4.43A). The mean plasma insulin concentrations had returned to basal levels with both insulins, by 6 to 8 h.

Following the subcutaneous injection of 'biosynthetic' NPH insulin at 0.15 U/kg body weight the plasma glucose fell from 5.3 ± 0.1 mmol/l to 4.3 ± 0.2 mmol/l at 3 h, followed by a brief recovery to 4.5 ± 0.1 mmol/l at 7 h before falling again to 4.4 ± 0.1 mmol/l by the end of the study (Figure 4.42C). The hypoglycaemic action of 'biosynthetic' human NPH insulin was significantly less than that of 'semi-synthetic' human NPH insulin at 4 h and 8 h ($p<0.05$) for the absolute and at 1 h, 2.5 h ($p<0.05$), 8 h ($p<0.01$) and 9 h ($p<0.05$) for the Δ values (Figures 4.42C, 4.43C). 'Biosynthetic' human insulin resulted in the lowering of the plasma C-peptide from 0.43 ± 0.05 nmol/l to 0.12 ± 0.02 nmol/l at 5 h, remaining at this level for the duration of the study. The suppression of the C-peptide levels was greater following 'semi-synthetic' than 'biosynthetic' human insulin between 5 and 10 h post-administration (Figures 4.42C, 4.43C). A rise in plasma insulin levels from 0.057 ± 0.01 nmol/l at 0 h to a peak mean level of 0.10 ± 0.01 nmol/l at 2.5 h was seen with 'biosynthetic' human insulin

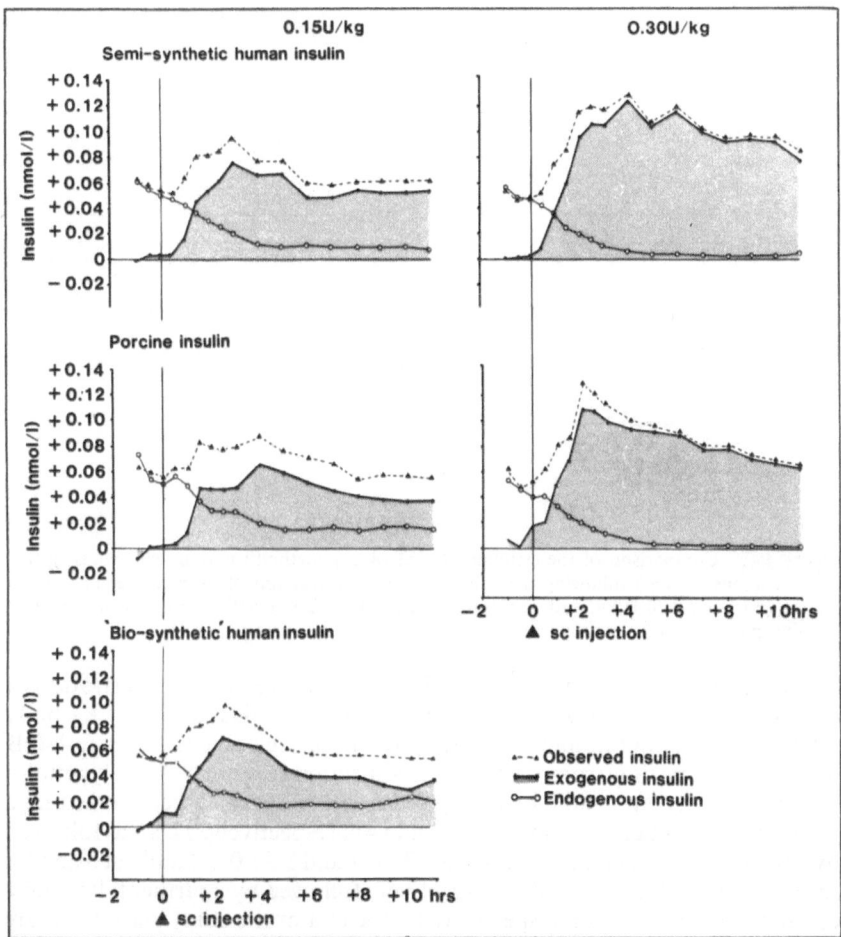

Figure 4.44 Effect of 'semi-synthetic' human, porcine (0.15 and 0.30 U/kg) and 'biosynthetic' human (0.15 U/kg) NPH insulins on plasma insulin (observed), and the estimated endogenous and exogenous ('control day method') insulin concentrations (means) in six subjects. Insulins injected subcutaneously (sc) at time 0

(Figure 4.42C). By 11 h the plasma insulin had returned to fasting levels of 0.058 ± 0.01 nmol/l. The plasma insulin profile was similar for the two human insulins except at 10h, when the level was significantly higher ($p<0.05$) with 'semi-synthetic' human NPH insulin (Figure 4.42C). The incremental insulin values were initially higher with 'biosynthetic' human insulin at 2.5 h ($p<0.05$). Thereafter the trend was reversed with the levels becoming significantly lower with 'biosynthetic' relative to 'semi-synthetic' human insulin at 10h ($p<0.05$; Figure 4.43C).

There was no significant difference in the plasma glucose, C-peptide and insulin responses between porcine NPH insulin and the 'biosynthetic' human NPH insulin.

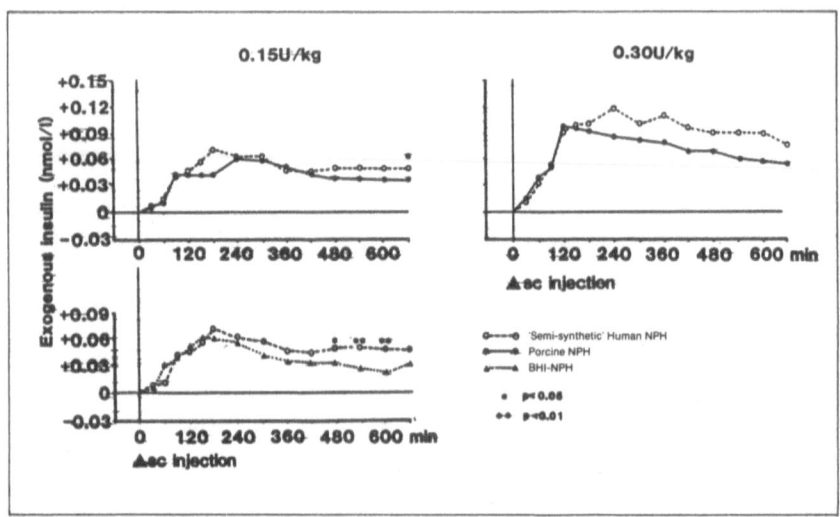

Figure 4.45 Comparison of the estimated ('control day method') plasma exogenous insulin concentrations (means) following the subcutaneous (sc) injection of porcine, 'semi-synthetic' human (0.15 and 0.30 U/kg) and 'biosynthetic' BHI (0.15 U/kg) NPH insulins in six subjects. Insulins injected subcutaneously (sc) at time 0

Dose: 0.30 U/kg. In comparison to the low dose level, the administration of both porcine and 'semi-synthetic' human NPH insulins at 0.30 U/kg body weight caused a more rapid and greater fall in plasma glucose (Figure 4.42B and 4.43A). Starting from a similar pre-injection level of 5.2 ± 0.1 mmol/l, porcine and human insulin promptly reduced the plasma glucose reaching a nadir of approximately 3.5 mmol/l at 3 and 4 h, respectively. This was followed by a relatively short-lived recovery to 3.9 ± 0.1 and 3.8 ± 0.2 mmol/l at 5 and 7 h for porcine and human insulin, respectively followed by a further fall to 3.6 ± 0.1 and 3.5 ± 0.1 mmol/l, respectively by the end of the study period (Figure 4.42B). There was no difference at the 0.30 U/kg dose level between the two species of NPH insulin throughout the 11 h post-injection observation period (Figures 4.42B, 4.43B).

The C-peptide levels were suppressed to approximately 10% of basal levels by 4 h with only a small recovery evident over the remainder of the study period. The response was nearly identical for the two insulins.

There was a sharp increase in plasma insulin levels over the initial 2 to 4 h period with peak levels of 0.132 ± 0.026 and 0.133 ± 0.023 nmol/l reached at 2 and 4 h with porcine and human insulin, respectively (Figure 4.42A). Thereafter there was an earlier fall in insulin levels with porcine insulin. Although the mean plasma insulin levels were higher on human insulin from 4 h onwards, the difference did not reach statistical significance (Figures 4.42B, 4.43B).

(iii) *Exogenous insulin estimations (Figures 4.44 and 4.45).* The plasma immunoreactive insulin (IRI) and estimated endogenous and exogenous insulin levels for the three insulin preparations are shown in Figure 4.44. Comparison of the estimated exogenous plasma insulin level between porcine and 'semi-synthetic' human NPH insulins at the low dose level revealed little difference, although the mean level was significantly higher ($p<0.05$) with human insulin at 11 h (Figure 4.45). The exogenous insulin concentration was also higher with the 'semi-synthetic' than the 'biosynthetic' human insulin from 5 h onwards, the difference reaching significance between 8 and 10 h ($p<0.05-0.01$). At the dose of 0.30 U/kg the exogenous insulin level was higher with 'semi-synthetic' human than porcine insulin after the first 4 h, although the difference did not reach statistical significance (Figure 4.45).

(iv) *Dose–response analysis and 'potency' estimations.* The dose–response relationship of 'semi-synthetic' human and porcine NPH insulin and the relative 'potency' (with 95% confidence limits) of human to the reference porcine insulin are summarised in Table 4.25 and Figures 4.46a, b, respectively. The hypoglycaemic 'potency' of 'semi-synthetic' human insulin is greater than its porcine counterpart for the 3 to 7, 7 to 11 and 0 to 11 h time intervals, although the difference did not reach significance (Table 4.25). A similar trend was observed in insulin 'bioavailability' which was significantly higher with human than porcine insulin during the 7 to 11 h period.

The 'potency' estimates for 'biosynthetic' relative to 'semi-synthetic' human insulin at the 0.15 U/kg dose level are included in Table 4.26. Whereas the mean area under the insulin curve is higher with 'biosynthetic' human insulin during the first 3 h, the reverse is true for the remainder of the study. This was reflected in the lower hypoglycaemic 'potency' of 'biosynthetic' human insulin, the difference reaching statistical significance ($p<0.05$) for the 7 to 11 h and the total study period (0 to 11 h).

Table 4.25 Dose–response analysis and 'potency' estimates (with 95% confidence limits) of human relative to porcine NPH insulin, determined using the parallel line model (Finney, 1978)

Response variable	Periods (area means)			
	0–3 h	*3–7 h*	*7–11 h*	*0–11 h*
Glucose	125 (87–168)	121 (89–156)	130 (98–166)	177 (94–150)
Δ Glucose	104 (59–198)	121 (93–168)	118 (90–163)	117 (90–160)
C-peptide	113 (77–180)	118 (74–228)	119 (80–203)	118 (81–191)
Δ C-peptide	—	—	—	—
% C-peptide	—	115 (64–280)	113 (75–192)	118 (69–267)
IRI	97 (30–267)	120 (76–243)	148 (98–350)	125 (86–214)
Δ IRI	102 (73–144)	118 (85–180)	137 (102–211)*	121 (96–161)
Exog IRI (1)	103 (66–164)	119 (85–184)	140 (103–225)*	123 (94–171)

Exog IRI (1): Exogenous insulin estimated by the 'control day method'
* The relative potencies are significantly different at the 5% level when the 95% interval does not contain the 100% value
— No estimates are given when the dose-response relationship was not significant at the 5% level

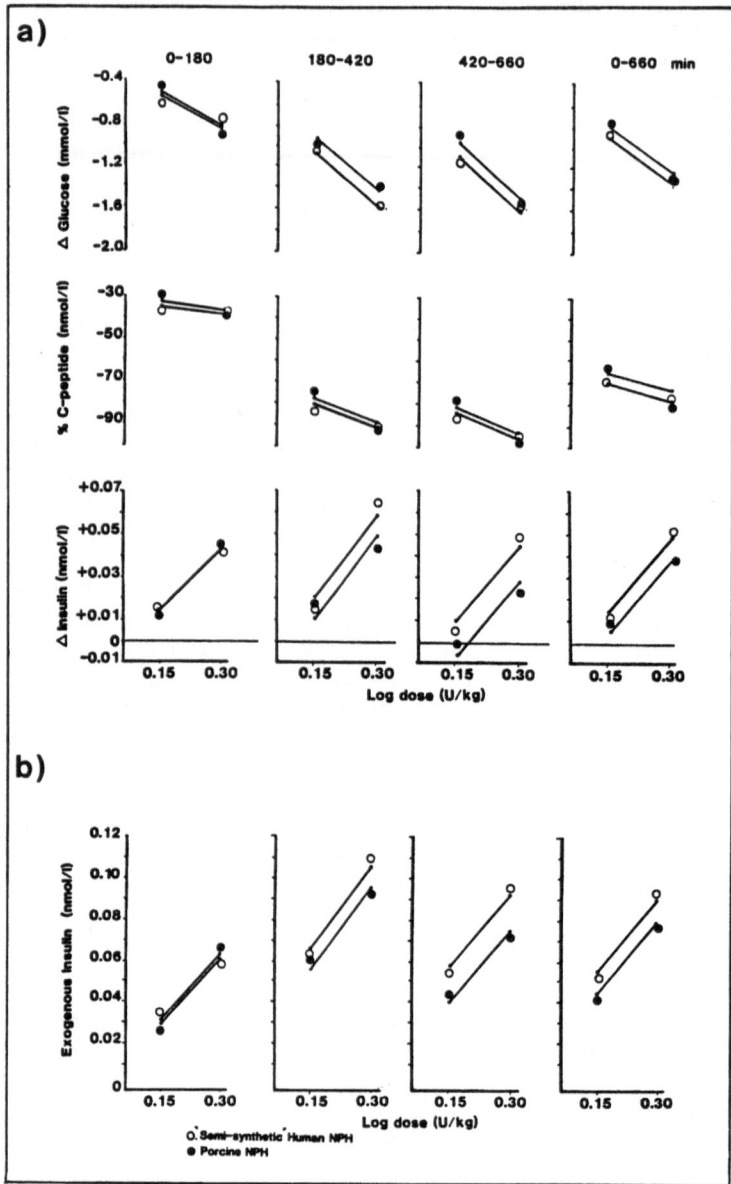

Figures 4.46a, b Dose–response analysis of effect of 'semi-synthetic' human and porcine NPH insulins on plasma glucose, C-peptide and insulin (IRI) concentrations in six subjects. Insulins (0.15 and 0.30 U/kg) given subcutaneously (sc) at time 0. Results shown as means of (**a**) Δ glucose, percentage C-peptide, Δ insulin and (**b**) estimated exogenous insulin ('control day method') values for the periods 0–180, 180–420, 420–660 and 0–660 min.

Table 4.26 Dose–response analysis and 'potency' estimates (with 95% confidence limits) of 'biosynthetic' relative to 'semi-synthetic' human insulin, determined using the parallel line model (Finney, 1978) .

Response variable	Periods (area means)			
	0–3 h	3–7 h	7–11 h	0–11 h
Glucose	64 (0–188)	80 (46–106)	62 (13–97)*	70 (29–100)*
Δ Glucose	—	73 (32–104)	53 (7–88)*	61 (15–94)*
C-peptide	—	—	—	—
Δ C-peptide	—	—	—	—
% C-peptide	—	—	—	—
IRI	—	88 (31–129)	82 (30–120)	90 (41–127)
Δ IRI	128 (71–201)	96 (56–129)	92 (57–121)	100 (70–125)
Exog IRI (1)	118 (1–288)	83 (36–118)	75 (32–107)	85 (45–115)

Exog IRI (1) Exogenous insulin estimated by the 'control day method'
* The relative potencies are significantly different at the 5% level when the 95% interval does not contain the 100% value
— No estimates are given when the dose-response relationship was not significant at the 5% level

Discussion

NPH (isophane) insulin is well established as an 'intermediate-acting' insulin used predominantly twice a day admixed with soluble insulin (Oakley et al, 1966), with only a relatively small number of patients treated with once-daily injection.

The hypoglycaemic action of subcutaneous NPH preparations has been studied in animals, normal subjects and insulin-requiring diabetics. The timing of action has been quoted as starting some 2 h after injection, reaching peak activity between 8 and 18h and with a total duration of effect of up to 30h (Izzo et al, 1953; Joslin et al, 1959; Ellenberg and Rifkin, 1962; Traisman and Newcomb, 1965; Oakley et al, 1968; Nelson and Vaughane, 1969; Malins, 1970; Bressler and Galloway, 1971; Dörzbach and Müller, 1971; Marble, 1971).

The majority of clinical–pharmacological studies have used ^{125}I-labelled NPH insulin preparations utilising external counting detectors to determine the absorption pattern of NPH insulin (Kølendorf et al, 1978; Koivisto and Felig, 1980; Kølendorf and Bojsen, 1982; Lauritzen et al, 1982).

The introduction of radioimmunological methods for the assay of insulin (Hales and Randall, 1963; Heding, 1972) has made it possible to study its appearance in plasma after parenteral administration.

Despite the fact that the 'intermediate-acting' insulins account for over 80% of insulin usage, there are still only comparatively few clinical-pharmacological studies with this group of insulin preparations (Galloway et al, 1981a). It is only in the last decade that data on plasma insulin levels following the subcutaneous administration of NPH (isophane) insulin preparations has become available (Ginsberg et al, 1973; Kølendorf et al, 1978;

Galloway et al, 1981a, b; Malone and Root, 1981; Lauritzen et al, 1982). The use of plasma insulin measurements to characterise the subcutaneous absorption of NPH insulin assumes that no protamine–zinc–insulin complexes are absorbed into the circulation. Using gel filtration, Bauman and Yalow have, however, demonstrated that some complexed insulin is in fact absorbed into the circulation (Bauman and Yalow, 1980).

The recent availability of human ('semi-synthetic' and 'biosynthetic') NPH insulin preparations has allowed comparisons to be made with the existing and established highly purified porcine NPH preparations both in normal man (Galloway et al, 1981b; 1982a; Bottermann et al, 1982; Weinges et al, 1982; Owens et al, 1984b) and diabetic patients (Clark et al, 1982; Galloway and Root, 1982; Galloway et al, 1982c, 1983; Mirouze et al, 1982b; Hildebrandt et al, 1984b; Richard et al, 1984).

Galloway and co-workers (1981b) did not demonstrate a difference in the hypoglycaemic response between purified porcine and 'biosynthetic' human insulin in normal subjects at 0.15 U/kg body weight following subcutaneous injection into the deltoid region. There was, however, a significantly higher serum insulin level with human insulin at 4 h after injection (Galloway et al, 1982a). Analysis of the observed glucose levels in this study of subcutaneous 'semi-synthetic' human NPH and porcine insulin at 0.15 and 0.30 U/kg agrees with this finding. However, comparing the Δ values indicates a significantly greater hypoglycaemic response with human insulin between 6 and 8 h after injection associated with a higher incremental insulin level at 8 h ($p < 0.05$). Whereas human NPH insulin can achieve higher plasma insulin levels than its porcine counterpart (Bottermann et al, 1982; Galloway et al, 1982a; Owens et al, 1984b), there is less agreement on the relative hypoglycaemic 'potency' of the two insulins. The relative 'bioavailability' estimations derived from the dose–response analysis indicates a trend towards higher insulin levels with human insulin, reaching significance for the 7 to 11 h period and associated with a greater hypoglycaemic response. There was no apparent difference between the insulins when comparing the individual pairs of treatments.

Interestingly, comparing the 'semi-synthetic' and 'biosynthetic' human NPH insulins at the 0.15 U/kg dose level revealed a greater hypoglycaemic response with the former. Whilst a similar glucose nadir was achieved with both insulins at 3 h after administration, a quicker recovery towards normoglycaemia was seen with 'biosynthetic' human NPH insulin. An extended period of observation would be necessary to see if this trend continued. The dose–response analysis confirms the greater hypoglycaemic 'potency' of 'semi-synthetic' human insulin during the 7 to 11 h and 0 to 11 h periods. It is not possible to offer an explanation for the discrepancy between the relative 'potency' and 'bioavailability' of the 'semi-synthetic' and 'biosynthetic' human insulin preparations based on the available data. The small variation in the protamine content is unlikely to explain the differences, although the proportion of protamine insulin complexes absorbed may, however, have been different for the two insulins. This was not measured in this study.

Recent clinical findings also suggest a trend towards a relatively shorter duration of hypoglycaemia with 'biosynthetic' human NPH insulin relative to porcine or bovine NPH insulin preparations (Clark et al, 1982; Galloway et al, 1982c, 1983; Galloway and Root, 1982).

The findings of this study underline the possible clinical relevance of insulin species and pharmaceutical formulation on the pharmacokinetic profile and hypoglycaemic action of the NPH insulin preparations examined. According to the experimental design adopted involving normal fasting subjects, the onset of the hypoglycaemia with NPH insulins is evident within the first hour, with the maximum effect occuring between 3 and 4 h and a duration of action in excess of 11 h. Critical clinical evaluation is, however, necessary to assess the relevance, if any, of the small differences observed between porcine and 'semi-synthetic' human NPH insulins and between 'semi-synthetic' and 'biosynthetic' human NPH insulin preparations in the management of the insulin-requiring diabetic patient.

4.2.1.3 Comparative study of Lente (Monotard) and NPH insulins ('semi-synthetic' human insulin: U-100, U-40; porcine insulin: U-40)

Introduction

Clinical use has resulted in Lente and NPH insulin preparations being regarded as similar 'intermediate-acting' insulins (Joslin et al, 1959; Oakley et al, 1968; Bressler and Galloway, 1978; Nabarro et al, 1979; Galloway et al, 1981a). Following the subcutaneous administration of Lente and NPH insulin the onset of hypoglycaemic action occurs between 0.5 and 4 h after injection, with a suggestion that NPH may have the earlier effect (Izzo et al, 1953; Ellenberg and Rifkin, 1962; Traisman and Newcomb, 1965). There appears to be little difference, however, in the timing of maximal effect (Bressler and Galloway, 1978) or total duration of activity (Schlichtkrull et al, 1975).

The subcutaneous absorption of these insulins, described as the rate of disappearance of radioactivity from the injection site when using ^{125}I-insulin preparations, has occasionally been shown to be different, with NPH having a relatively faster absorption (Kølendorf et al, 1978, 1982, 1983a, b; Pedersen, 1978; Kølendorf and Bojsen, 1982) than Lente insulin (Binder, 1969; Faber et al, 1975). Others using the same technique have not been able to demonstrate a difference in the resorption of NPH (porcine, bovine, human) and Lente (porcine, human) insulins when administered at the same dose level (Schlichtkrull, 1977; Lauritzen et al, 1979; Sestoft et al, 1982; Hildebrandt et al, 1983c, 1984c). As the rate of absorption is dose-dependent, decreasing with increasing doses (Lauritzen et al, 1982; Hildebrandt et al, 1984a), this factor could account for the reported differences between Lente and NPH insulins in the early studies.

Little or no difference has been demonstrated, however, between the plasma insulin profiles following the administration of Lente and NPH insulins in diabetic patients (Faber et al, 1975; Schlichtkrull, 1977; Griffin et al, 1980; Werther et al, 1980; Galloway et al, 1981a, b, 1982a; Fukumoto et al, 1982).

The above studies refer to 'intermediate-acting' insulins at a concentration of 40 IU/ml and prepared from porcine and/or bovine insulin.

The purpose of this study was to compare the recently available 'semi-synthetic' human Lente (Monotard HM) and NPH (Protaphane HM) insulin preparations at a 'potency' of 100 IU/ml in normal subjects. As a supplement, analysis of the results from earlier studies involving porcine and human Lente (Monotard HM) and NPH (Protaphane HM) insulins at the lower strength of 40 IU/ml are included.

Lente and NPH insulin: U–100 (100 IU/ml) 'semi-synthetic' human insulin preparations

The main aim of this study was to compare the plasma glucose, C-peptide and insulin levels after subcutaneous administration of Lente (Monotard HM) and NPH (Protaphane HM) human insulin preparations (100 IU/ml) at a dose level of 0.30 U/kg body weight in normal fasting subjects. Diluting medium was used in the control studies.

Subjects, materials and methods

Six healthy normal male subjects aged 23–30 years, weighing between 59 and 75 kg, all within 20% of their ideal body weight (Metropolitan Life Insurance Co. 1960) were entered into the study. The comparative insulin preparations were given in a dose range of 18–22 units (~0.30 U/kg body weight) with an equivalent volume of Lente diluting medium as the control preparation. The studies were carried out at 1–3-week intervals, with the order of the preparations randomised. Details of the test preparations are included in Table 4.27.

Table 4.27

	Lente (Monotard HM)	NPH (Protaphane HM)	Diluting medium
Nitrogen (mg/ml)	0.638	0.631	—
Potency[a] (IU/ml)	97.6[a]	102.4[b]	—

[a] Theoretical potency: 185 IU/mgN
[b] Potency determinations were performed by a quantitative HPLC gel permeation chromatography method with monocomponent porcine insulin as standard

Each study commenced at 0800 h after a 10 h overnight fast, the volunteers having a standard diet containing a high-carbohydrate content on the previous day. Venous blood samples were collected $\frac{1}{2}$-hourly during the 1 h basal (pre-insulin) period, and for the first 3 h after subcutaneous injection of the test preparations. Thereafter, samples were taken hourly to 8 h and then 2-hourly up to the end of the 24 h study. The insulins were administered using a Becton-Dickinson LO-Dose 0.5 ml syringe.

Blood was taken into fluoride for glucose determination (glucose oxidase:

Yellow Springs glucose analyser, Ohio, USA) and heparin for the measurement of immunoreactive insulin (modification of Heding, 1972) and C-peptide (modification of Heding, 1975) concentrations.

Statistical methods

The results are represented as means ± SE unless stated otherwise. The individual pairs of data were compared using the Student's t-test. This method was preferred to analysis of variance as it does not require assumptions about variance homogeneity. The analyses were carried out on the raw data and Δ values. The Δ values were used in an attempt to take into account changes observed during the prolonged fasting and the inter- and intra-individual differences observed during the basal period, and were calculated by subtracting firstly the control from the insulin study days and then the mean basal value from all subsequent levels.

An approximate estimate of the exogenous plasma insulin (IRI_{EXOG}) was made based on the 'control day method' (cf. 4.2.1.1).

Results

The mean absolute and Δ plasma glucose, C-peptide and insulin values are shown in Figures 4.47a and 4.47b, respectively.

During the control day the plasma glucose fell from a level of 5.1 ± 0.1 mmol/l at the beginning to 3.9 ± 0.3 mmol/l at the end of the 25 h study period. This was accompanied by a reduction in C-peptide and insulin concentrations from 0.41 ± 0.04 to 0.19 ± 0.02 nmol/l and 0.07 ± 0.02 to 0.022 ± 0.010 nmol/l, respectively.

Approximately 1 h after administration of the NPH insulin the plasma glucose began to fall, becoming significantly lower than controls from 2.5 h onwards ($p<0.05$–0.001). The maximal hypoglycaemic effect was achieved at 5 h post-injection when the glucose level was reduced by about 1.7 mmol/l. The glucose concentration then gradually recovered to within 1 mmol/l of the controls at 24 h. In comparison, the glucose lowering action of Lente insulin, although quantitatively similar, was delayed by approximately 1 h during the first 5 h after injection. This early difference did not reach statistical significance (Figure 4.47). Thereafter, there was no difference between the two preparations.

Following NPH insulin the C-peptide level fell from a pre-injection value of 0.34 ± 0.05 nmol/l to 0.01 nmol/l between 6 and 12 h. Although there was some increase in plasma C-peptide level after 14 h, the level was still only 0.07 ± 0.02 nmol/l at 24 h. In comparison after the injection of Lente insulin, the plasma C-peptide concentration fell from 0.42 ± 0.08 nmol/l to a nadir of 0.02 ± 0.01 nmol/l reached much later at 18 h.

The levels were significantly lower than controls from 2 h after administration ($p<0.05$–0.001) with both NPH and Lente insulin. An earlier suppression of C-peptide levels was seen with NPH compared to Lente insulin, the difference reaching statistical significance at 2 h ($p<0.05$). From 6 h

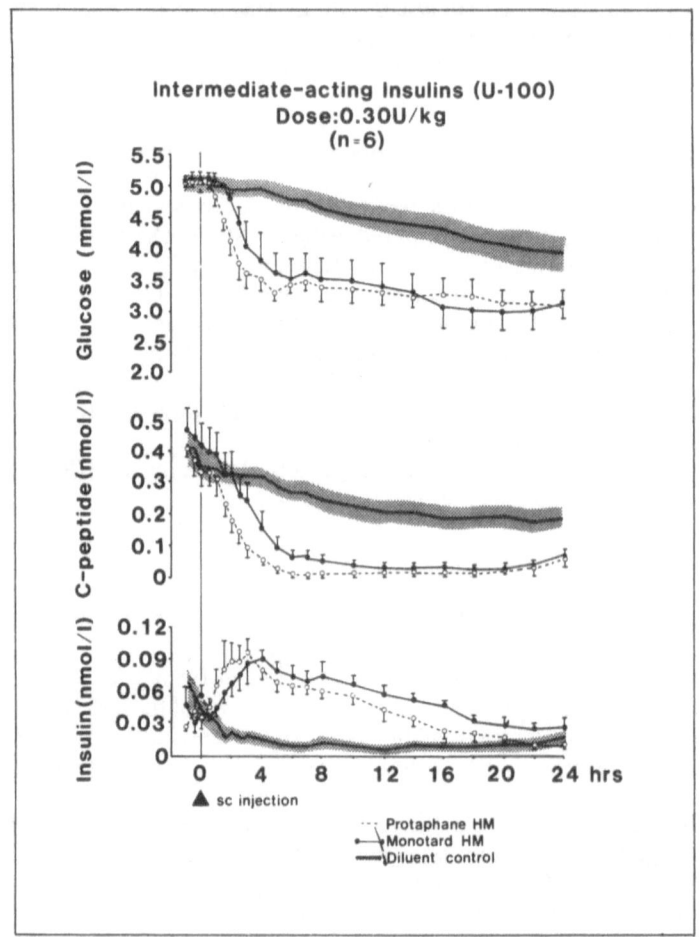

Figure 4.47a Comparison of the effect of human NPH (Protaphane HM) and lente (Monotard HM) insulins on plasma glucose, C-peptide and insulin (IRI) concentrations (means ± SE) in six subjects. Insulins (0.30 U/kg) or diluent (control) given subcutaneously (sc) at time 0

onwards, however, the trend was reversed although the difference between the insulins was not significant.

In response to the administration of NPH insulin the plasma insulin level increased from a fasting pre-insulin level of 0.038 ± 0.012 nmol/l to a peak of 0.1 ± 0.01 nmol/l at 3 h. Following Lente insulin there was a slower increase in the plasma insulin levels from 0.057 ± 0.012 nmol/l to a lower and slightly later peak of 0.09 ± 0.01 nmol/l at 4 h (Figure 4.47a). The incremental insulin values were significantly higher ($p < 0.05$) with NPH insulin at 1 and 2 h after injection. In contrast, from 8 h onwards the mean incremental insulin level was lower with NPH insulin (Figure 4.47b).

Similar peak plasma exogenous insulin concentrations of 0.089 ± 0.022 and

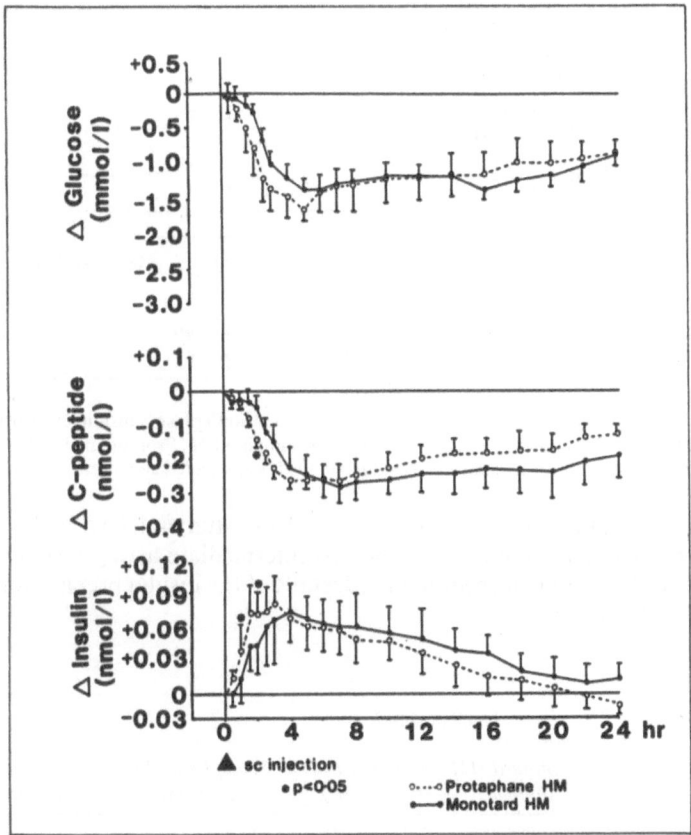

Figure 4.47b Comparison of the effect of human NPH (Protaphane HM) and lente (Monotard HM) insulins on plasma glucose, C-peptide and insulin (IRI) concentrations (means ± SE) in six subjects. Insulins (0.30 U/kg) or diluent (control) given subcutaneously (sc) at time 0. Results shown as means of Δ values

0.088 ± 0.022 nmol/l were achieved at 3 and 4 h with NPH and Lente insulin, respectively (Figure 4.48). The level was also significantly higher with NPH insulin 1 h after injection ($p<0.05$). From about 4 h onwards the level was higher with Lente insulin and, whereas there was no detectable exogenous insulin at 22 h with NPH insulin, the level was still 0.03 ± 0.01 nmol/l ($\sim$ 30% of peak level) following Lente insulin.

Supplement:
Lente and NPH insulin: U–40 (40 IU / ml) porcine and 'semi-synthetic' human insulin preparations

The plasma glucose, C-peptide and insulin levels following the subcutaneous administration of human and porcine Lente and NPH insulins at the lower concentration of 40 IU/ml have been compared. The data for the Lente and

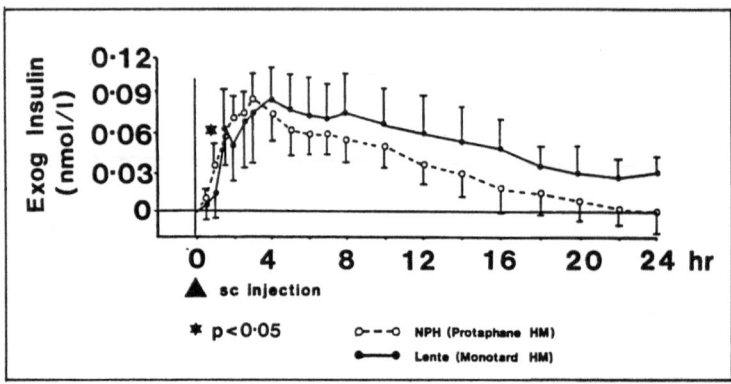

Figure 4.48 Comparison of the estimated ('control day method') plasma insulin concentrations (means ± SE) following subcutaneous (sc) injection of human NPH (Protaphane HM) and lente (Monotard HM) insulins in six subjects. Insulins (0.30 U/kg) injected subcutaneously at time 0

NPH human and porcine insulins originate from studies 4.2.1.1 and 4.2.1.2, respectively. Comparisons between the two 'intermediate-acting' insulins were made for the 0.30 U/kg dose level only. Details of the insulin preparations are included in Table 4.28.

Table 4.28

	Lente insulins[a]		NPH insulins[b]	
	Monotard HM (human)	Monotard MC (porcine)	Protaphane HM (human)	Protaphane MC (porcine)
Nitrogen (mg/ml)	0.217	0.210	0.247	0.253
Potency[a] (IU/ml)	40.1	38.9	40.9	39.6

[a] Theoretical potency 185 IU/mgN
[b] Determined by quantitative HPLC gel permeation chromatography method with monocomponent porcine insulin as standard

Statistical methods

The results are represented as means ± SE unless stated otherwise. The individual pairs of data were compared using the unpaired Student's t-test. The analysis was carried out on the Δ values, derived by subtracting the mean basal value from all subsequent levels for each parameter on each study day. An estimate of the plasma exogenous insulin level was made according to the 'control day method' as described under study 4.2.1.1.

Results

The mean ± SE Δ plasma glucose, C-peptide and insulin levels for the two comparative formulations (Lente, NPH) of human and porcine insulin are shown in Figures 4.49a and 4.49b, respectively.

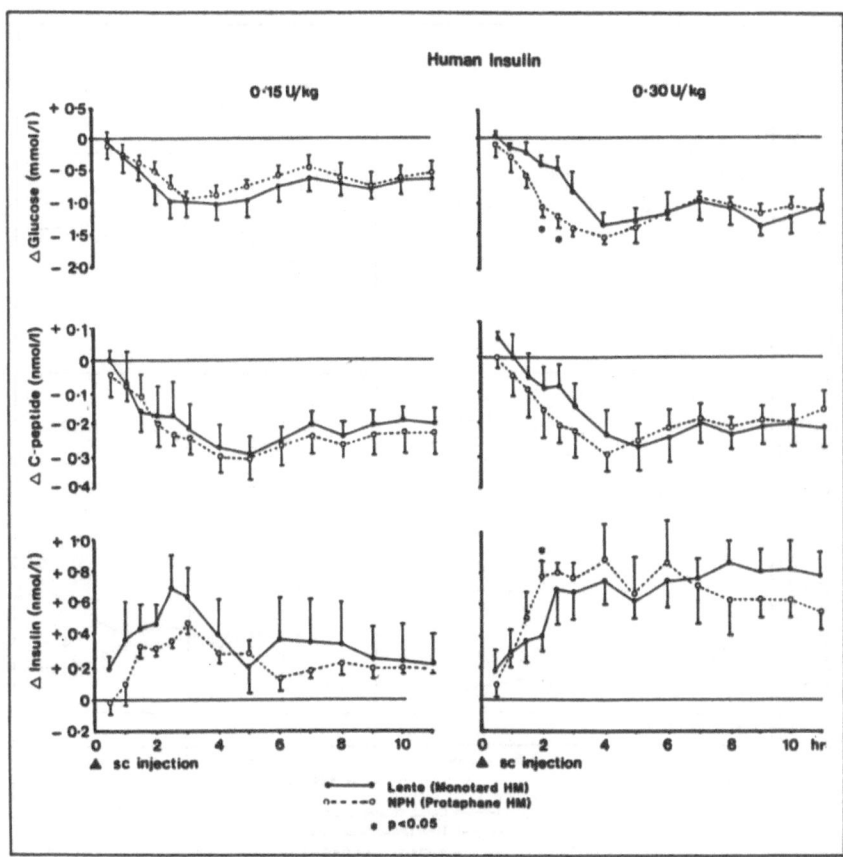

Figure 4.49a Comparison of the effect of human lente (Monotard HM) and NPH (Protaphane HM) insulins on plasma glucose, C-peptide and insulin (IRI) concentrations in six subjects. Insulins (0.15, 0.30 U/kg) given subcutaneously (sc) at time 0. Results shown as means of Δ values

At the low dose level of 0.15 U/kg there was no true difference in the Δ glucose, C-peptide and insulin levels throughout the 11 h study period comparing Lente and NPH insulin of both species. In contrast, at the 0.30 U/kg dose level there was an earlier fall in plasma glucose with human NPH compared to human Lente insulin. The hypoglycaemic response to the NPH insulin was significantly greater ($p<0.05$) at 2 h and 2.5 h after injection. The early difference in the hypoglycaemic response between the 'intermediate-acting' insulins reflected the higher incremental insulin levels with NPH insulin during the first hour after injection. The plasma insulin level continued to increase slowly with the Lente insulin to reach a plateau at 10 h in contrast to NPH insulin where the levels started to fall after 6 h. The C-peptide responses mirrored the plasma glucose profiles, although the difference between the two human insulin preparations did not reach significance.

Similar differences were observed between the NPH and Lente formulations

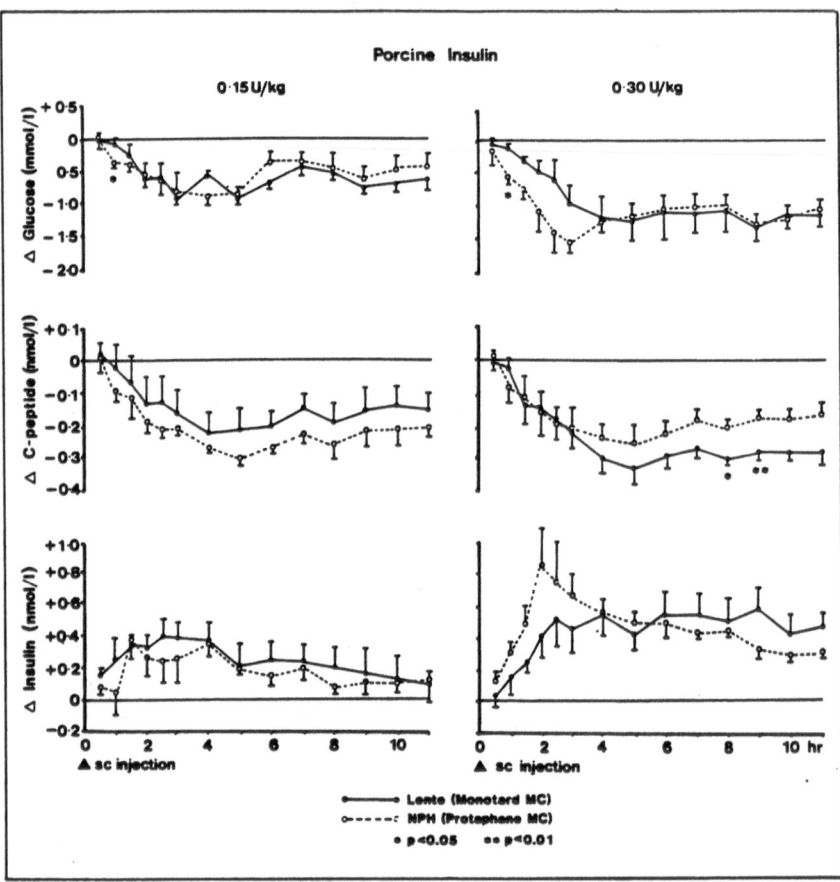

Figure 4.49b Comparison of the effect of porcine Lente (Monotard MC) and NPH (Protaphane MC) insulins on plasma glucose, C-peptide and insulin (IRI) concentrations in six subjects. Insulins (0.15, 0.30 U/kg) given subcutaneously (sc) at time 0. Results shown as means of Δ values

of porcine insulin. At the 0.30 U/kg dose level a more marked hypoglycaemic response was observed with NPH insulin during the first 3 h, the difference reaching significance at 1 h ($p < 0.05$). Thereafter from 4 h onwards the hypoglycaemic effect was identical for the two insulins. An early peak incremental insulin level was observed at 2 h with NPH insulin in contrast to the slowly increasing concentrations on Lente insulin, reaching a maximum level at 9 h. The difference between the insulin profiles, however, did not reach statistical significance. Despite an equivalent hypoglycaemic effect towards the end of the study the C-peptide level was more suppressed with Lente insulin at 8 to 9 h ($p < 0.05 - 0.01$) (Figure 4.49b).

The estimated exogenous plasma insulin levels also indicated that at the high dose level of 0.30 U/kg, NPH insulin of both species tended to result in earlier and higher peak insulin levels compared to the Lente insulins (Figure 4.50).

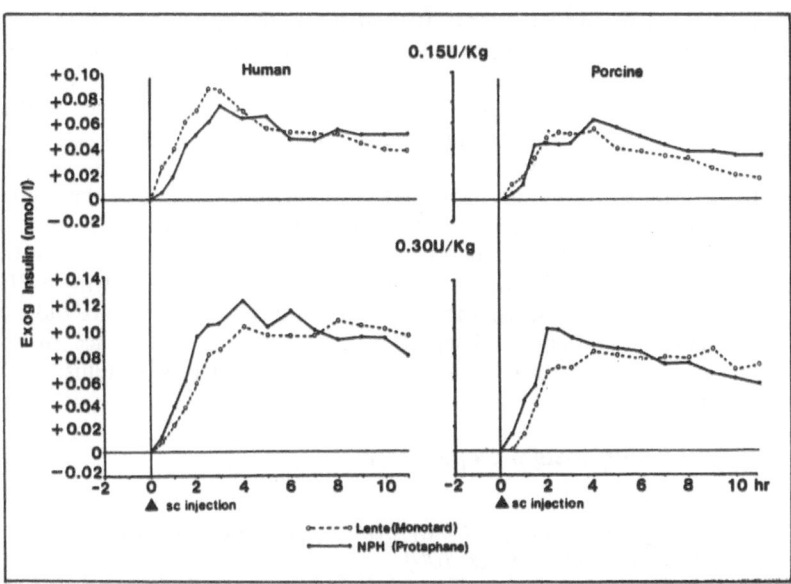

Figure 4.50 Comparison of the estimated ('control day method') plasma exogenous insulin concentrations (means) following the subcutaneous (sc) injection of human and porcine lente (Monotard HM, Monotard MC) and NPH (Protaphane HM, Protaphane MC) insulins (0.15, 0.30 U/kg) in six subjects. Insulins or diluent (control) injected subcutaneously (sc) at time 0

The trend was reversed during the second half of the study, with the levels falling with NPH insulin whilst remaining relatively stable on Lente insulin up to the end of the 11 h post-injection period. At no time was the difference statistically significant between the two formulations of human or porcine insulin.

Discussion

The results of the studies demonstrate differences between NPH and Lente 'semi-synthetic' human (U–40 and U–100) and porcine insulin (U–40) preparations following subcutaneous administration to normal man.

In the 'between' subject analysis involving the 40 IU/ml human insulin preparations, there was a more marked hypoglycaemic response to NPH insulin within the first 4 h after injection, which reflected the higher insulin levels achieved during this period on NPH insulin. A similar but less impressive difference was seen between the two formulations of porcine insulin. When employing radiolabelled Lente and NPH insulins some studies demonstrated a shorter disappearance time to 50% of the initial activity with NPH relative to Lente insulin (Binder, 1969; Faber et al, 1975; Kølendorf and Bojsen, 1982) whilst others demonstrate similar absorption rates for the two 'intermediate-acting' insulins (Lauritzen et al, 1979; Hildebrandt et al, 1984a, c). At the high dose level of 0.30 U/kg the plasma insulin profiles show that NPH insulin achieves peak insulin levels within 4 h of injection, followed by a gradual fall from about 6h onwards. In contrast, with Lente insulin there was a slower appearance rate in plasma reaching a plateau between 4 and 10h. The early difference in the insulin levels was reflected in the greater hypoglycaemic response with NPH insulin during the first 4h. Thereafter, despite higher insulin levels with Lente insulin, there was no difference in the hypoglycaemic effect up to 11h after injection.

In the 'within' subject study using NPH and Lente insulins at the higher concentration of 100 IU/ml similar trends were observed. NPH insulin achieved significantly higher incremental insulin levels at 1 and 2h after injection. Consequently the onset of hypoglycaemia was earlier with NPH, with lower glucose levels during the first 5h although the difference did not reach statistical significance. Thereafter, there was no difference in the hypoglycaemic effect of the comparative 'intermediate-acting' insulins.

4.2.2 'Long-acting' insulin preparations

4.2.2.1 A study of human ('semi-synthetic') porcine and bovine Ultralente insulins (U-100)

There is compelling evidence to suggest that there is a relationship between diabetic complications and the degree of metabolic derangement that exists in diabetes mellitus (Cahill et al, 1976; Tchobroutsky, 1978; Pirat, 1977; Brownlee and Cahill, 1979; Skyler, 1979). Several studies have demonstrated that improvement in glycaemic control can result in morphological and functional changes (Camerini-Davalos et al, 1983; Holman et al, 1983; Lauritzen et al, 1983b; Raskin et al, 1983; Siperstein, 1983) emphasising the need to strive for the best possible metabolic control in the insulin-requiring diabetic patient.

Attempts to achieve normoglycaemia have involved a multiplicity of insulin preparations, regimens, and delivery systems to provide both basal and meal-related insulin requirements (Tattersall, 1979; Tattersall and Gale, 1981; Skyler et al, 1982; Watkins, 1982). The most common subcutaneous insulin regimen currently used involves twice daily mixtures of 'short-' and 'intermediate-acting' insulin preparations (Oakley et al, 1966; Galloway and Bressler, 1978; Skyler et al, 1981, 1982). One limitation of this treatment is nocturnal hypoglycaemia necessitating delaying the evening 'intermediate-acting' insulin (Tattersall and Gale, 1981; Schiffrin and Belmonte, 1982; Francis et al, 1983) therefore giving a pre-evening meal injection of 'short-acting' insulin with the 'intermediate-acting' insulin at bedtime. Recent attempts to fulfil the need to provide both basal and meal-related insulin requirements have resulted in the introduction of continuous subcutaneous insulin infusion (CSII) using a portable pump with adjustable rates (Pickup et al, 1978, 1979; Tamborlane et al, 1979; Champion et al, 1980). Comparable glycaemic control can, however, be achieved with intensively applied 'conventional' treatment involving 'long-acting' Ultralente insulin plus multiple pre-prandial injections of soluble insulin (Rizza et al, 1980; Reeves et al, 1982). The use of Ultralente-based insulin regimens offers an alternative to insulin delivered by pumps (Phillips et al, 1979; Saibene et al, 1981; Skyler et al, 1981; Ward et al, 1981; Gwinup and Elias, 1982; Hosker and Turner, 1982; Reeves et al, 1982; Turner et al, 1982, 1983).

Limited data are available on the absorption characteristics of bovine Ultralente, and what is available is restricted to studies of the disappearance of the ^{125}I isotope from the site of injection (Binder, 1969; Hildebrandt et al, 1984b), from which estimates of the plasma insulin concentrations have been derived (Schlichtkrull, 1977).

Concern has recently been expressed about the immunogenicity of highly purified bovine Ultralente insulin (Reeves and Kelly, 1982) which may explain the relatively high dose requirements (Turner et al, 1982). Others have failed to confirm an immunological basis for these high requirements, proposing instead that reduced bioavailability could be the main reason (Home et al, 1983).

The purpose of this study was to compare the plasma glucose, C-peptide and insulin levels in response to equivalent pharmaceutical formulations of human, bovine and porcine Ultralente insulin administered subcutaneously to normal subjects.

Subjects, materials and methods

Six healthy normal male volunteers aged 21–28 years with no family history of diabetes mellitus and within 20% of their ideal body weight (Metropolitan Life Insurance Co., 1960) were entered into the study. Details of the human, bovine and porcine Ultralente (U–100; 100 IU/ml) insulins are included in Table 4.29. The insulin dose was approximately 0.30 U/kg body weight (18–24 U), with an equivalent volume of diluting medium used in the control studies.

Table 4.29

| | Ultralente U–100 | | |
	Human	*Bovine*	*Porcine*
Nitrogen (mg/ml)	0.543	0.529	0.518
Potency (IU/ml)*	100.46	97.87	95.83
Crystal size (μ)	28.0	28.5	28.0
Methyl parahydroxy- benzoate (mg)	0.96	0.97	0.98
Zinc (mg)			
Total	0.152	0.151	0.144
In solution	0.059	0.060	0.056
Sodium chloride (mg)	7	7	7
Sodium acetate (mg)	1.4	1.4	1.4
pH	7.34	7.44	7.36

* Theoretical potency: 185 IU/mgN

Each subject was involved on four separate study days 1 to 3 weeks apart. For 2 days prior to each study the subjects were advised to consume a high-carbohydrate intake. Each study consisted of a 1h basal and a 32h post-injection observation period. The comparative preparations were administered subcutaneously into the anterior abdominal wall. Venous blood samples were taken ½-hourly during the basal period and the first 3h after injection, followed by hourly samples up to 8h and then 2-hourly up to 32h.

Blood samples were aliquoted into fluoride for glucose estimation (glucose oxidase: Yellow Springs glucose analyser, Ohio, USA), heparin for immunoreactive insulin (IRI) (Heding, 1972) and C-peptide (Heding, 1975) determinations.

Statistical methods

The results are expressed as means ± SE except where otherwise stated. Individual pairs of treatments were compared using the paired Student's *t*-test.

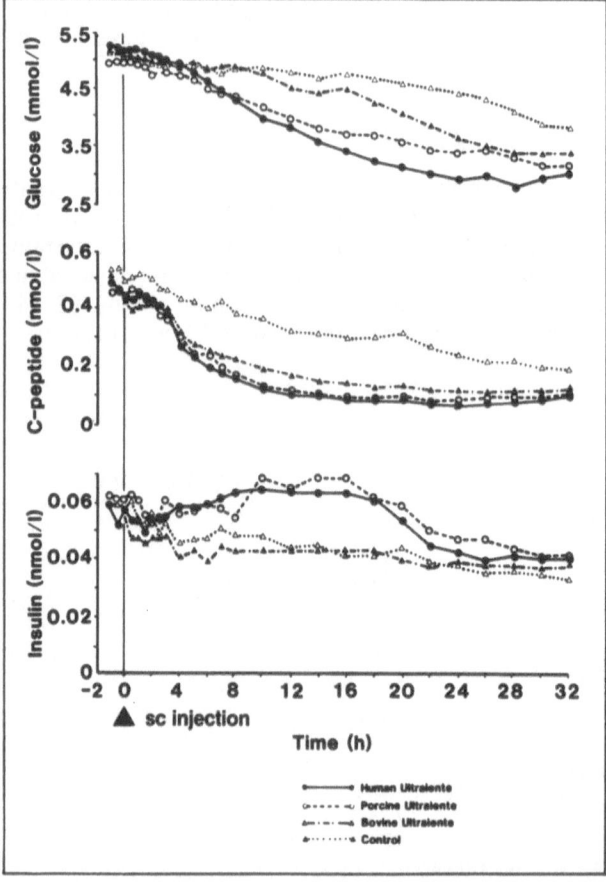

Figure 4.51a Effect of human, porcine and bovine Ultralente insulins on plasma glucose, C-peptide and insulin (IRI) concentrations (means) in six subjects. Insulin (0.30 U/kg) or diluent (control) given subcutaneously (sc) at time 0

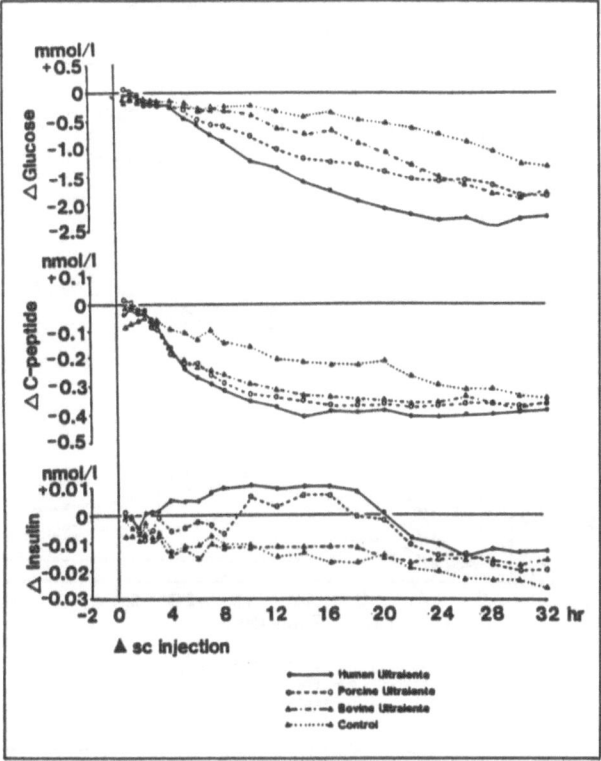

Figure 4.51b Effect of human, porcine and bovine Ultralente insulins on plasma glucose, C-peptide and insulin (IRI) concentrations in six subjects. Insulin (0.30 U/kg) or diluent (control) given subcutaneously (sc) at time 0. Results shown as means of Δ values

This method was preferred to analysis of variance as it does not require assumptions about variance homogeneity. The analysis was conducted on the absolute and Δ glucose, C-peptide and 'exogenous' insulin values (see below). The Δ glucose and C-peptide levels were determined by subtracting the corresponding control day levels and then the mean basal level from all subsequent post-injection levels.

An approximate estimate of the exogenous plasma insulin levels was calculated based on the 'control day method' referred to in study 4.2.1.1. As the ratio does not take into consideration the different clearance rates of insulin and C-peptide, only a crude approximation can be derived which will underestimate the exogenous insulin level during the early phase of hypoglycaemia.

Results

The mean absolute and Δ plasma glucose, C-peptide and insulin levels following the subcutaneous injection of human, bovine and porcine Ultralente

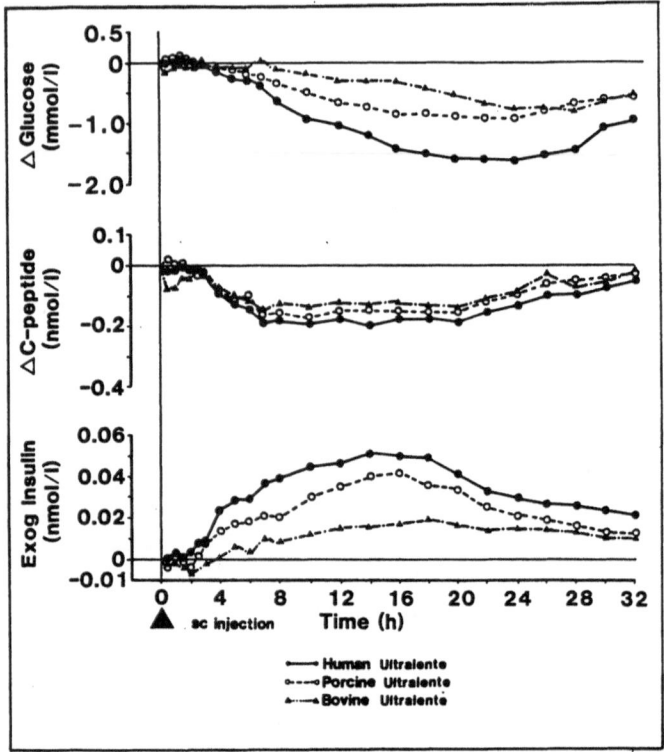

Figure 4.52 Effect of human, porcine and bovine Ultralente insulins on plasma glucose, C-peptide and estimated ('control day method') exogenous insulin concentrations (means) in six subjects. Insulin (0.30 U/kg) given subcutaneously (sc) at time 0. Results for glucose and C-peptide shown as means of Δ values

insulin in normal subjects are shown in Figures 4.51a, b and 4.52.

During prolonged fasting (control) the plasma glucose levels gradually fell from 5.1 ± 0.2 mmol/l at 0800h to 3.8 ± 0.2 mmol/l 32h later. Similarly, the plasma C-peptide and insulin levels fell from 0.54 ± 0.02 nmol/l and 0.06 ± 0.005 nmol/l at the beginning to 0.20 ± 0.02 and 0.03 ± 0.003 nmol/l respectively at the end of the 32h study period (Figure 4.51a). After the administration of bovine Ultralente insulin there was little, if any, change in the plasma glucose level up to 8h, after which there was a gradual fall. The maximum hypoglycaemic effect was achieved at 28h with a reduction of 0.8 ± 0.2 mmol/l. In contrast to bovine insulin, an earlier onset of hypoglycaemia was observed with both human and porcine Ultralente commencing at about 3 to 4h after administration and achieving a maximum reduction from basal levels of 1.6 ± 0.3 mmol/l and 0.95 ± 0.4 mmol/l at 20 and 24h, respectively. Subsequently, the glucose levels recovered slowly to within 0.49 ± 0.1 mmol/l and 0.55 ± 0.2 mmol/l of the controls by the end of the study period with bovine and porcine insulin, respectively.

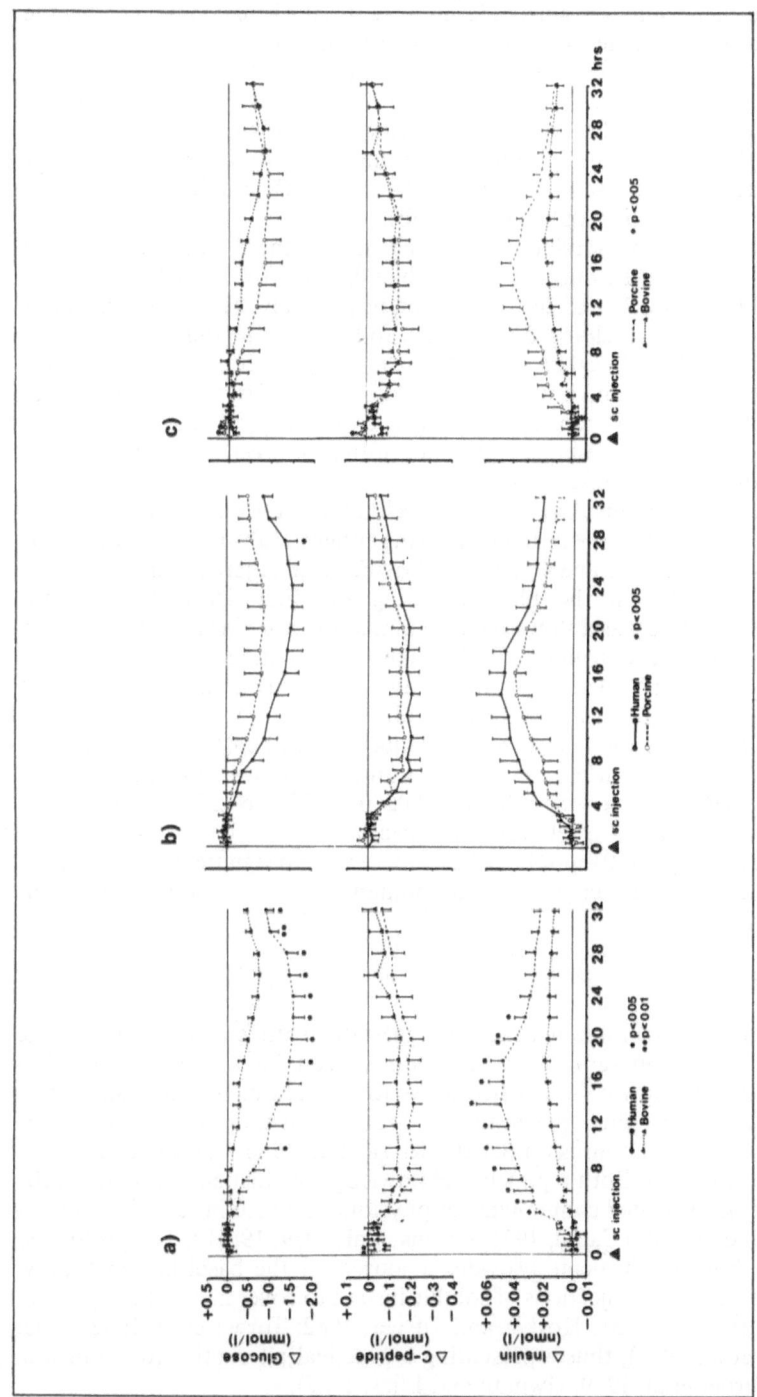

Figure 4.53 Comparison of the effect of (**a**) human and bovine, (**b**) human and porcine, and (**c**) porcine and bovine Ultralente insulins on plasma glucose, C-peptide and estimated ('control day method') exogenous insulin concentrations (means) in six subjects. Insulin (0.30 U/kg) given subcutaneously (sc) at time 0. Results for glucose and C-peptide shown as means (± SE) of Δ values

175

With human insulin the glucose levels were still 0.93 ± 0.2 mmol/l below the control values at 32 h despite a faster recovery rate from nadir values.

The hypoglycaemic response was greater with human compared to bovine insulin at 10, and from 18 to 32 h ($p < 0.05$–0.01; Figure 4.53a). An 'intermediate' effect was observed with porcine insulin which did not differ significantly from bovine insulin throughout the study (Figure 4.53c). The hypoglycaemic response was significantly less with porcine than human insulin at 28 h only ($p < 0.05$) (Figure 4.53b).

Following human, porcine and bovine insulin there was a decrease in plasma C-peptide levels during the first 7 h of 0.2 ± 0.06, 0.16 ± 0.05 and 0.14 ± 0.06 nmol/l i.e. a 43, 28 and 26% reduction, respectively. Thereafter, the levels remained relatively unchanged up to 20 h, followed by a gradual recovery to within 0.12 ± 0.06, 0.08 ± 0.04 and 0.07 ± 0.06 nmol/l of control values at 24 h, with human, porcine and bovine insulin, respectively. However, at 32 h there was no difference in C-peptide levels between the control and insulin study days. The C-peptide responses did not differ between the three insulin preparations (Figures 4.52, 4.53).

Comparison of the insulin responses was limited to the estimated exogenous insulin levels in view of the difficulty in using either the absolute or Δ values, as seen from Figures 4.51a and 4.51b. With bovine insulin there was no detectable exogenous insulin in the plasma during the first 4 h after injection. Subsequently there was a slow rise in insulin levels reaching a peak of 0.025 ± 0.04 nmol/l at 18 h returning to 0.013 ± 0.04 nmol/l at 32 h (Figure 4.52). In comparison, human insulin resulted in an earlier appearance of exogenous insulin in the plasma at about 2 h post-administration, increasing to a peak level of 0.054 ± 0.02 nmol/l at 14 h and falling to 0.022 ± 0.01 nmol/l by the end of the study. The insulin levels were significantly higher with human compared to bovine insulin between 4 and 22 h ($p < 0.05$–0.01; Figure 4.53a). With porcine Ultralente the insulin level reached a peak of 0.04 ± 0.01 nmol/l at 16 h returning to 0.013 ± 0.01 nmol/l at 32 h. There was no significant difference in the insulin levels between porcine and human or porcine and bovine insulin (Figures 4.53b, c).

Discussion

There is now considerable evidence to suggest that with few exceptions (Home et al, 1982c) comparable glycaemic control can be achieved in insulin-dependent diabetics with intensified conventional treatment comprising once-daily Ultralente plus pre-prandial soluble insulin and continuous subcutaneous insulin infusion (CSII) (Rizza et al, 1980; Saibene et al, 1981; Reeves et al, 1982). Both regimens acknowledge the distinction between the basal and meal-related components of physiological insulin secretion in non-diabetic individuals (Cahill, 1971; Owens et al, 1979; 1981b). The prolonged action of bovine Ultralente provides a source for the basal insulin supply, requiring additional injections of soluble insulin to cover meals (Phillips et al, 1979; Ward et al, 1981; Hosker and Turner, 1982; Turner et al, 1982, 1983; Holman et al, 1983), thus representing a practical alternative to the insulin pump (Turner et al, 1979; Gwinup and Elias, 1982).

As the immunogenicity of highly purified bovine Ultralente insulin may present a problem in some patients (Reeves and Kelly, 1982; Turner and Holman, 1982; Walford et al, 1982) the introduction of 'semi-synthetic' human Ultralente insulin offers theoretical advantages. Holman and co-workers (1984) recently demonstrated that the substitution of bovine by human Ultralente in insulin treated non-insulin-dependent diabetics and insulin-dependent diabetics was accompanied by a reduction in insulin binding antibody levels within 6 weeks. Human Ultralente was considered equally effective as bovine Ultralente in controlling basal plasma glucose concentrations (Holman et al, 1984), both in the non-insulin-dependent and insulin-dependent diabetics who require additional 'short-acting' insulin.

The results from this study indicate that with subcutaneous bovine insulin at 0.30 U/kg, little or no exogenous insulin appeared in the plasma during the first 4 h after administration. Thereafter there was a gradual rise to a relatively flat peak of approximately 0.023 nmol/l at 18 h with only a small reduction occurring over the following 14 h. This was in contrast to human Ultralente insulin, after which there was an earlier appearance of insulin in plasma reaching a peak of about 0.054 nmol/l at 14 h followed by a more rapid clearance from plasma. The insulin levels remained significantly higher with human than bovine Ultralente insulin between 4 h and 22 h after administration (Owens et al, 1984c). These results support the findings of Hildebrandt and co-workers (1984b), who demonstrated a faster disappearance of human compared to bovine Ultralente from the site of injection using ^{125}I-labelled insulin.

In agreement with the plasma insulin data, there was no discernible change in plasma glucose for the first 8–10 h after bovine insulin, whereas the onset of hypoglycaemic occurred at 4 to 6 h with human. There was a significantly greater hypoglycaemic response to human than to bovine Ultralente between 10 and 32 h after injection. Porcine Ultralente insulin occupied an intermediate position between human and bovine insulin with respect to 'bioavailability' and hypoglycaemic 'potency'. The transfer of patients from bovine to human Ultralente may require dosage adjustments (Holman et al, 1984) due to the greater antigenicity and/or poorer and delayed 'bioavailability' of the bovine insulin (Reeves and Kelly, 1982; Home et al, 1983; Owens et al, 1984c). Consequently, the use of a high initial loading dose of bovine Ultralente in new insulin-requiring patients (Holman and Turner, 1977; Turner et al, 1983), should not be as necessary with human Ultralente insulin. The subcutaneous absorption of human insulin also appears to be less dose-dependent than bovine insulin (Hildebrandt et al, 1984b).

Human Ultralente-based intensified conventional treatment regimens should be clinically evaluated along with other regimens and techniques of insulin delivery in the quest for normoglycaemia, in the hope of delaying or preventing acute and chronic diabetic complications.

4.3 FACTORS INFLUENCING SUBCUTANEOUS ABSORPTION OF HUMAN INSULIN

General introduction

Whereas subcutaneous insulin replacement therapy became generally available soon after its first clinical use in 1922 (Banting et al, 1922b), little attention has been paid until relatively recently to factors that influence the absorption process (Binder, 1969; Cüppers, 1981; Galloway et al, 1981a; Berger et al, 1982; Binder et al, 1984). Several variables known to influence insulin absorption from subcutaneous tissue are listed in Table 4.30.

Table 4.30   Factors influencing subcutaneous insulin absorption

Insulin
Pharmaceutical formulation
Species
Concentration
Dose
Admixing
Site of injection
'Within' and 'between' subject variation

Methods involving the determination of local clearance of insulin labelled with a γ-emitting isotope (^{125}I-insulin) by counting the residual radioactivity with a crystal detector (Binder, 1969; Schlichtkrull, 1977; Hansen et al, 1979; Kølendorf et al, 1983a) and/or the measurement of plasma insulin levels (Galloway et al, 1981a; Berger et al, 1982) have been employed to study the influence of many factors on the subcutaneous absorption of insulin.

The variation in subcutaneous absorption between different insulin formulations, concentrations, doses, sites of administration, injection techniques, the influence of exercise and ambient temperature are reviewed by Schlichtkrull (1977); Galloway et al, (1981a); Berger et al, (1982) and Binder et al, (1984).

In addition to the earlier studies utilising various formulations of the different species of insulin administered by different routes, a further series of studies was conducted to examine certain of the other factors that may influence the subcutaneous absorption of human insulin. The following studies were conducted to evaluate the influence of injection site, the addition of a protease inhibitor to insulin, insulin concentration and mixing of insulins on absorption as well as assessing the 'within' and 'between' subject variation in both absorption and the hypoglycaemic response to subcutaneously administered 'semi-synthetic' human insulin.

4.3.1 Site of administration and influence of a protease inhibitor, aprotinin (Trasylol)

Introduction

This study was conducted to explore any differences between the absorption of neutral, soluble 'semi-synthetic' human insulin when administered subcutaneously into the anterior abdominal wall and thigh region. Within the same study the protease inhibitor, aprotinin, was used to enhance insulin absorption from the thigh in an attempt to achieve parity with the abdominal region.

Regional differences in the absorption of soluble insulin (porcine and bovine) are well documented, with higher rates of absorption from the abdominal and deltoid areas compared to the femoral and gluteal regions (Binder et al, 1967; Koivisto and Felig, 1980; Galloway et al, 1981a; Berger et al, 1982; Süsstrunk et al, 1982). This may be related to regional differences in blood flow (Kølendorf et al, 1979; Lauritzen et al, 1980; Hildebrandt et al, 1982, 1983a; Kølendorf et al, 1979, 1983a).

Aprotinin, a protease inhibitor (Offord et al, 1979), has been used with some success in a variety of patients with severe insulin resistance when added either directly to the insulin or by separate intravenous administration; this has been attributed to the inhibition of insulin degradation locally (Freidenberg et al, 1980; Gunnarsson et al, 1980; Müller et al, 1980; Pickup et al, 1980b; Misbin et al, 1981) or systemically (Maberley et al, 1982). Other studies in insulindependent diabetics do not show an additive effect of aprotinin (Linde and Gunnarsson, 1983; Lunetta et al, 1984).

Berger et al (1980) demonstrated in normal subjects that when aprotinin was admixed with soluble insulin and injected into the thigh region, higher plasma insulin levels were observed between 15 and 45 min after injection compared to a saline/insulin mixture. The observation that the subcutaneous injection of aprotinin causes local hyperaemia offers another basis for enhanced insulin absorption when admixed with aprotinin (Williams et al, 1983).

Subjects, materials and methods

Six normal healthy male subjects aged 20–29 years, none of whom had a family history of diabetes mellitus, history of atopy, or allergy, were taking any other medication nor had received aprotinin previously were entered into the study.

The insulin used in the study was neutral, soluble 'semi-synthetic' human insulin (nitrogen content 0.218 mg/ml; potency 40.3 IU/ml). The aprotinin employed was Trasylol® (Bayer AG, Leverkusen, West Germany: 20,000 KIU per ml).

The study was commenced at approximately 0800 h (–120 min) after a 10 h overnight fast. Two intravenous cannulae were sited in contralateral antecubital veins, one for the purpose of frequent blood sampling and the other for the infusion of somatostatin (100 μg/h) to suppress endogenous beta-cell secretion (Alberti et al, 1973). The latter was commenced after a 30 min basal period at –90 min, and continued for the remainder of the study. After 90 min human insulin was administered subcutaneously into (i) the anterior abdominal wall, (ii) upper thigh and (iii) upper thigh immediately after admixing with 0.5 ml aprotinin equivalent to 10,000 KIU referred to in the text as 'thigh plus aprotinin'. The order of the comparative groups was according to a randomisation schedule. The dose of insulin was 6 U (~0.075 U/kg body weight) with no volume adjustment for the injections without aprotinin. The preparations were administered using a Becton-Dickinson SFP 1 ml disposable syringe.

Venous blood samples were obtained at –120, 105, 90, 60, 30, 0, 10, 20, 30, 40, 50, 60 and every 30 min thereafter up to 360 min. Aliquots were taken into fluoride for plasma glucose determination (hexokinase), heparin for the measurement of immunoreactive insulin (Heding, 1972) and C-peptide (Heding, 1975) concentrations.

Statistical methods

The results are expressed as means ± SE except where stated otherwise. The individual pairs of treatments were compared using the Student's paired t-test for the Δ values calculated by subtracting the level immediately prior to injection (time 0 min) from all subsequent values on each study day.

Results

Figures 4.54a and 4.54b illustrate the mean absolute and Δ plasma glucose and insulin levels for the three comparative treatment groups. Figures 4.55a–c show the paired comparisons of the Δ values between the three groups, i.e.

(i)   abdomen versus thigh,
(ii) thigh versus 'thigh plus aprotinin',
(iii) abdomen versus 'thigh plus aprotinin'.

The mean plasma C-peptide concentration decreased during the first 90 min of the somatostatin infusion in the three comparative groups from 0.33 ± 0.04, 0.26 ± 0.05, and 0.29 ± 0.02 nmol/l (–90 min) to 0.08 ± 0.02, 0.06 ± 0.01 and 0.08 ± 0.01 nmol/l (0 min) for the 'abdomen', 'thigh' and 'thigh plus aprotinin' treatment groups, respectively, i.e. a mean reduction from basal values of approximately 75% (range 72–77%). After insulin administration there was a further fall to 0.01 nmol/l in all groups.

(i) Abdomen versus thigh (Figure 4.55a)

Following subcutaneous injections into the abdomen and thigh regions, peak incremental insulin levels of 0.12 ± 0.01 and 0.09 ± 0.02 nmol/l, respectively, were reached at 90 min. Between 30 and 50 min the levels were significantly higher ($p<0.05$) after administration into the anterior abdominal wall compared to the thigh. Subsequently, a more rapid fall in plasma insulin was observed when using the abdomen compared to the thigh, the levels becoming significantly lower between 240 and 300 min ($p<0.05$).

Following insulin administration the plasma glucose continued to rise for 30 min before falling to reach a nadir of 1.4 ± 0.4 and 1.0 ± 0.3 mmol/l below pre-injection levels at 150 min for both the abdomen and thigh regions, respectively. Thereafter, in agreement with the trends in plasma insulin, a quicker recovery to pre-insulin levels was observed with the abdominal site of

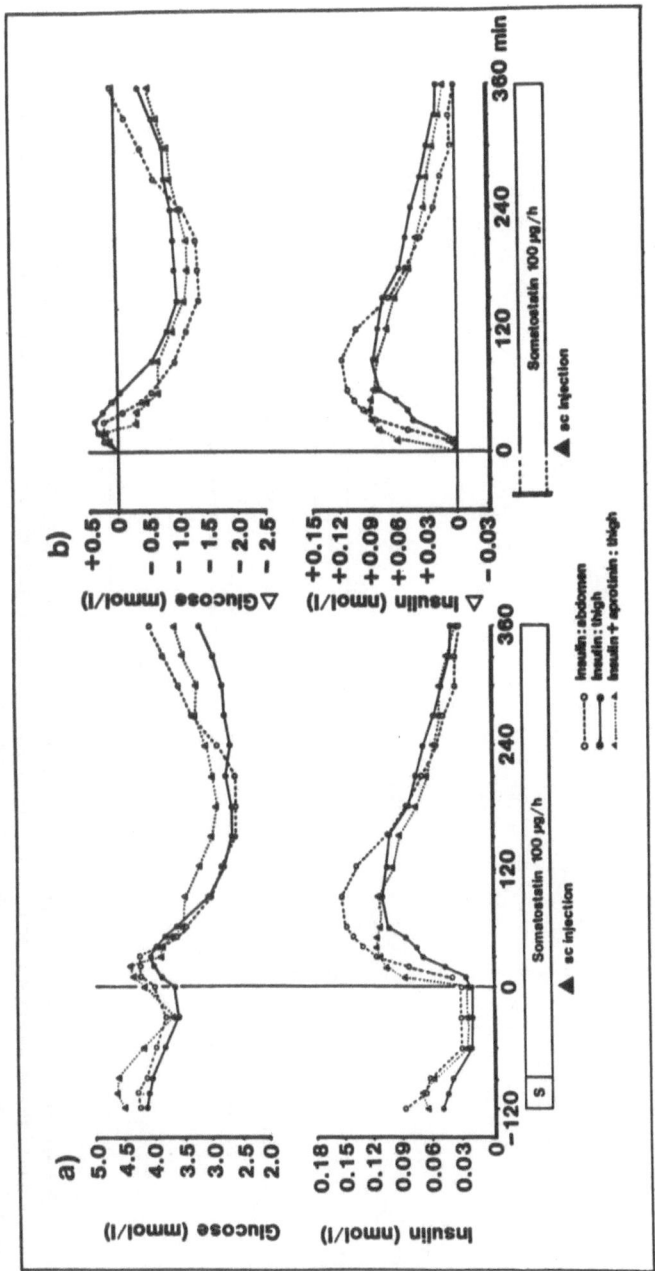

Figure 4.54 **(a)** Effect of human insulin on plasma glucose and insulin concentrations (means) in six subjects. Somatostatin infused from −90 to 360 min. Insulin (0.075 U/kg) given at time 0. **(b)** Results shown as means of Δ values

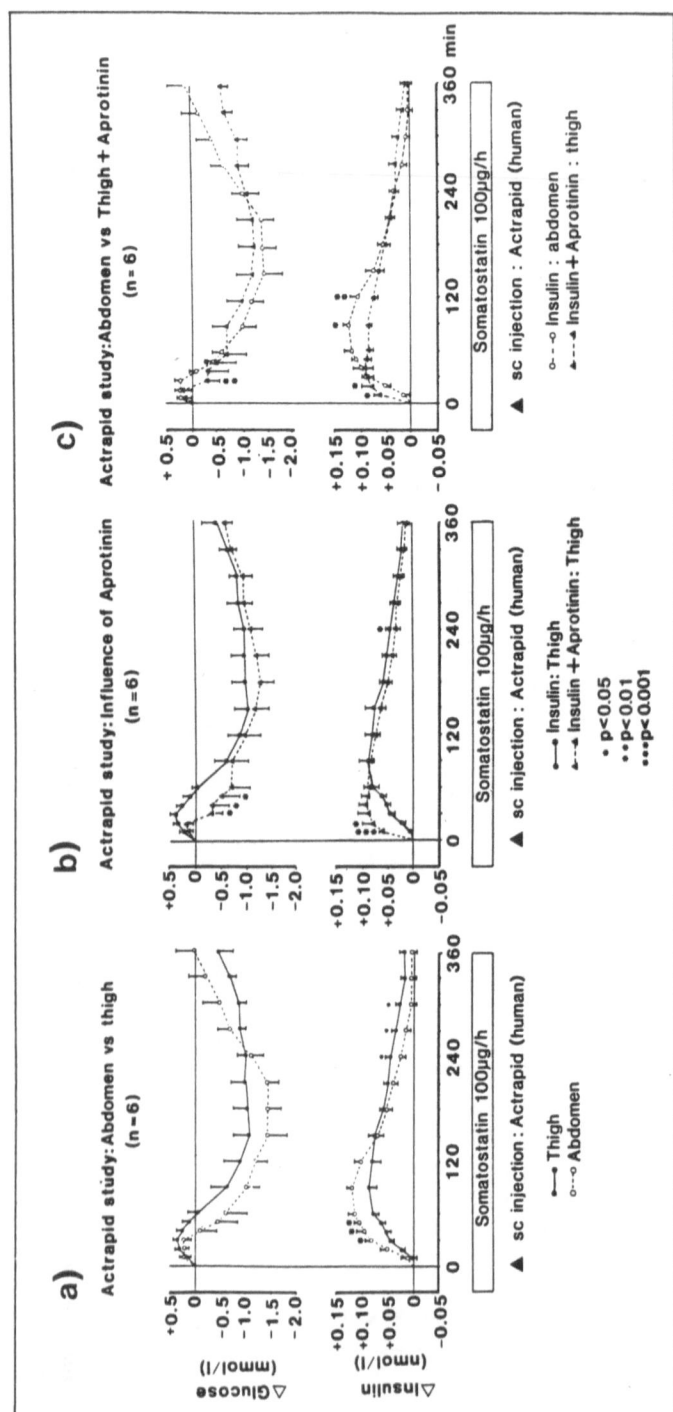

Figure 4.55 Comparison of the effect of human insulin, given subcutaneously (sc) into (**a**) thigh and abdomen, (**b**) thigh, with and without aprotinin, (**c**) abdomen alone and thigh after mixing with aprotinin, on plasma glucose and insulin concentrations in six subjects. Somatostatin infused from –90 to 360 min. Insulin (0.075 U/kg) given at time 0. Results shown as means ± SE of Δ values

injection compared to the thigh. The tendency towards an earlier and shorter-lived hypoglycaemic response with insulin administered into the abdomen compared to the thigh did not, however, reach statistical significance.

(ii) Thigh versus 'thigh plus aprotinin' (Figure 4.55b)

Subcutaneous injection of insulin admixed with aprotinin resulted in a steep increase in incremental insulin levels during the first 30 min after administration. The levels achieved were significantly higher than those with insulin alone injected into the same region at 10 min ($p<0.001$) and 20 min ($p<0.05$).

Insulin admixed with aprotinin achieved peak insulin levels of 0.93 ± 0.02 nmol/l at 40 min, followed by a gradual fall to near pre-insulin levels at 360 min. A slower increase in plasma insulin levels was observed with insulin alone reaching a similar but delayed peak of 0.91 ± 0.02 nmol at 90 min. Thereafter, the insulin levels were the same for the two comparative groups except at 240 min when the insulin concentration was lower with the admixture ($p<0.05$).

Plasma glucose fell acutely after 10 min with insulin plus aprotinin, the hypoglycaemic response becoming significantly greater than with insulin alone between 30 min and 50 min ($p<0.05$). Thereafter, from 90 min onwards there was no difference in the hypoglycaemic profiles between the two groups.

(iii) Abdomen versus 'thigh plus aprotinin' (Figure 4.55c)

There was an earlier increase in plasma insulin levels with the admixture of insulin and aprotinin injected into the thigh compared to insulin alone administered into the abdominal region. The incremental insulin level was significantly higher with the admixture at 10 and 20 min ($p<0.05$). Subsequently, the levels plateaued at about 0.09 nmol/l between 40 to 90 min following insulin plus aprotinin.

After a relatively slower initial rise in plasma insulin following injection into the abdomen the mean insulin level was higher from 40 to 120 min, the difference reaching statistical significance at 90 min ($p<0.05$) and 120 min ($p<0.01$). From 150 min onwards, however, there was a tendency for the plasma insulin level to fall more rapidly following injection into the abdominal wall compared to insulin plus aprotinin into the thigh, although the difference did not reach statistical significance.

Within 30 min of injection of the admixture of insulin and aprotinin into the thigh region, the hypoglycaemic response was significantly greater ($p<0.01$) than that observed following insulin injected alone into the abdomen. From 40 min to the end of the study there were no further significant differences between the hypoglycaemic action of the two regimens. Despite the very early hypoglycaemic response to insulin plus aprotinin, the duration of hypoglycaemia was still longer than that observed with insulin injected into the anterior abdominal wall.

Discussion

This study demonstrates that subcutaneous neutral, soluble ('semi-synthetic') human insulin is absorbed quicker into the systemic circulation from the anterior abdominal wall compared to the thigh region. The reputed faster absorption of human compared to porcine insulin, when injected into the thigh (Sundermann et al, 1981; Sestoft et al, 1982), and the lack of a difference between the species, when administered into the abdomen (Owens et al, 1981a), did not negate a regional difference in the absorption of human insulin. The earlier rise and fall of plasma insulin with the abdomen relative to the thigh was reflected in the tendency towards a quicker and shorter-lived hypoglycaemic response with the former site of injection. The relationship to subcutaneous blood flow may explain the regional differences in absorption from a subcutaneous depot (Kølendorf et al, 1979; Hildebrandt et al, 1982, 1983a).

Recently, Linde and Gunnarsson (1983) and Williams et al (1983) have, using different techniques, demonstrated increased skin blood flow with subcutaneous aprotinin. The local hyperaemic response may be the basis for enhanced insulin absorption in insulin-dependent diabetics when mixing insulin with aprotinin (Freidenberg, et al, 1980, 1981; Gunnarsson et al, 1980; Müller et al, 1980). Other environmental factors, such as high or low ambient temperature, massage of injection site and exercise, also markedly alter insulin absorption rates by virtue of local subcutaneous blood flow changes (Koivisto and Felig, 1978; Berger et al, 1979, 1982; Koivisto, 1980; Koivisto et al, 1981).

In healthy normal subjects aprotinin has been shown to enhance subcutaneous insulin absorption (Berger et al, 1980). This study, utilising human instead of porcine insulin at the same dose, site of administration, volume and formulation of aprotinin, but without adjusting the volume of comparative insulin injection, gave results identical to those of Berger et al (1980). The addition of aprotinin enhanced the early absorption of subcutaneously injected soluble human insulin. This effect was apparent during the first hour after injection, with the incremental insulin levels significantly higher at 10 min and 20 min, resulting in a more marked early hypoglycaemic response between 30 min and 50 min with insulin plus aprotinin compared to insulin alone, when both were administered into the thigh region. The brief enhancement of insulin absorption by aprotinin could be consistent with a short-lived local hyperaemic response.

Similar acute differences were present when comparing the response to insulin plus aprotinin into the thigh, and insulin alone injected into the anterior abdominal wall. However, during the second hour after administration the plasma insulin level was significantly higher with insulin injected into the abdomen. Following the rapid increase in plasma insulin during the first 30 min with the insulin/aprotinin mixture injected into the thigh, there was a slow decrease in plasma levels during the remaining 5 h causing a more prolonged hypoglycaemic response than that seen with insulin given into the abdominal wall.

The observed insulin profiles do not support the suggestion that the protease inhibitor aprotinin enhances insulin 'bioavailability' by the inhibition of subcutaneous insulin degradation (Freidenberg et al, 1980, 1981; Gunnarsson et al, 1980; Müller et al, 1980).

The findings do, however, indicate that mixing insulin with substances capable of stimulating local blood flow in order to achieve an earlier increase in plasma insulin levels with possible therapeutic benefits, deserves further investigation (Berger et al, 1982; Williams et al, 1984).

4.3.2 Insulin concentration: U–40 versus U–100 'short-' and 'intermediate-acting' insulin preparations

Introduction

The first unit of insulin 'potency' was established by Banting et al (1922c) as the number of cubic centimetres of pancreatic extract that lowered the blood sugar to 2.5 mmol/l in 2 to 4 h, sometimes considered as the minimal dosage required to cause convulsions in normal rabbits and referred to as the '*rabbit unit*' (Table 4.31). Later in the same year a '*mouse unit*' was introduced, being the smallest dose required to cause convulsions in half the mice injected under specific conditions. In the following year the Standardisation Committee of the League of Nations Health Organisation defined a unit as 'that amount which is capable of lowering the blood glucose to the convulsive level, within three hours, in rabbits of approximately 2 kg weight from which food has been withheld for twenty four hours and referred to as the '*Toronto unit*'. It was soon realised that the variability of response to insulin in rabbits did not allow a rigid statement of the relationship of blood sugar and symptoms. Therefore, a method based on the hypoglycaemic response in rabbits was recommended with the introduction of the '*physiological unit*', which was divided by three to give the '*clinical unit*'. In 1925, the First International Standard was defined as 8 units of insulin per mg of dry insulin standard (or 1 unit = 0.125 mg) prepared by the Medical Research Council of Great Britain (League of Nations, 1926).

Following advances in the preparation and purification of insulin, a new standard was prepared and the unit of insulin was redefined in 1935 as 1/22 part of the latest standard establishing the Second International Standard (League of Nations, 1936). This was followed in 1952 by the introduction of the Third

Table 4.31   Insulin potency (units)

1922	Rabbit unit	
	Mouse unit	
1923	Toronto unit	
	Physiology unit	
	Clinical unit	
International Unit (IU per mg)		
1925	First Standard	8
1935	Second Standard	22
1952	Third Standard	24.5
1958	Fourth Standard	24

International Standard determined as the activity contained in 0.04082 mg, i.e. 24.5 IU/mg (Miles et al, 1952). In 1958 the Fourth International Standard was established, and defined as the activity contained in 0.04167 mg of the Fourth International Standard preparation of 24 IU/mg which is in use today (Bangham and Mussett, 1959). The Fourth International Standard consisting of 52% bovine and 48% porcine insulin will eventually be replaced by the appropriate insulin standard of bovine, porcine and human insulin, respectively (WHO, 1982). This will avoid errors in biological 'potency' determinations of the individual insulins due to time-dependent variations when measured against a mixed porcine/bovine insulin standard (Pingel et al, 1985).

Table 4.32 Concentration of insulin preparations:

1922	5 IU/ml
1923	10 and 20 IU/ml
1924	40 IU/ml
1925	80 IU/ml
1973	100 IU/ml

The first insulins available for clinical use were produced in a strength of 5 IU/ml (Table 4.32). The concentration of insulin was rapidly increased to 10 and 20 IU/ml in 1923, 40 IU/ml in 1924 and 80 IU/ml in 1925. The availability of different insulin strengths led to countless dosage errors (Watkins et al, 1967; Brearley and Mackie, 1978). The American Diabetes Association's Committee on the Use of Therapeutic Agents recommended, in the early 1970s, the adoption of a single strength of insulin, i.e. U-100 (100 IU/ml) (American Diabetes Association, 1972a, b), which was introduced in 1973. A few clinical trials were conducted in different countries confirming the safety and acceptability of U-100, both in children and adults with insulin-dependent diabetes (Rosenbloom, 1974; McKinley and Farquhar, 1976; Sheldon et al, 1976). In Canada the change-over to U-100 was achieved in just over a year during 1974 and 1975. Five years later the USA Food and Drug Administration (FDA) recommended the withdrawal of insulin preparations containing 80 IU/ml, which became law in 1980.

Many other countries have since followed recommendations by the International Diabetes Federation (IDF) to withdraw 80 IU/ml from clinical use whilst ensuring the parallel introduction of more accurate re-usable and disposable syringes for the higher-strength insulin. Whereas the adoption of a single strength of insulin, 100-unit insulin, should reduce dosage errors (Bloom et al, 1981) several countries, especially in Europe, still retain the 40 IU/ml insulin preparations.

The effect of concentration on the absorption of soluble insulin has been studied by Binder (1969), using radiolabelled insulin (0.4, 4 and 40 IU/ml), demonstrating a slower absorption rate with increasing concentrations. Galloway and co-workers (1981a) also observed higher peak insulin levels with U-40 compared to U-100 and U-500 soluble insulin. Both groups postulated that either a greater depression of the microcirculation and/or a smaller surface area exposed to tissue fluids could possibly account for these differences. Recently, however, it has been shown that the slower absorption of U-100 insulin occurs irrespective of injection volume (Hildebrandt et al, 1983b). Insulin concentration may therefore be of potential clinical significance in patients when changed from one strength of insulin to another. In general, conversion to U-100 has been accomplished with minimal problems when associated with adequate patient education (Bonnici, 1983; Cartwright et al, 1983; Parr, 1983; Swift et al, 1983). There is, however, only very limited clinical information available comparing U-40 and U-100 strengths of the 'short-' and 'intermediate-acting' insulin preparations (McKinley and Farquhar, 1976; Rosenbloom, 1974; Parr, 1983).

In view of the continuing international debate, a number of studies have been carried out for the purpose of comparing the U-40 (40 IU/ml) and U-100 (100 IU/ml) 'short-acting' (cf. 4.3.2.1) and 'intermediate-acting' insulin preparations (cf. 4.3.2.2) following subcutaneous administration.

4.3.2.1   U-40 versus U-100: 'short-acting' insulins

Purpose, subjects, materials and methods

The purpose of this study was to compare the U-40 and U-100 strengths of 'semi-synthetic' neutral, soluble human insulin in a group of six subjects aged 20–30 years (mean, 26 years) within 20% of ideal body weight (mean, 71 kg, range 61–85 kg) given the same dose, i.e. 6 units of each preparation. Details of the comparative insulin preparations are included in Table 4.33.

Table 4.33

	Actrapid HM[a] 1 ml	
	U–40	U–100
Nitrogen content (mg/ml)	0.209	0.531
Potency (IU/ml)[b]	38.8	98.2
Phenol (mg)	2.0	2.0
Glycerol (mg)	16.0	16.0
pH	7.5	7.5

[a] USP formulation
[b] Theoretical potency: 185 IU/mgN

The study was conducted according to a randomised block design with each subject receiving, either 6 U of U–40 (0.15 ml) or 6 U of U–100 (0.06 ml) insulin, each on two separate days, viz. 4 study days 1 week apart. The replicated identical injections into the same subject enable the estimation and comparison of the variability of the response to the two preparations to be made, as well as testing whether a significant interaction exists between subjects and preparations.

On each of the study days, after a 30 min basal period, insulin was injected subcutaneously into the anterior abdominal wall mid-way between the umbilicus and left or right anterior superior iliac spines using the Becton-Dickinson LO-Dose 0.5 ml syringe. Blood samples were obtained at –30 min, immediately prior to injection, and every 10 min during the first hour reverting to ½-hourly for the remaining 300 min post-insulin period.

All the blood samples were centrifuged within 5 min of sampling and plasma was aliquoted into fluoride for glucose estimation (glucose oxidase: Yellow Springs glucose analyser, Ohio, USA), heparin for immunoreactive insulin and C-peptide determinations (modification of methods of Heding 1972, 1975, respectively).

Statistical methods

The results are expressed as means ± SE unless otherwise stated. The data were analysed both according to a method of analysis of variance for a cross-over design, making it possible to check for 'order of treatment' or 'trend' effects, and the analysis of variance of a randomised block design (a two-way analysis of variance) with replicates. In addition, the data of the U–40 and U–100 insulins were also analysed separately by one-way analysis of variance to estimate the 'within' subject variation for each preparation. The analyses of variance were carried out on the absolute and Δ values. The Δ values were derived by subtracting the mean level of the –30 and 0 min samples from all subsequent values for each of the following variables: insulin, exogenous insulin*, C-peptide and glucose and the integrated mean levels over 0 to 60, 60 to 120, 120 to 240, 240 to 360 and 0 to 360 min (trapezoid method).

Results

The means ± SE absolute and Δ plasma glucose, C-peptide and insulin levels for the U–40 and U–100 study days are shown in Figures 4.57a and 4.57b, respectively. The day-to-day variation in the response to U–40 and U–100 insulins are illustrated in Figures 4.58 and 4.59, respectively.

(i) *Results of cross-over analysis of variance:* After the injection of the two insulins a steep rise in plasma insulin levels was evident during the first hour with levels reaching 0.187 ± 0.01 nmol/l at 90 min with U–40 compared to 0.18 ± 0.01 nmol/l, 30 min later with U–100 insulin. The plasma insulin level was higher with U–40 compared to U–100 insulin betwen 30 min and 90 min after injection with the difference reaching significance at 50 min ($p<0.05$). During the last 180 min, however, the reverse was true, showing lower concentrations with U–40 insulin between min 270 and 360 min ($p<0.05-0.001$). Also the insulin levels – which underestimate the exogenous insulin level – were

---

* The plasma levels of exogenous insulin were estimated according to the 'initial ratio method' described earlier (cf. 4.2.1.1). As there was no control day, the initial insulin and C-peptide measurements before the injection of insulin on all study days were used to derive individual factors, being a ratio between the mean insulin and C-peptide concentrations. The individual pairs of insulin and C-peptide levels at –30 and 0 min for all six subjects on the four study days are illustrated in Figure 4.56.

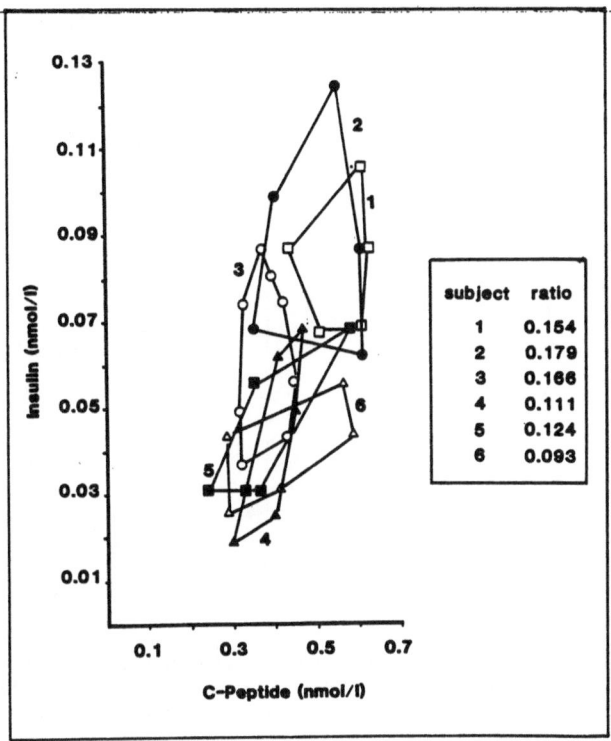

Figure 4.56 Relationship between insulin (IRI) and C-peptide concentrations during the basal period (–30 and 0 min) in all six subjects

significantly higher on U–40 relative to U–100 insulin during the initial 120 min (Figure 4.57b). This difference was reflected in the higher ($p < 0.05$) integrated mean insulin level (AUC_{0-60}) with U–40 insulin during this early phase after injection. There was no difference, however, between the two insulins for the total post-insulin period (AUC_{0-360}).

Analysis of the approximate exogenous insulin levels clearly demonstrates that U–40 insulin results in higher plasma insulin levels than U–100 insulin during the first 120 min, the difference reaching significance at 50 min ($p < 0.01$) and 90 min ($p < 0.05$) (Figure 4.57c). The trend was reversed during the last 90 min period when the insulin levels became significantly lower with U–40 compared to U–100 insulin ($p < 0.05-0.01$).

The mean fasting glucose levels were similar at 5.0 ± 0.1 mmol/l and 5.2 ± 0.1 mmol/l for the U–40 and U–100 insulin study days. After insulin, the plasma glucose levels fell reaching a nadir of about 3 mmol/l at 120 min and 150 min, followed by a recovery to within 0.5 mmol/l of basal values at 360 min with U–40 and U–100 insulin, respectively. Although there was no statistically significant difference in the hypoglycaemic response between the two preparations, the glucose tended to fall and later recover more rapidly after U–40 than after U–100 insulin.

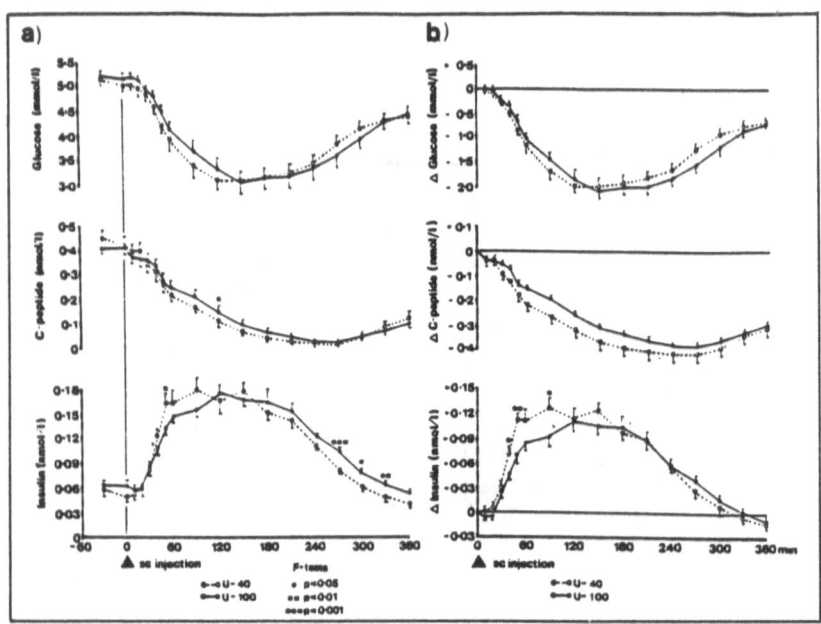

Figure 4.57a,b (a) Comparison of the effect of U–40 and U–100 human insulin on plasma glucose, C-peptide and insulin concentrations (means ± SE) in six subjects ($n = 6 \times 2$). Insulin (6 U) given subcutaneously (sc) at time 0. **(b)** Results shown as means ± SE of Δ values

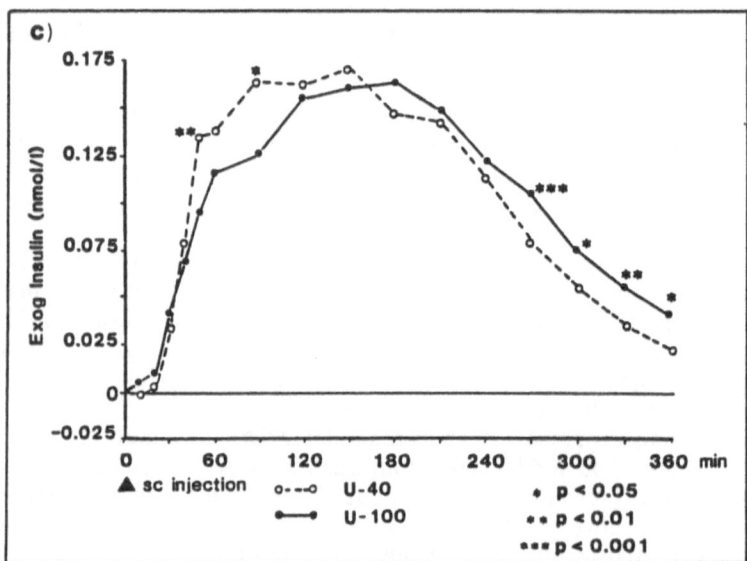

Figure 4.57c Comparison of the estimated ('initial ratio method') plasma exogenous insulin concentrations (means) in six subjects following the subcutaneous (sc) injection of 6 U U–40 and U–100 human insulin at time 0

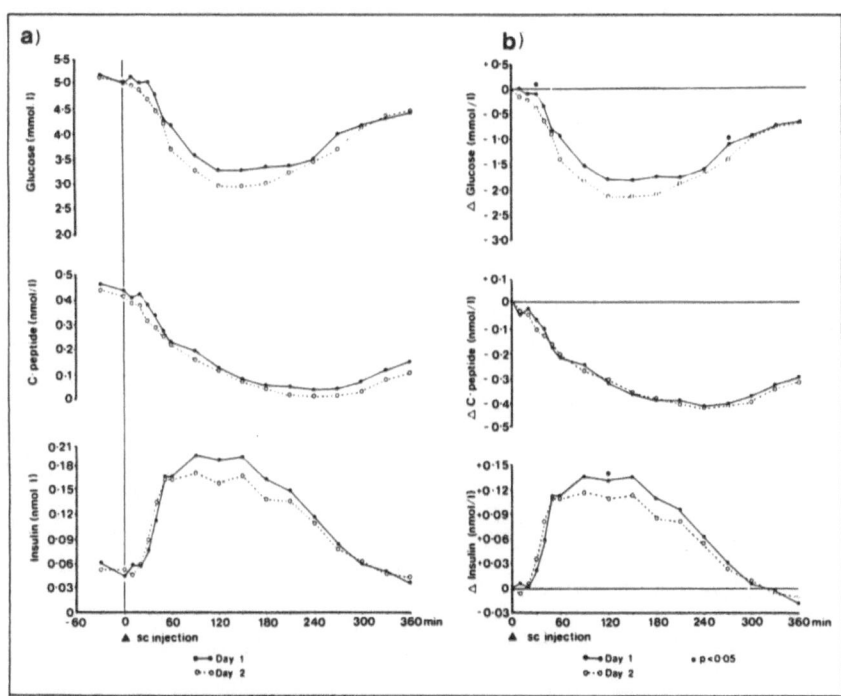

Figure 4.58a, b (a) Comparison of the effect of U–40 human insulin on plasma glucose, C-peptide and insulin concentrations (means) on two separate days in six subjects. Insulin (6 U) given subcutaneously at time 0. (b) Results shown as means of Δ values

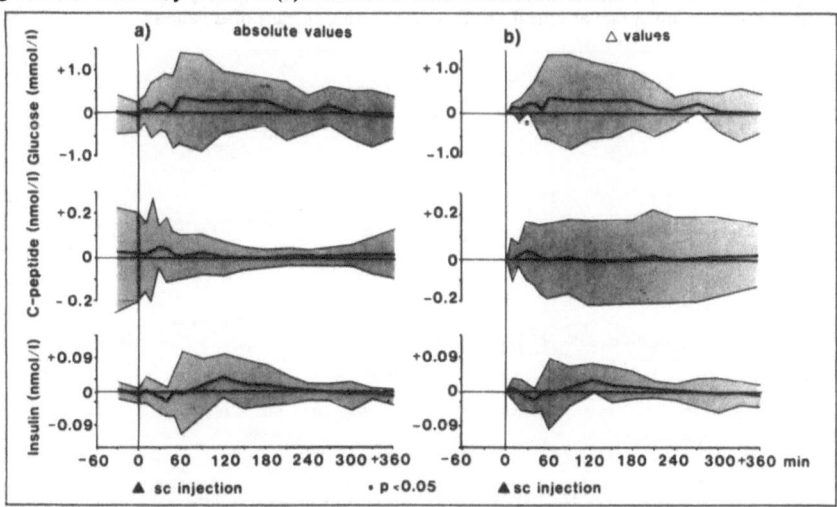

Figure 4.58c, d (c) Comparison of the effect of U–40 human insulin on plasma glucose, C-peptide and insulin concentrations in six subjects. Insulin (6 U) given subcutaneously (sc) at time 0. Results shown as means of differences (with 95% confidence limits) between responses on two separate days. (d) Results shown as means of differences (with 95% confidence limits) between Δ values

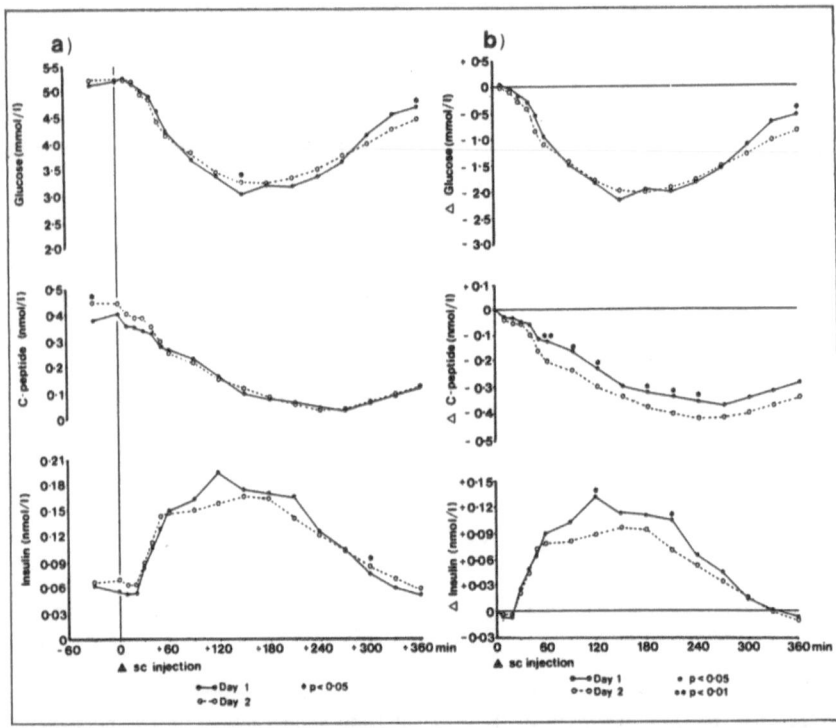

Figure 4.59a, b (**a**) Comparison of the effect of U–100 human insulin on plasma glucose, C-peptide and insulin (IRI) concentrations (means) in six subjects on two separate days. Insulin (6 U) given subcutaneously (sc) at time 0. (**b**) Results shown as means of Δ values

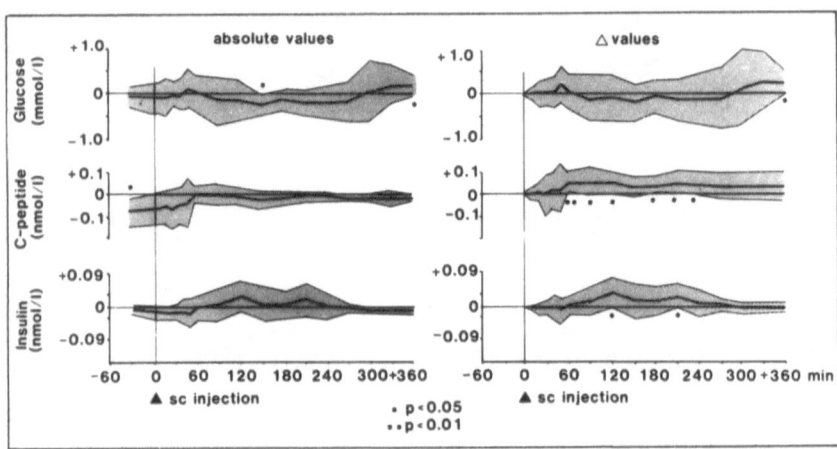

Figure 4.59c, d (**c**) Comparison of the effect of U–100 human insulin on plasma glucose, C-peptide and insulin (IRI) concentrations in six subjects on two separate days. Insulin (6 U) given subcutaneously (sc) at time 0. Results shown as means of differences (with 95% confidence limits) between responses for the two separate days. (**d**) Results shown as means of differences (with 95% confidence limits) between Δ values

The fall in C-peptide levels was similar with the two insulin preparations reaching a level of about 5% of basal values at 240 and 270 min followed by a small recovery during the last 90 to 120 min of the study.

(ii) *Results of randomised block analysis of variance (Tables 4.34a, b).* The randomised block analysis is a two-way analysis of variance with replicates within blocks (subjects), meaning that the underlying linear model is a sum of subject, treatment and interaction parameters plus a random term which describes the variation between identical treatments. The interaction parameters describe the possibility that the differences between U–40 and

Table 4.34 Randomised block analysis of variance: means (F1, 17)

(a)

Time (min)	Glu (mM)	CP (nM)	IRI (nM)	Glu† (mM)	CP† (nM)	IRI† (nM)	Exog. IRI (nM)
−30	0.00	1.48	1.55	—	—	—	—
0	2.87	0.05	4.65*	—	—	—	—
10	2.60	0.64	0.52	1.55	0.07	0.60	1.77
20	1.92	0.73	0.00	1.78	0.30	1.98	0.60
30	0.43	0.23	0.34	0.01	1.64	0.71	0.08
40	2.58	0.21	1.78	1.45	2.29	6.54*	1.36
50	2.59	0.13	5.25*	1.51	1.38	15.59**	6.27*
60	1.03	3.20	0.78	0.45	3.35	2.71	1.32
90	1.70	5.01*	3.03	0.96	4.92*	7.84*	5.04*
120	1.74	6.26*	0.25	0.65	3.31	0.12	0.02
150	0.02	4.00	0.41	0.35	2.84	2.46	1.01
180	0.00	3.54	1.44	0.33	2.32	0.20	0.88
210	0.33	1.54	0.67	1.30	1.31	0.01	0.36
240	0.62	0.92	1.77	1.81	1.03	0.02	1.52
270	2.59	0.00	26.78***	4.37*	0.64	2.51	24.72***
300	1.26	0.07	5.59*	2.37	0.83	0.79	4.49*
330	0.02	0.81	14.57**	0.39	0.09	0.68	11.20**
360	0.16	0.61	5.12*	0.20	0.11	0.24	5.41*

(b)

Time (min)	Glu (mM)	CP (nM)	IRI (nM)	Glu† (mM)	CP† (nM)	IRI† (nM)	Exog. IRI (nM)
0–60	2.90	0.00	0.63	1.69	2.17	7.80*	1.43
60–120	1.73	6.00*	1.32	0.86	4.34*	4.74	2.58
120–240	0.00	4.30	0.30	0.45	2.13	0.35	0.05
240–360	1.11	0.13	18.91***	2.66	0.51	1.25	14.20**
0–360	0.18	0.12	0.43	0.23	1.85	2.31	0.11

Glu = Glucose
CP = C-peptide
IRI = Insulin
Exog. IRI = Exogenous insulin
F-tests of significant differences: *$p < 0.05$; **$p < 0.01$; ***$p < 0.001$
†Δ values

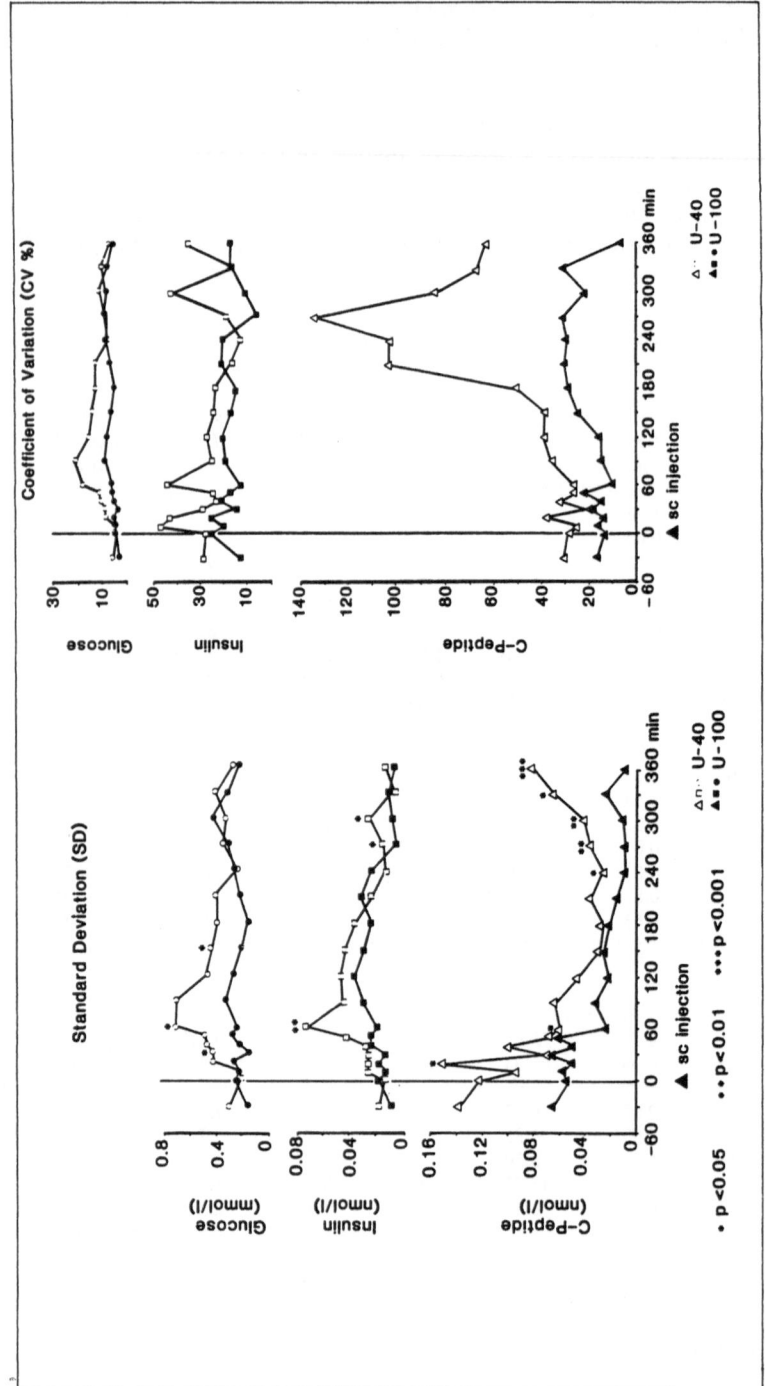

Figure 4.60 The mean standard deviation (SD) and coefficient of variation (CV%) estimates for the plasma glucose, C-peptide and insulin (IRI) concentrations following the subcutaneous (sc) injection at time 0 of U−40 and U−100 human insulin in six subjects on two separate days

Table 4.35 Comparison of variance estimates (SD, F = 6)

Time	Glucose (mM)		C-peptide (nM)		Insulin (nM)	
(min)	U–40	U–100	U–40	U–100	U–40	U–100
–30	0.29	0.15	0.137	0.065	0.017	0.008
0	0.24	0.24	0.122	0.054	0.014	0.016
10	0.22	0.22	0.097	0.056	0.025	0.011
20	0.42	0.27	0.151*	0.050	0.026	0.016
30	0.43*	0.14	0.070	0.068	0.025	0.013
40	0.48	0.23	0.099	0.047	0.029	0.024
50	0.53	0.27	0.069	0.061	0.041	0.024
60	0.72*	0.24	0.060*	0.023	0.074*	0.019
90	0.71	0.34	0.063	0.031	0.046	0.030
120	0.49	0.26	0.046	0.022	0.048	0.036
150	0.44	0.20	0.029	0.025	0.045	0.029
180	0.40*	0.15	0.025	0.021	0.036	0.024
210	0.41	0.21	0.036	0.015	0.024	0.032
240	0.24	0.25	0.025*	0.009	0.014	0.024
270	0.38	0.31	0.036**	0.008	0.015*	0.005
300	0.34	0.44	0.041**	0.011	0.026*	0.008
330	0.41	0.31	0.065*	0.024	0.008	0.011
360	0.26	0.21	0.081***	0.007	0.014	0.009

*$p<0.05$; **$p<0.01$; ***$p<0.001$

U–100 may vary more between subjects than can be accounted for by the random variation between the same preparation. If the interaction is non-significant it may be regarded as random and pooled with random variation between replicates and used for a more powerful test of differences between U–40 and U–100 insulin. As the interaction exceeded the 5% level in only a single value, i.e. insulin level at 360 min, it is reasonable to conclude that there was no significant interaction. Therefore the interaction and error terms were pooled to give better estimates of the random variation. The analyses for treatment differences are summarised in Tables 4.34a, b. The results are similar to those seen earlier using the cross-over analysis of variance, although there is a single significant difference, which did not appear earlier between the Δ plasma glucose levels at 270 min, indicating a greater hypoglycaemic effect with U–100 than U–40 (Figure 4.57b; Table 4.34a).

(iii) *Analysis of 'within' subject variation:* Figures 4.58 and 4.59 illustrate the day-to-day variability in the plasma glucose, C-peptide and insulin concentrations with the U–40 and U–100 insulins, respectively. There appears to be a systematic tendency to higher 'within' subject SDs with the U–40 than with the U–100 insulin preparation especially during the first and last 1 to 2h (Tables 4.35 and 4.36). The estimated 'within' subject standard deviation and coefficient of variation (CV%) for each parameter for the two preparations are illustrated in Figures 4.60 and 4.61. The CV for plasma glucose levels with U–100 insulin remained below 10% throughout the study period, whereas with U–40 it increased above 10% between 40 min and 210 min reaching a peak of 21% at 90 min. For insulin levels the CV was relatively steady at about 15%

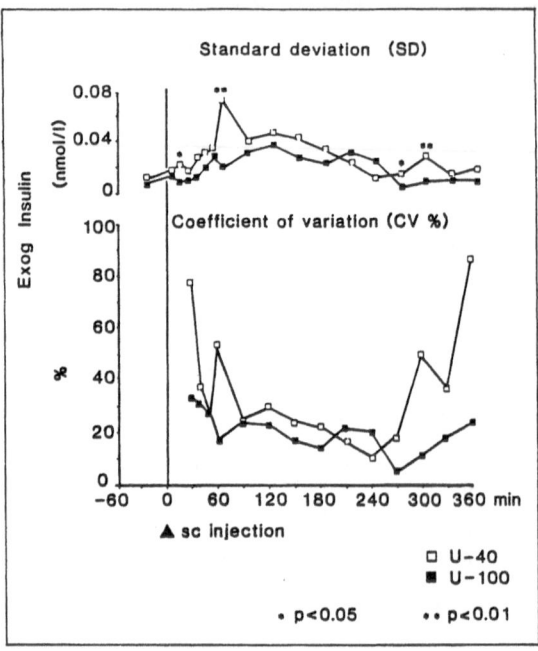

Figure 4.61 The mean standard deviation (SD) and coefficient of variation (CV%) for the estimated ('initial ratio method') plasma exogenous insulin concentrations following the subcutaneous (sc) injection at time 0 of U–40 and U–100 human insulin in six subjects on two separate days

Table 4.36 Comparison of variance estimates (SD, $F = 6$) : Δ values

Time	Glucose (mM)		C-peptide (nM)		Insulin (nM)		Exog Insulin (nM)	
(min)	U–40	U–100	U–40	U–100	U–40	U–100	U–40	U–100
–30	—	—	—	—	—	—	—	—
0	—	—	—	—	—	—	—	—
10	0.15	0.10	0.068**	0.020	0.024**	0.006	0.022*	0.008
20	0.22	0.20	0.033	0.033	0.026	0.012	0.016	0.010
30	0.29	0.19	0.090	0.062	0.027	0.012	0.028	0.013
40	0.37	0.23	0.093	0.048	0.027	0.022	0.031	0.020
50	0.39	0.29	0.099	0.065	0.030	0.019	0.036	0.028
60	0.68*	0.24	0.109	0.058	0.063*	0.018	0.072**	0.019
90	0.71	0.31	0.104	0.066	0.034	0.030	0.040	0.031
120	0.57	0.31	0.122	0.057	0.039	0.041	0.047	0.036
150	0.54	0.29	0.118*	0.038	0.036	0.032	0.041	0.027
180	0.45	0.22	0.116	0.049	0.027	0.026	0.033	0.022
210	0.38	0.30	0.135	0.062	0.016	0.033	0.023	0.032
240	0.20	0.37	0.118	0.059	0.014	0.024	0.012	0.024
270	0.25	0.43	0.120	0.052	0.028*	0.011	0.015*	0.004
300	0.27	0.56	0.110	0.057	0.032**	0.008	0.028**	0.008
330	0.40	0.44	0.097	0.056	0.018	0.009	0.013	0.010
360	0.26	0.26	0.086	0.054	0.020*	0.006	0.019	0.009

*$p<0.05$; **$p<0.01$; ***$p<0.001$

(4–25%) with the U–100 insulin, whereas with U–40 the values were twice as high (41–46%) during the first and last 90 min periods. The CV for plasma C-peptide concentrations with U–100 insulin ranged from 6 to 31%, whereas with U–40 it was twice as high up to 180 min and increasing up to 133% at 270 min. The use of the analysis of variance in the cross-over analysis and randomised block analysis is therefore not strictly correct, since it requires that the variation is homogeneous for the U–40 and U–100 preparations. The analysis of variance, however, is regarded as being able to accomodate moderate deviations from variance homogeneity.

Discussion

With regard to the primary purpose of comparing the plasma insulin levels and effects on glucose and C-peptide after injection of the same dose of U–40 and U–100 insulin, the results appear quite conclusive in that U–40 insulin is absorbed more rapidly than U–100 insulin. This is reflected in higher insulin concentrations in the first hours and lower concentrations towards the end of the 6 h study with U–40 insulin. In agreement with this, the glucose tends to fall more rapidly and recover earlier than with U–100 insulin. In addition, the C-peptide level is suppressed more with U–40 than after U–100 in the beginning, and less towards the end, of the study period.

Therefore, these results agree with previous data showing that the absorption rate of soluble insulins is inversely correlated with the concentration of the injected insulin (Binder, 1969; Galloway et al, 1981a; Kølendorf et al, 1983b) and directly correlated with the injection volume (Binder, 1969).

Others have been unable to detect any difference in blood glucose profiles after subcutaneous administration of U–40 and U–100 soluble insulin when given at the same dose (Swift et al, 1983; Lauritzen et al, 1984).

The higher 'within' subject variability in the response to U–40 compared to U–100 insulin may be related to the absorption process but also to a number of other factors, e.g. the different syringes used for the administration of the insulin preparations compared.

4.3.2.2   U-40 versus U-100: 'intermediate-acting' insulin study

Data from three separate studies were used to compare the responses between U–40 and U–100 human and porcine Lente (Monotard) and human NPH (Protaphane) insulin preparations at the 0.30 U/kg dose level.

Details of the 'intermediate-acting' insulins used in the three reference studies are combined in Table 4.37.

Details of the experimental procedures involved in the individual studies are included in the following sections:
  (i) Lente insulin: Monotard HM, MC (human and porcine)
                                U–40: cf. section 4.2.1.1
                                U–100: cf. section 4.2.1.3.

Table 4.37 'Intermediate-acting' insulins (1 ml)

	Lente (Monotard)				NPH (Protaphane)	
	HM (human)		MC (porcine)		HM (human)	
	U–40	U–100	U–40	U–100	U–40	U–100
Nitrogen content (mg/ml)	0.217	0.529	0.210	0.546	0.247	0.634
Potency (IU)	40.45[a]	97.6[a]	38.85[a]	100.4[a]	40.9[b]	102.3[b]
Protamine sulphate (mg/ml)	—	—	—	—	0.142	0.36
Glycerol (mg)	—	—	—	—	16.0	16.0
m-Cresol (mg)	—	—	—	—	1.5	1.5
Phenol (mg)	—	—	—	—	0.65	0.65
Methyl hydroxyparabens (mg)	1.0	1.0	1.0	1.0	—	—
Amorphous (%)	35.8	33.7	31.9	35.2	—	—
Crystalline (%)	64.2	66.3	68.1	64.8	—	—
pH	7.46	7.32	7.42	7.37	7.35	7.32

[a] 185 IU/mg nitrogen
[b] Determined by quantitative HPLC gel permeation chromatography method using monocomponent porcine insulin as standard

(ii) NPH insulin: Protaphane HM (human)
U–40: cf. section 4.2.1.2
U–100: cf. section 4.2.1.3.

Statistical methods

For the comparisons of U–40 and U–100 human and porcine Lente and U–40 and U–100 human NPH insulin, the plasma glucose, C-peptide and insulin levels obtained during a 1 h basal and 10 h post-insulin period were employed. The unpaired Student's t-test was used to compare the individual pairs of treatments. The analysis was carried out on both the raw data and Δ values – derived by subtracting the mean basal value from all subsequent levels for each study day.

An approximate estimate of the exogenous plasma insulin level was calculated using the 'control day method' referred to in 4.2.1.1.

The results are expressed as means ± SE unless stated otherwise.

Results

The mean absolute and Δ plasma glucose, C-peptide and insulin levels for human and porcine Lente (Monotard) and human NPH (Protaphane) insulins are illustrated in Figures 4.62 and 4.63, respectively. There was no real difference in the glucose, C-peptide response and insulin levels between the U–40 and U–100 strengths of the three 'intermediate-acting' insulin preparations.

Comparing the estimated exogenous insulin levels demonstrated very

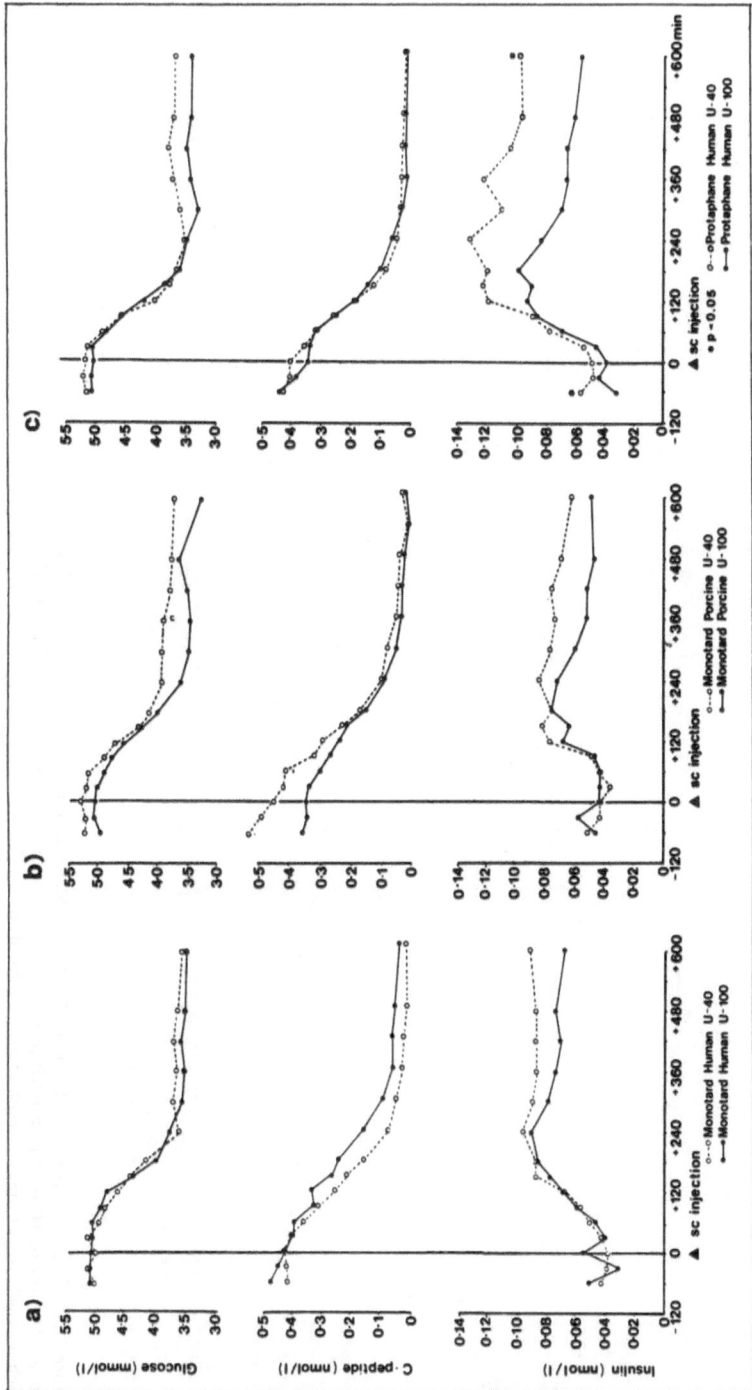

Figure 4.62 Comparison of the effect of U−40 and U−100 strengths of (**a**) human Monotard (Monotard HM), (**b**) porcine Monotard (Monotard MC) and (**c**) human Protaphane (Protaphane HM) insulins on plasma glucose, C-peptide and insulin (IRI) concentrations (means) in six subjects. Insulin (0.30 U/kg) given subcutaneously (sc) at time 0

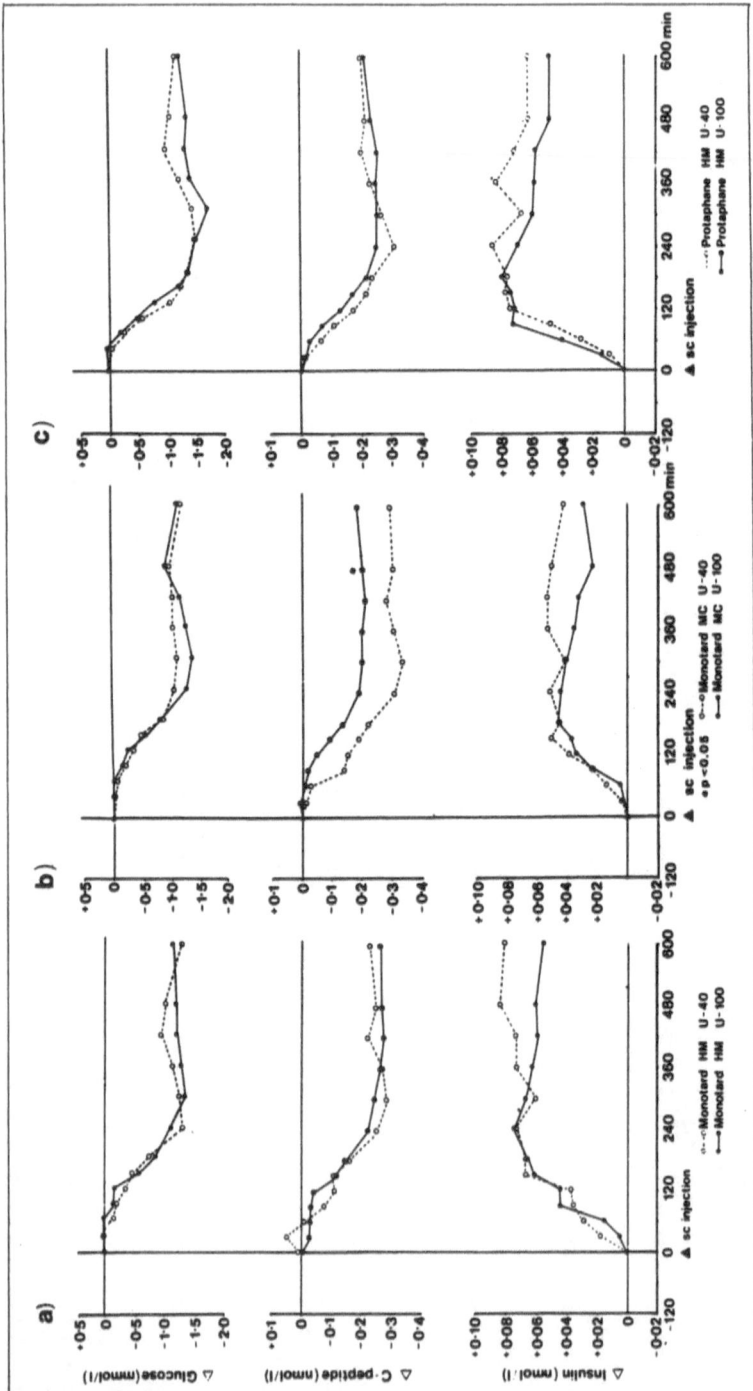

Figure 4.63 Comparisons of the effect of U–40 and U–100 strengths of (**a**) human Monotard (Monotard HM), (**b**) porcine Monotard (Monotard MC) and (**c**) human Protaphane (Protaphane HM) insulins on plasma glucose, C-peptide and insulin (IRI) concentrations in six subjects. Insulin (0.30 U/kg) given subcutaneously (sc) at time 0. Results shown as means of Δ values

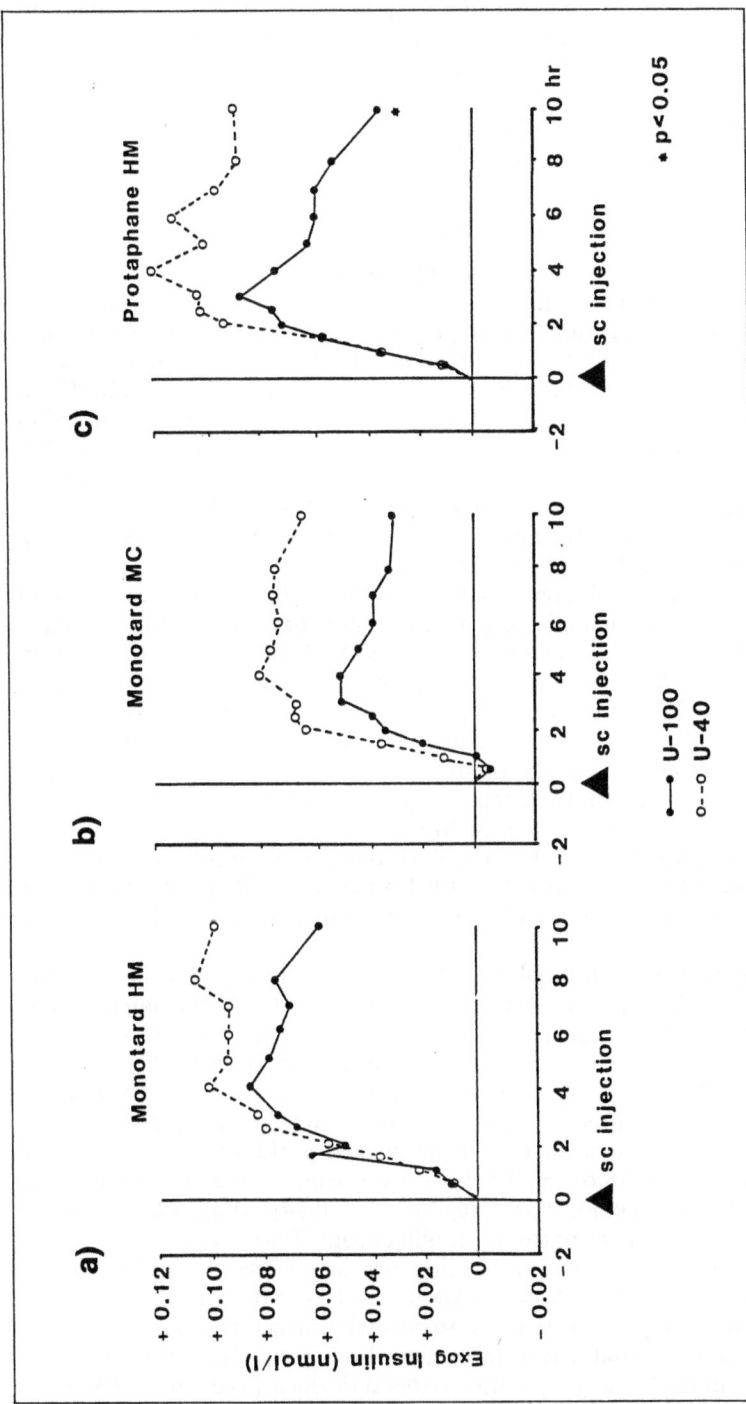

Figure 4.64 Comparison of the estimated ('control day method') plasma exogenous insulin concentrations (means) following the injection of U–40 and U–100 strengths of (a) human Monotard (Monotard HM), (b) porcine Monotard (Monotard MC) and (c) human Protaphane (Protaphane HM) insulins. Insulin (0.30 U/kg) given subcutaneously (sc) at time 0

similar plasma levels for the two concentrations up to 3 to 4 h after injection (Figure 4.64). Thereafter, the mean levels tended to be higher with the U–40 preparations, although the difference between U–40 and U–100 human and porcine Lente insulin did not reach statistical significance. With human NPH insulin, however, the estimated exogenous insulin level was significantly higher with U–40 than U–100 insulin at 10 h only ($p < 0.05$; Figure 4.64).

4.3.2.3 General discussion and summary

At the present time insulins are available for clinical use in various strengths ranging from 40 to 500 IU/ml for the 'short-acting' and from 40 to 100 IU/ml for the 'intermediate-acting' insulin preparations. To minimise life-threatening dosage errors (Joslin, 1946) the American Diabetes Association (1972a, b) and, latterly, the British Diabetic Association, recommended that 100 IU/ml should be the sole insulin strength (Bloom et al, 1981). Since the introduction of U–100 insulin into the USA in 1973 it has been adopted in several other countries, e.g. Canada 1974, Australia/New Zealand 1981 and Britain 1983, whereas most of Europe still uses predominantly U–40 insulin preparations. It is therefore important to be aware of any differences that may exist between the two main strengths of insulin: U–40 and U–100.

There is a measure of agreement between the studies comparing U–40 and U–100 soluble insulins indicating a slower absorption rate with the higher strength (Binder, 1969; Galloway et al, 1981a; Hildebrandt et al, 1983b; Lauritzen et al, 1984). This study demonstrates more clearly that U–40 neutral, soluble human insulin is absorbed more rapidly than its U–100 counterpart, consistent with the observed quicker onset and shorter duration of hypoglycaemia and C-peptide suppression. Interestingly, the 'within' subject variability is greater with U–40 relative to U–100 insulin, possibly a reflection of the more rapid absorption of the former.

The differences between U–40 and U–100 soluble insulin appear to be clinically insignificant (Swift et al, 1983; Lauritzen, 1984) despite the more rapid absorption rate and earlier hypoglycaemic response with the U–40 insulin.

There appears to be little or no difference in the hypoglycaemic response, C-peptide and insulin levels between the two strengths of the 'intermediate-acting' insulin when comparing the response to a single injection of either in different subjects. There appears, however, to be a trend towards higher insulin levels with the U–40 preparations. Further studies are necessary with the 'intermediate-acting' preparations before any reasoned opinion can be formed.

Some studies observed slightly higher glucose profiles and/or glycosylated haemoglobin levels following the changeover from U–40 and U–80 to U–100 insulins (Cartwright et al, 1983; Langdon et al, 1984), whilst others observed no change in glycaemic control or insulin dosage (Parr, 1983).

In conclusion, there is a clear difference in the plasma insulin profiles between the U–40 and U–100 'short-acting' (Actrapid HM) insulin when given subcutaneously at a dose level of 6 U to normal subjects. The magnitude of the difference suggests that it is of little clinical relevance. However, the slower absorption of the U–100 preparation is theoretically a disadvantage (Berger et al, 1982). With hindsight, standardisation at the lower strength of U–40 might have been the best solution for this and other reasons.

Accepting the need for a single strength of insulin, the transfer of patients from U–40 to U–100 insulin should not place the diabetic patient at any greater risk of hypoglycaemia when used at the same dosage level for the same preparations.

4.3.3 Insulin mixtures

Introduction

It was soon realised that one daily injection of the first unmodified 'short-acting' insulin (Banting and Best, 1922b) was inadequate in the majority of patients. The need for multiple injections stimulated the search for insulins with prolonged effect. This resulted in the introduction of a series of 'intermediate-' and 'long-acting' insulin preparations, including protamine insulin (Hagedorn et al, 1936), Protamine Zinc Insulin (Scott and Fisher, 1936), Globin insulin (Bauman, 1939; Reiner et al, 1939), Surfen insulin (Umber et al, 1938), Iso-insulin (Hallas-Møller and Hey, 1944), NPH insulin (Krayenbühl and Rosenburg, 1946) and the Lente insulins (Hallas-Møller et al, 1952).

The inadequacy of Protamine Zinc Insulin (PZI) as a once-a-day insulin (Lawrence and Archer, 1937) prompted clinicians to add soluble insulin to the syringe (Campbell et al, 1936; Lawrence and Archer, 1937; Peck, 1946; Colwell, 1947; Izzo et al, 1953). A ready-made mixture of PZI and soluble insulin (75:25) was suggested but found to be unstable and therefore abandoned (Peck and Schechter, 1944). In 1946, NPH (*N*eutral *P*rotamine *H*agedorn) insulin was introduced to replace such mixtures (Krayenbühl and Rosenberg, 1946). Theoretically, NPH contains stoichiometric quantities of protamine and insulin so that the soluble insulin remains in solution and is available to exert an independent initial effect (Deckert, 1980). The Lente insulins (Semilente, Lente and Ultralente) were developed in an attempt to satisfy the requirements with one daily injection, as the Lente preparations can be mixed with any other member of the Lente trilogy, in any ratio, to give a physically stable mixture. Also mixtures of the biphasic insulin, Rapitard, a suspension of bovine insulin crystals in a neutral solution of porcine insulin (Schlichtkrull et al, 1961) and soluble insulin are physically stable.

In an attempt to achieve glycaemic control as close to physiological as possible, multiple-component insulin regimens have been used in an attempt to provide both meal and basal insulin requirements.

During the late 1970s many considered the maintenance of normal blood glucose an impossible task in practice (Siperstein et al, 1977). However, the introduction of 'closed-loop' insulin infusion devices has clearly demonstrated that plasma glucose concentrations even in unstable insulin-dependent diabetics, with rare exceptions, can be controlled by intravenously delivered insulin (Albisser et al, 1974; Pfeiffer et al, 1974; Kraegen et al, 1977; Mirouze et al, 1977; Santiago et al, 1979). Similar success has been achieved using pre-programmed 'open-loop' insulin infusions *intravenously* (Slama et al, 1974;

Deckert and Lorup, 1976; Santiago et al, 1979; Mirouze et al, 1980; Poulsen et al, 1980; Mirouze and Selam, 1983), *intraperitoneally* (Erwald et al, 1974; Schade et al, 1979; Irsigler et al, 1981; Selam et al, 1983) and *subcutaneously* (Pickup et al, 1978, 1979, 1980a; Slama et al, 1979; Champion et al, 1980; Rizza et al, 1980; Tamborlane et al, 1980) with the aid of blood-glucose monitoring (Walford et al, 1978; Sönksen et al, 1980; Alberti and Home, 1982).

Comparable glycaemic control can also be achieved by the optimisation of conventional subcutaneous insulin therapy on an in-patient basis (Champion et al, 1980; Rizza et al, 1980; Saibene et al, 1981). The results from out-patient studies have been less consistent, demonstrating either an equivalent (Nathan et al, 1982; Reeves et al, 1982; Schiffrin and Belmonte, 1982) or poorer degree of control with multiple-injection regimens compared to subcutaneous insulin infusion (Champion et al, 1980; Home et al, 1982c).

Intensified conventional therapy (ICT) offers the potential to achieve acceptable glycaemic control with the use of multi-component subcutaneous regimens (Skyler et al, 1982). The most popular regimen is the 'split-and-mixed' regimen involving the twice-daily injection of combinations of 'short-' and 'intermediate-acting' NPH or Lente insulin (Oakley et al, 1966; Brownlee, 1979; Skyler et al, 1981, 1982; Ward et al, 1981; Forsham, 1982; Reeves et al, 1982). These commonly used mixtures are physically unstable *in vitro*; the soluble insulin binding to free zinc ions or protamine insulin crystals in Lente or NPH insulins, respectively (Galloway et al, 1982b; Nolte et al, 1982, 1983; Grootendorst et al, 1983). The loss of soluble insulin in such mixtures is seen to increase with increasing proportions of the 'intermediate-acting' insulin and time (Galloway et al, 1982b; Nolte et al, 1983). The interaction is minimised by injecting the admixtures immediately after preparation (Berger et al, 1982; Kølendorf et al, 1983b; Heine et al, 1984a,b). The use of pre-mixed insulin preparations containing soluble and NPH insulins in fixed proportions is advocated for certain categories of patients (Watkins, 1982; Roland, 1984). The insulin in solution in such mixtures, although quoted as being 30%, may be as little as 13% (Galloway et al, 1982b) although the biological effect appears unchanged (Ho and Jawadi, 1984). Recently pre-mixed human insulin preparations have been introduced (Sailer et al, 1982), but no similar analytical data are yet available.

It has been demonstrated recently that there is decreased solubility of 'short-acting' human insulins when mixed with 'intermediate-acting' human insulins *in vitro*, which appears to be much greater in the presence of Lente compared to NPH insulin (Misawa et al, 1984).

Two separate studies were therefore conducted to examine the possible clinical relevance of admixing:

Neutral, soluble and NPH human insulin (study 4.3.3.1),
Neutral, soluble and Lente human insulin (study 4.3.3.2)

in a ratio of 30:70 for the 'short-' and 'intermediate-acting' insulins respectively.

4.3.3.1 Soluble and NPH mixtures

The purpose of this study was to examine the plasma glucose, C-peptide and insulin levels after the subcutaneous administration of the following insulin regimens:

(a) Soluble (Actrapid HM) and NPH (Protaphane HM) 'semi-synthetic' human insulins, in a ratio of 30:70, administered either by:
  - (i) separate injections (Regimen 1),
  - (ii) admixed and injected immediately (Regimen 2),
  - (iii) admixed and injected after 30 min (Regimen 3).
(b) Premixture of soluble and NPH 'semi-synthetic' human insulin (Actra-phane HM, a 30:70 mixture of Actrapid HM and Protaphane HM) (Regimen 4).
(c) Diluting medium as control (Regimen 5).

Subjects, materials and methods

Six volunteer subjects aged 22–31 years were entered into the study. One subject had a family history of diabetes mellitus (father had non-insulin-dependent diabetes) but a pre-study oral glucose tolerance test (75 g) was normal. Each subject was involved in 5 study days separated by 1–4 weeks with the total study period extending over 5 months.

Each study day consisted of a 1 hour basal and 24 hour post-injection period with blood samples taken ½-hourly during the basal and first 3 hours, hourly up to 8 hours and then 2-hourly for the remainder of the study.

The test preparations were administered subcutaneously into the anterior abdominal wall, both sides being used for the separate injections, using a LO-Dose Becton-Dickinson disposable syringe. The total insulin dose per regimen was 20 U, consisting of 6 U of the soluble and 14 U NPH (U-100) insulin, respectively. An equal volume of diluting medium was used during the control days. Details relating to the test materials are included in Table 4.38.

Table 4.38

	Actrapid HM[a]	Protaphane HM[b]	Actraphane HM[b]	Diluent
Nitrogen (mg/ml)	0.531	0.618	0.609	—
Potency[a] (IU/ml)	98	100.9	102	—
Protamine sulphate (mg/ml)	—	0.35	0.25	—
m-Cresol (mg/ml)	—	1.5	1.5	1.5
Phenol (mg/ml)	2.0	0.65	0.65	0.65
pH	7.4	7.3	7.3	7.5

[a] Theoretical potency 185 IU/mgN – Actrapid HM
[b] Potency of NPH-containing preparations (Protaphane HM, Actraphane HM) determined by quantitative high-performance liquid chromatography gel permeation method with monocomponent porcine insulin as standard

The procedures for the preparation and administration of the test materials (Regimens 1–5) were as follows:

Regimen 1 Actrapid HM (6 U) and Protaphane HM (14 U) were administered by separate injections into opposite sides of the anterior abdominal wall. The Protaphane HM vial was gently rolled between the fingers prior to withdrawal of the insulin and injecting immediately.

Regimen 2 Actrapid HM (6 U) and Protaphane HM (14 U) were withdrawn in that order into the same syringe and then injected immediately. The procedure for mixing was standardised for Regimens 2 and 3, i.e. the vial containing Protaphane HM was gently rolled between the fingers prior to withdrawal of the insulin. The same syringe was rolled between the fingers for approximately 2 seconds before injection.

Regimen 3 The Actrapid HM (6 U) and Protaphane HM (14 U) were withdrawn into the same syringe and admixed as described above. The syringe was then allowed to stand for 30 min before injection.

Regimen 4 The vial containing the pre-mixture, Actraphane HM, was gently rolled between the fingers before withdrawing 20 U and injecting immediately.

Regimen 5 0.2 ml of Actrapid HM diluting medium was injected as a control.

At each sampling time venous blood was withdrawn and taken into fluoride for subsequent glucose analysis (glucose oxidase: Yellow Springs glucose analyser, Ohio, USA), and heparin for insulin (modification of Heding, 1972) and C-peptide (modification of Heding, 1975) determinations.

Statistical methods

The results are represented as means ± SE unless stated otherwise. The paired comparisons were made using the Student's t-test on the Δ glucose, C-peptide and insulin values derived by initially correcting for the control day and then subtracting the mean basal ($-1, 0.5, 0$ h) from all subsequent values.

An estimate of the plasma exogenous insulin level was made according to the 'control day method' as described earlier (cf. 4.2.1.1).

The paired comparisons were carried out between the following 'treatments':

   (i)   separate injections (1) vs admixture injected immediately (2),
   (ii) separate injections (1) vs admixture injected after 30 min (3),
   (iii) separate injections (1) vs pre-mixed insulin (4),
   (iv) admixture injected immediately (2) vs after 30 min (3),
   (v)   admixture injected immediately (2) vs pre-mixed insulin (4),
   (vi) admixture injected after 30 min (3) vs pre-mixed insulin (4).

Results

The mean absolute and Δ plasma glucose, C-peptide and insulin levels for the

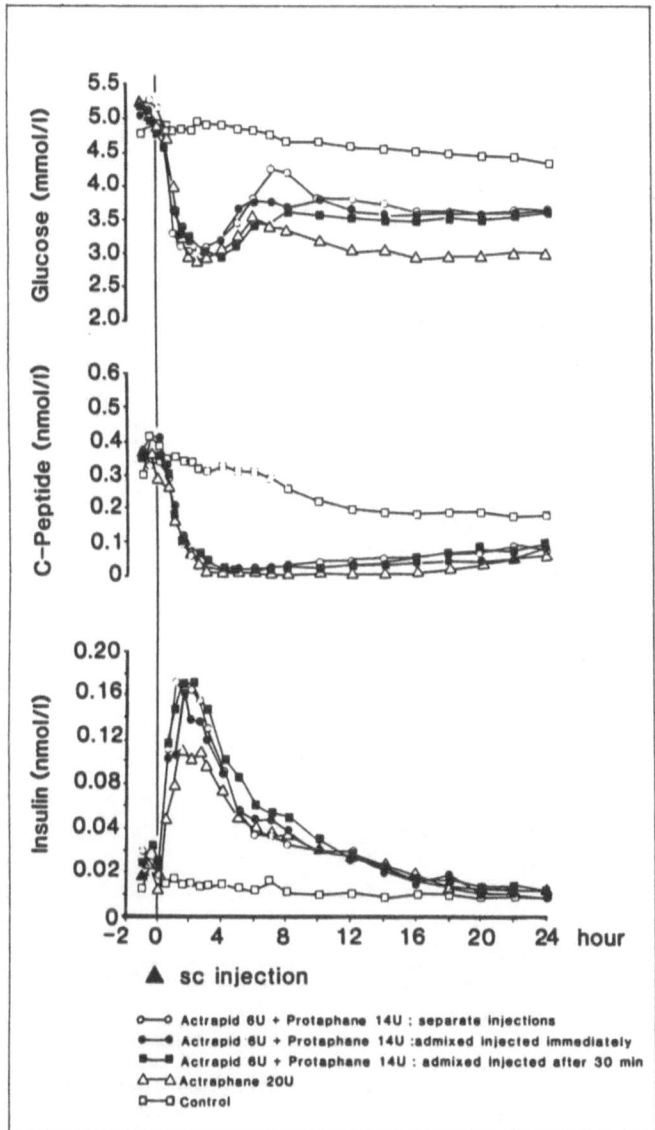

Figure 4.65a Effect of neutral, soluble (Actrapid HM: U–100), NPH (Protaphane HM: U–100) and pre-mixed soluble/NPH (30:70; Actraphane HM: U–100) insulins on plasma glucose, C-peptide and insulin (IRI) concentrations (means) in six subjects. Actrapid (6 U) and Protaphane (14 U) given either by separate injections, admixed and injected immediately or 30 min after preparation. Insulins including Actraphane (20 U) or diluent (control) given subcutaneously (sc) at time 0

five regimens are shown in Figures 4.65a and 4.65b, with the paired comparisons illustrated in Figures 4.66–4.68.

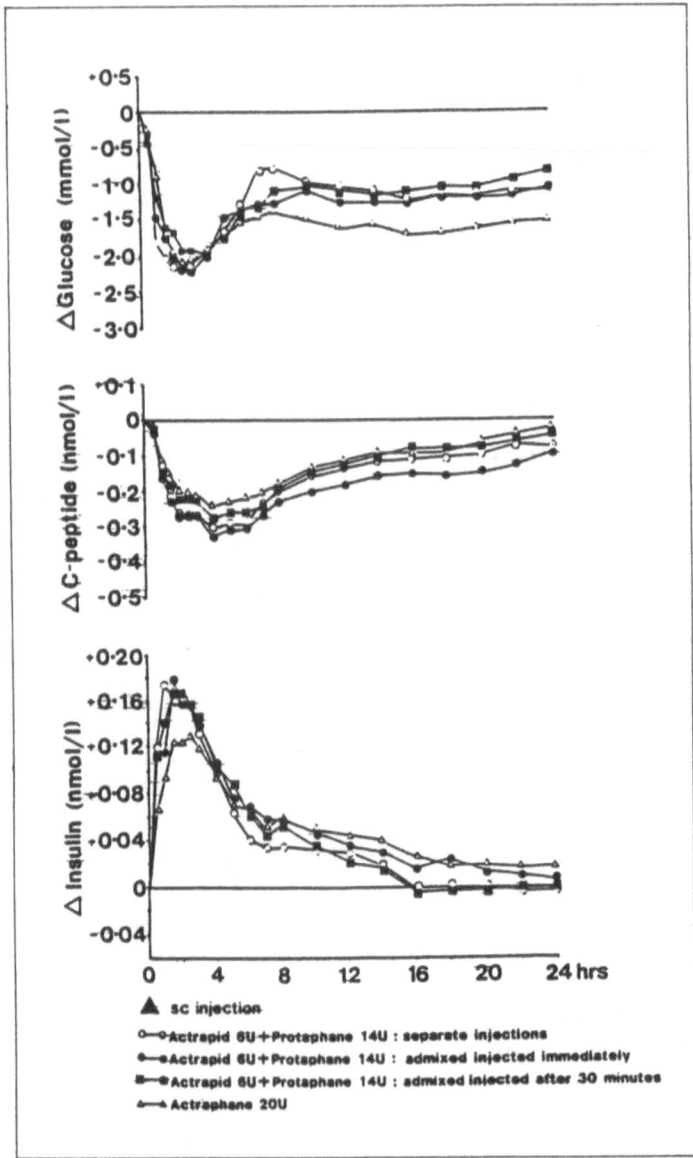

Figure 4.65b Effect of neutral, soluble (Actrapid HM: U–100), NPH (Protaphane U–100) and pre-mixed soluble/NPH (30:70; Actraphane HM: U–100) insulins on plasma glucose, C-peptide and insulin concentrations in six subjects. Actrapid (6 U) and Protaphane (14 U) given either by separate injections, admixed and injected immediately or 30 min after preparation. Insulins including Actraphane (20 U) or diluent (control) given subcutantously (sc) at time 0. Results shown as means of Δ values

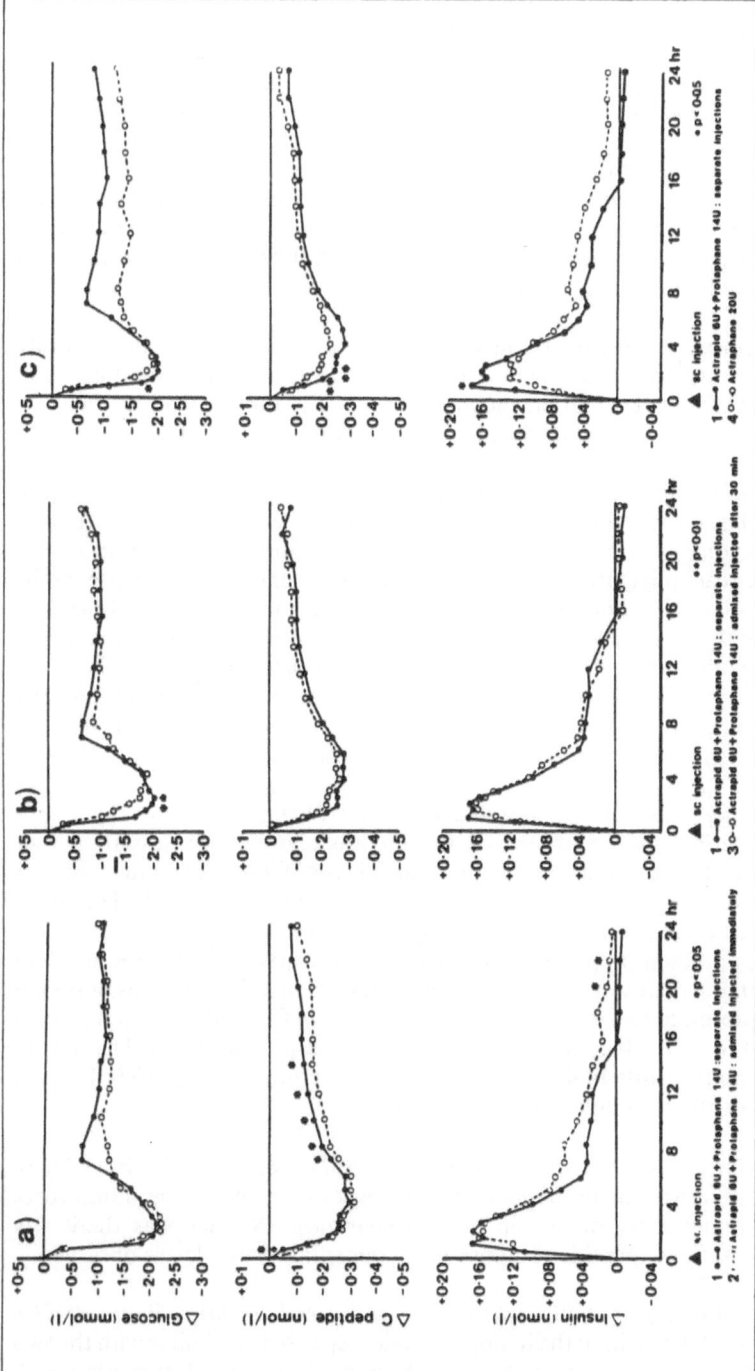

Figure 4.66 Comparison of effect of Actrapid HM: U–100 (6 U) plus Protaphane HM: U–100 (14 U) administered (1) by separate injections, (2) admixed and injected immediately, (3) admixed and injected 30 min after preparation, and (4) pre-mixed (Actraphane HM: U–100; 20 U) on plasma glucose, C-peptide and insulin (IRI) concentrations in six subjects. Insulins given subcutaneously (sc) at time 0. Results shown as means of Δ values

(i) *Separate injections vs admixture injected immediately (Figure 4.66a).* The hypoglycaemic effect was similar with the two regimens, the plasma glucose falling by 2.2 ± 0.3 mmol/l between 2 and 3 h after administration. Over the ensuing 4 to 5 h period the plasma glucose recovered to within 1 mmol/l of the control day values. No further change was observed during the remainder of the study.

The time course of the C-peptide suppression was also similar for the two comparative treatments, with the values reaching a nadir at 4 h followed by a slow recovery to within 0.1 nmol/l of the controls at 24 h. The reduction in plasma C-peptide levels was significantly less ($p<0.05$) between 7 and 14 h with the separate injections, possibly reflecting the trends observed in the glucose levels.

A sharp rise in incremental insulin levels was observed with the separate injections and admixture reaching peak levels of about 0.18 nmol/l at 1 and 1.5 h, respectively. Thereafter, the levels fell equally rapidly over the next 4 h followed by a slower decline during the remainder of the study.

(ii) *Separate injections vs admixture injected after 30 min (Figure 4.66b).* The early reduction in plasma glucose was greater with the separate injections compared to the admixture injected 30 min after preparation, the difference reaching statistical significance at 2 h ($p<0.01$). The glucose nadir, whilst similar with both regimens, occurred 2 h later with the admixture. Subsequently, a rapid recovery in glucose levels was observed over the next 4 to 5 h reaching a plateau approximately 1 mmol/l below control levels.

The C-peptide levels were similar in both studies. The plasma insulin profile with the admixture injected almost immediately after preparation did not differ from that observed with the separate injections.

(iii) *Separate injections vs pre-mixed insulin (Figure 4.66c).* The hypo-glycaemic effect of the pre-mixed insulin was significantly less than that achieved with the separate injections at 1 h ($p<0.05$). Thereafter, similar glucose nadirs were reached at 2.5 h followed by a slower, less marked recovery on the pre-mixed insulin. The degree of C-peptide suppression was also less with the pre-mixed preparation compared to the separate injections at 1.5 to 2.5 h ($p<0.01$). A slower rise in incremental plasma insulin levels was observed with the pre-mixed insulin, reaching a peak level of 0.13 ± 0.03 nmol/l at 2.5 h compared to 0.18 ± 0.03 nmol/l at 1 h for the separate injections. The insulin level was significantly higher on the separate injections at 1 h ($p<0.05$). From 4 h onwards the insulin levels were similar.

(iv) *Admixture injected immediately vs after 30 min (Figure 4.67a).* There was no difference in the hypoglycaemic response between the admixtures injected immediately or 30 min after preparation. Neither was there any difference in the C-peptide response or incremental insulin levels observed.

(v) *Admixture injected immediately vs pre-mixed insulin (Figure 4.67b).* The early part (0 to 8 h) of the hypoglycaemic response was similar with the two comparative insulin regimens. After 8 h the hypoglycaemic effect was less with

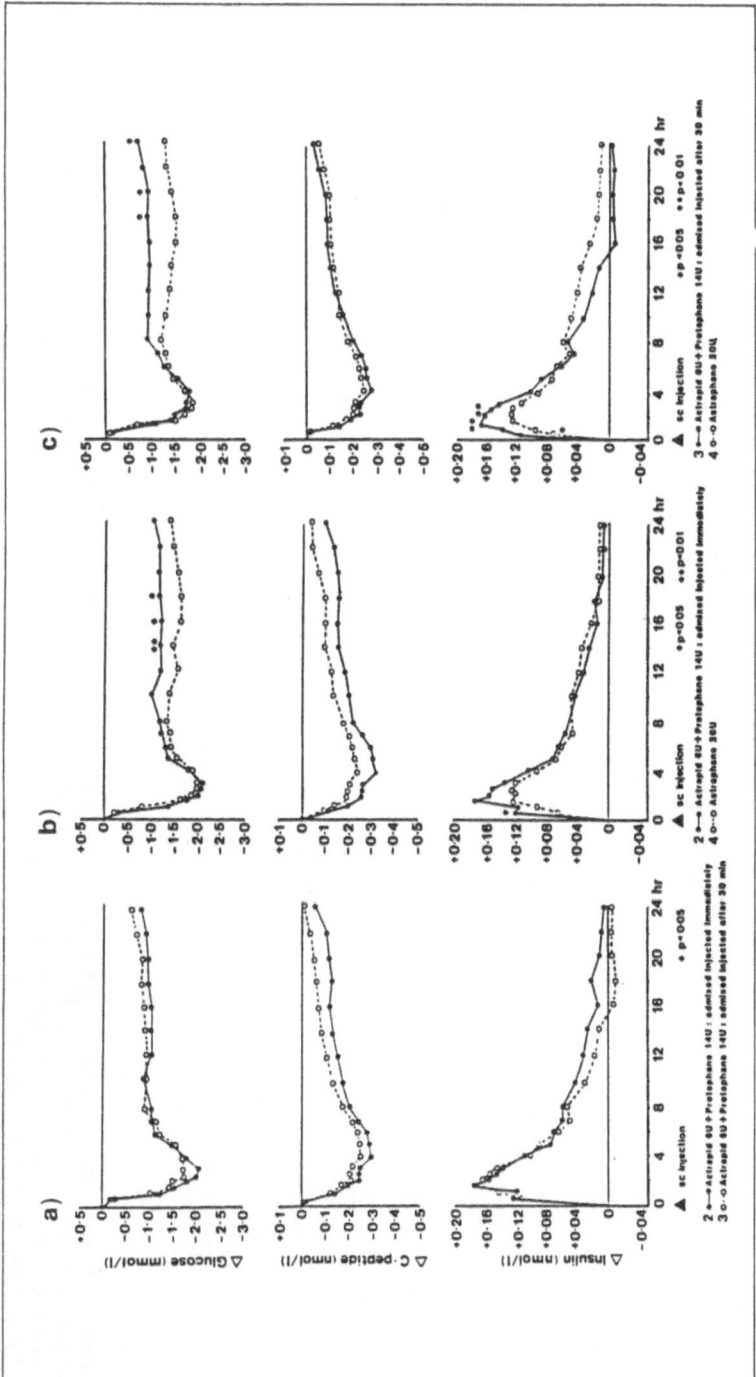

Figure 4.67 Comparison of effect of Actrapid HM: U–100 (6 U) plus Protaphane HM: U–100 (14 U) administered (1) by separate injections, (2) admixed and injected immediately, (3) admixed and injected 30 min after preparation, and (4) pre-mixed (Actraphane HM: U–100; 20 U) on plasma glucose, C-peptide and insulin (IRI) concentrations in six subjects. Insulins given subcutaneously (sc) at time 0. Results shown as means of Δ values

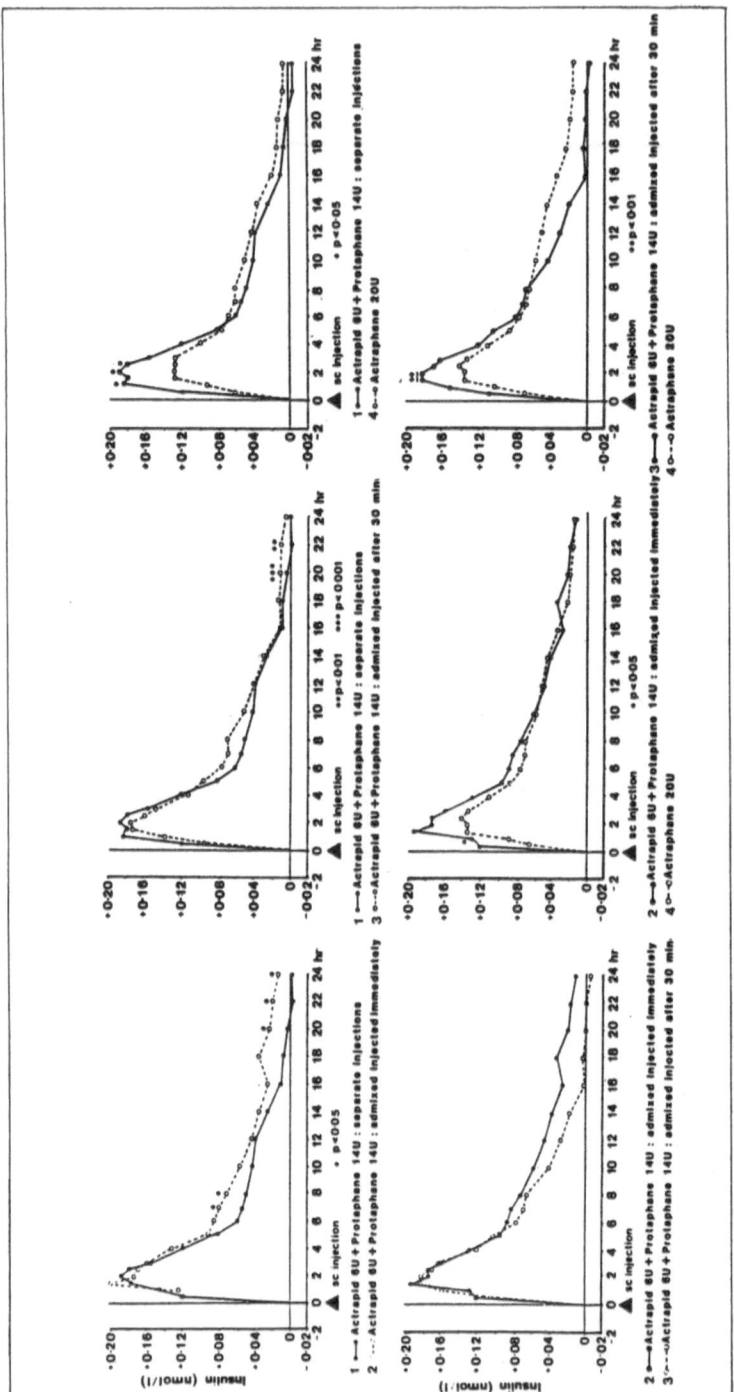

Figure 4.68 Comparison of the estimated ('control day method') exogenous plasma insulin concentrations (means) following the subcutaneous injection of Actrapid HM: U–100 (6 U) plus Protaphane HM: U–100 (14 U) administered (1) by separate injections, (2) admixed and injected immediately, (3) admixed and injected 30 min after preparation, and (4) pre-mixed (Actraphane HM: U–100; 20 U) on plasma insulin, C-peptide and insulin (IRI) concentrations in six subjects. Insulins given subcutaneously (sc) at time 0

the insulin admixture compared to the pre-mixed insulin, the difference reaching statistical significance between 14 and 18 h ($p<0.05$–0.01). There was no difference in the C-peptide levels between the two regimens. A greater incremental insulin level was observed with the admixture at 1 h post-injection ($p<0.05$) compared to the pre-mixed insulin preparation. Thereafter, at 1 to 2 h peak insulin levels of approximately 0.18 nmol/l and 0.13 nmol/l were observed with the separate injections and the pre-mixed insulin, respectively, whereas from 3 h onwards the levels were almost identical.

(vi) *Admixture injected after 30 min vs pre-mixed insulin (Figure 4.67c).* The hypoglycaemic profile was similar with the two comparative treatments up to 8 h after injection. Subsequently, the hypoglycaemic effect was less with the admixture compared to the pre-mixed insulin preparation, the difference reaching statistical significance at 18, 20 and 24 h ($p<0.05$). No differences were evident in the C-peptide levels. The incremental insulin levels were significantly higher with the admixture at 0.5 h ($p<0.05$), 1.5 and 2.0 h ($p<0.01$).

The mean plasma exogenous insulin levels for the four insulin regimens, including the comparison between the groups, are shown in Figure 4.68. The paired comparisons of the estimated exogenous insulin levels between the various 'treatment' regimens are in agreement with the above (i–vi). Significantly higher exogenous insulin levels were observed with the separate injections and admixtures of soluble and NPH insulins compared to the pre-mixed preparation between 1 and 3 h after administration. Similar peak insulin levels were achieved with the soluble and NPH admixtures injected immediately or 30 min after preparation and the separate injections of the individual insulins.

Discussion

The results did not reveal any difference in the hypoglycaemic response between soluble and NPH insulins given by separate injections or admixed and injected immediately after preparation. The early hypoglycaemic response, however, was significantly less at 2 h when the admixture was allowed to stand for 30 min prior to administration. A similar difference was observed between the pre-mixed insulin and the separate injections also during the first 2 h after injection. There was no significant difference, however, in the maximal hypoglycaemic effect achieved with the four insulin regimens compared. In all groups the glucose nadir was achieved within 4 h, followed by a relatively rapid recovery during the subsequent 4 to 6 h period reaching a plateau approximately 1 mmol/l below control values for the remainder of the study. During the second phase of the hypoglycaemic response the glucose levels were lower on the pre-mixed insulin.

Although an earlier peak insulin level was achieved with the separately administered insulins, there was no real difference in the incremental plasma insulin levels between this regimen and the two admixtures when administered immediately or 30 min after preparation. In contrast, the incremental insulin levels observed with the pre-mixed insulin were significantly lower than with the other three insulin regimens during the first 2.5 h. However, from 4 h onwards there was no real difference in the insulin levels between the different insulin regimens, although the effect of dilution on the absorption of the soluble insulin component in the admixtures could not be separated out in these experiments.

The results therefore confirm that soluble and NPH insulins, admixed in a 30:70 ratio and injected either immediately or 30 min after preparation, achieved similar incremental plasma insulin levels to the constituent insulins administered by separate injections (Galloway et al, 1981a; Berger et al, 1982; Galloway et al, 1982b). An increasing proportion of NPH to soluble insulin in such admixtures may, however, lower the peak insulin levels (Galloway et al, 1981b) due to the loss of the soluble insulin fraction as demonstrated *in vitro* (Galloway et al, 1982b; Nolte et al, 1983; Misawa et al, 1984). Binding is minimised by using NPH insulins containing 0.3mg or less of protamine per 100 units of insulin (Galloway et al, 1982b). These findings and previous clinical investigations establish that the binding of soluble insulin to protamine is of no clinical significance when the admixtures are injected immediately after preparation or even allowed to stand for 30 min in the syringe prior to administration (Kølendorf et al, 1978, 1983b; Heine et al, 1984a,b, 1985; Ho and Jawadi, 1984).

Pre-mixed, soluble and NPH porcine, and human insulin preparations are widely used (Renner et al, 1982; Sailer et al, 1982; Roland, 1984). This study clearly demonstrates that a pre-mixed soluble, NPH human insulin preparation results in significantly lower insulin levels during the first 3 h after administration when compared with the individual insulins given by separate injection or admixed and given immediately or 30 min after preparation. The loss of solubility of the 'short-acting' insulin in such pre-mixtures may result in poorer post-prandial glycaemic levels in patients previously mixing the individual insulins prior to administration. The clinical relevance of this observation needs to be established.

4.3.3.2 Soluble and Lente mixtures

The purpose of this study was to examine the interaction of U–100 neutral, soluble (Actrapid HM) and Lente (Monotard HM) human insulin preparations in normal man following bolus subcutaneous administration. The plasma glucose, C-peptide and insulin responses were determined for the following insulin regimens:

Regimens

1. Admixture of *soluble insulin* with its *own diluting* medium
2. Admixture of *soluble insulin* plus *Lente medium* injected *immediately* after preparation
3. Admixture of *soluble insulin* plus *Lente medium* injected *5 min* after preparation
4. Admixture of *soluble* and *Lente insulin* injected *immediately* after preparation

5. Admixture of *soluble* and *Lente insulin* injected *5 min* after preparation
6. Separate injections of *soluble* and *Lente insulins*

Subjects, materials and methods

The study involved 10 normal male volunteer subjects aged 19–26 years, weighing 62–81 kg. Each volunteer received 6 insulin regimens in random order, each on separate days 1 to 3 weeks apart.

Details of the regimens employed are represented schematically in Figure 4.69.

Regimens	Preparations				Administration		
	Insulins (U – 100)		Diluting Media		* Time of admixture (min.)		Separate injection
	ACT	MT	ACT	MT	−5	0	
1	6U		(0.14)			x	
2	6U			(0.14)		x	
3	6U			(0.14)	x		
4	6U	14U				x	
5	6U	14U			x		
6	6U	14U				x	x

ACT = Actrapid HM; MT = Monotard HM.
Values in ( ) = volume (ml)
* Time of admixture prior to administration

Figure 4.69

The admixtures were prepared by withdrawing the soluble insulin into the syringe, followed by either its own medium (1) Lente medium (2, 3) or Lente insulin (4, 5). Prior to withdrawal of the Lente insulin the vial was gently rolled between the fingers for approximately 1 min. For schedules 1, 2 and 4 the admixtures were administered after both preparations had been withdrawn into the syringe, which was then rolled twice between the fingers prior to injection. For schedules 3 and 5 the syringe containing the admixture was also gently rolled between the fingers and then placed on the bench for 5 min. Immediately prior to administration (5 min after completing the initial withdrawal of the soluble and Lente insulin) the syringe was again rolled between the fingers.

Details of the study materials are included in Table 4.39. The dose of soluble insulin (Actrapid HM) was 6 U and of Lente insulin (Monotard HM) 14 U with the volume of either the soluble or Lente diluting medium at 0.14 ml for admixtures 1, 2, 3 (Figure 4.69). The insulins were injected into the anterior abdominal wall using the LO-Dose 0.5 ml Becton-Dickinson syringe. When giving separate injections of the two insulin preparations (6) both sides of the abdomen were used.

Table 4.39

	Actrapid HM (U–100)	Actrapid medium	Monotard HM (U–100)	Lente medium
Nitrogen (mg/ml)	0.537	—	0.543	—
Potency[a] (IU/ml)	99.3	—	100.5	—
Zinc (μg/ml)				
Total	15	—	144	—
Solution	—	—	60.2	47
pH	7.2	7.4	7.3	7.4

[a] Theoretical potency 185 IU/mgN

Venous blood samples were taken at –30, –15, 0 min during the basal period and every 15 min during the first hour, $\frac{1}{2}$-hourly up to 360 min and hourly up to 480 min for all treatment schedules, continuing to 720 min for the Lente insulin regimens (4, 5, 6). Aliquots were taken into fluoride for plasma glucose determination (glucose oxidase, Yellow Springs, glucose analyser, Ohio, USA), and heparin for the measurement of immunoreactive insulin (modification of Heding, 1972) and C-peptide (modification of Heding, 1975) concentrations.

Statistical methods

The results are expressed as means ± SE except where stated otherwise. The statistical analysis was carried out on the absolute and Δ glucose, C-peptide and insulin values. The Δ values were determined by subtracting the mean basal value (–30, 15, 0 min) from all the subsequent levels during each study day. Individual pairs of treatments for the Δ values only were compared using the Student's t-test.

Results

The results are presented in three parts, relating to:

(i)   soluble insulin plus diluting media,
(ii) soluble plus Lente insulin admixtures and separate administration,
(iii) soluble insulin versus soluble plus Lente insulin admixtures and separate administration.

(i) *Soluble insulin plus diluting media (Figures 4.70 and 4.71).* The mean absolute and Δ plasma glucose, C-peptide and insulin levels for soluble insulin admixed with its own diluting medium, and soluble insulin admixed with Lente medium and injected either immediately or after 5 min are shown in

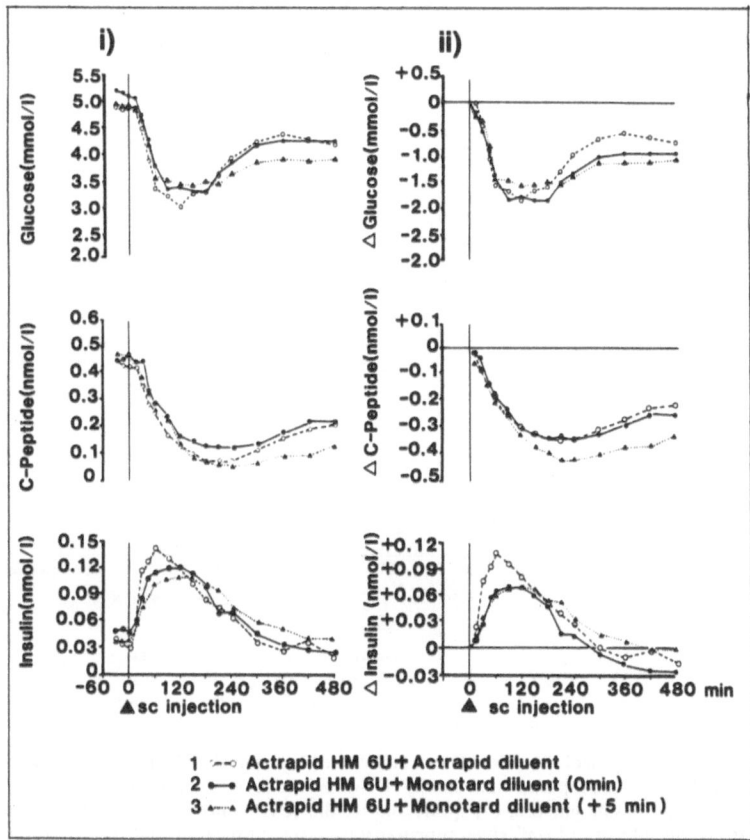

Figure 4.70 Effect of neutral, soluble (Actrapid HM: U-100) insulin admixed with Actrapid diluent and injected immediately (1), Monotard diluent injected immediately (2) or after 5 min (3) on plasma glucose, C-peptide and insulin (IRI) concentrations in ten subjects. Insulin (6 U) plus diluent (0.14 ml) given subcutaneously (sc) at time 0. Results shown as **(i)** means and **(ii)** means of Δ values

Figure 4.70. Paired comparisons between the three regimens (1, 2, 3) are illustrated in Figure 4.71.

(a) Plasma glucose. A similar hypoglycaemic response was observed during the first 120 min after injection of soluble insulin admixed with its own or the Lente diluting medium and injected immediately, leading to a maximal fall of 1.85 ± 0.2 and 1.83 ± 0.2 mmol/l at 120 and 150 min, respectively. A slightly weaker hypoglycaemic effect was observed when the soluble insulin was mixed with the Lente medium 5 min prior to injection achieving a nadir of 1.4 ± 0.2 mmol/l at 180 min. There was a delay in the recovery of plasma glucose towards basal values with the soluble insulin and Lente medium admixtures, the difference reaching significance at 240 min for the admixture injected immediately after preparation. The glucose levels did not differ statistically between the two insulin/Lente medium admixtures, although there was a

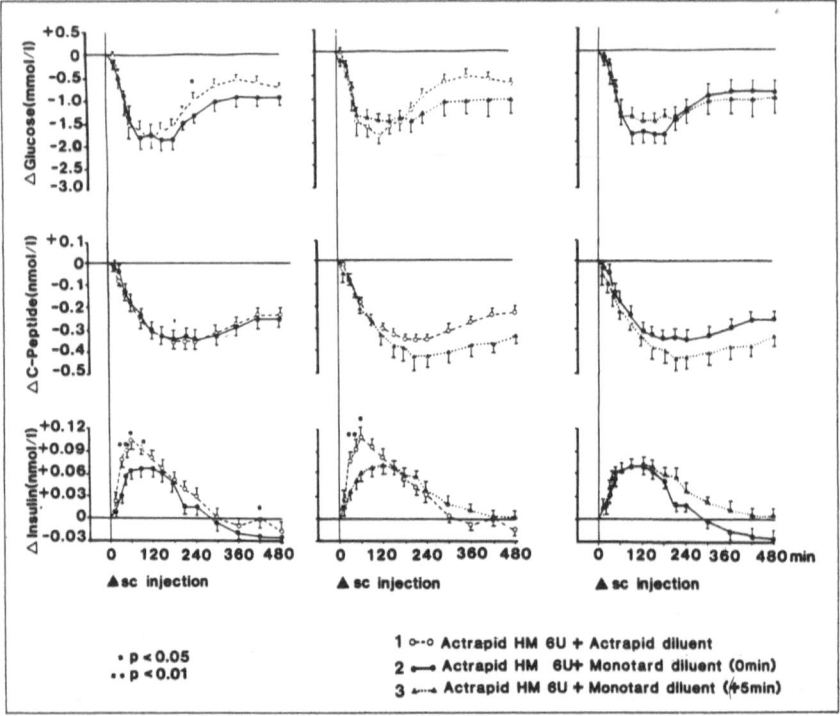

Figure 4.71 Comparison of the effect of neutral, soluble (Actrapid HM: U–100) insulin admixed with Actrapid diluent and injected immediately (1), Monotard diluent injected immediately (2) or after 5 min (3) on plasma glucose, C-peptide and insulin (IRI) concentrations in ten subjects. Insulin (6 U) plus diluent (0.14 ml) given subcutaneously (sc) at time 0. Results shown as means ± SE of Δ values

tendency to a weaker and more delayed hypoglycaemic response with the admixture injected 5 min after preparation.

(b) Plasma C-peptide. The plasma C-peptide response was similar following the injection of soluble insulin after admixing with either its own or Lente medium and injected immediately. A more prolonged suppression of C-peptide was observed with the admixture of soluble/Lente medium allowed to stand for 5 min prior to injection. There was, however, no statistically significant difference between the three comparative regimens.

(c) Plasma insulin. Following the injection of soluble insulin diluted with its own medium, the incremental plasma insulin level reached an early peak of 0.11 ± 0.02 nmol/l at 60 min. In contrast, when the insulin was admixed with Lente medium and injected immediately or after 5 min there was a slower increase in plasma insulin with delayed peaks of 0.073 ± 0.01 and 0.075 ± 0.01 nmol/l at 90 to 120 and 120 min, respectively. The insulin levels were significantly lower with the soluble/Lente medium admixtures between 60 and

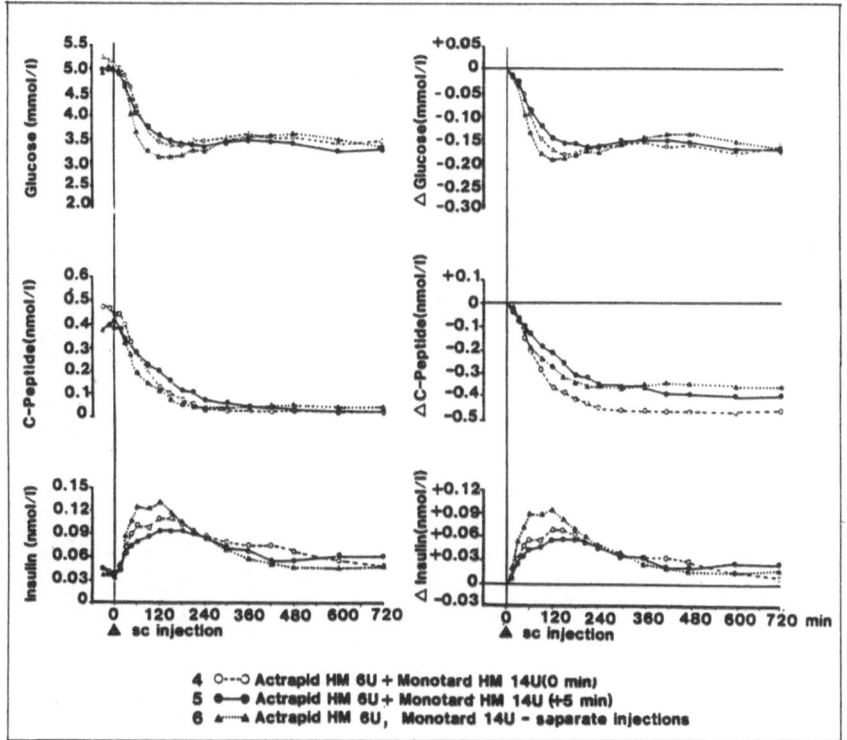

4 ○---○ Actrapid HM 6U + Monotard HM 14U(0 min)
5 ●—● Actrapid HM 6U + Monotard HM 14U (+5 min)
6 ▲┄┄▲ Actrapid HM 6U, Monotard 14U – separate injections

Figure 4.72 Effect of neutral, soluble (Actrapid HM: U–100) plus lente (Monotard HM: U–100) insulins admixed and injected immediately (4) and after 5 min (5) or administered by separate injections (6) on plasma glucose, C-peptide and insulin (IRI) concentrations in ten subjects. Insulins (Actrapid HM 6 U, Monotard HM 14 U) given subcutaneously (sc) at time 0. Results shown as (i) means and (ii) means of Δ values

90 min ($p<0.05$–0.001) compared to the soluble insulin plus its own medium. There was no difference in the plasma insulin profiles between the two soluble and Lente medium admixtures although, from 120 min onwards, the insulin level tended to be higher with the soluble/Lente medium admixture allowed to stand for 5 min before administration.

(ii) *Soluble plus Lente insulin admixtures and separate administration (Figures 4.72 and 4.73).*   The mean absolute and Δ plasma glucose, C-peptide and insulin levels following the subcutaneous administration of soluble and Lente insulin admixed and injected either immediately or 5 min after preparation, and the simultaneous but separate injections of the soluble and Lente insulin are shown in Figure 4.72. The paired comparisons between the three insulin regimens (4, 5, 6) are illustrated in Figure 4.73.

(a) Plasma glucose.   Following the simultaneous but separate injections of the soluble and Lente insulin a maximum fall in plasma glucose of 1.9 ± 0.2

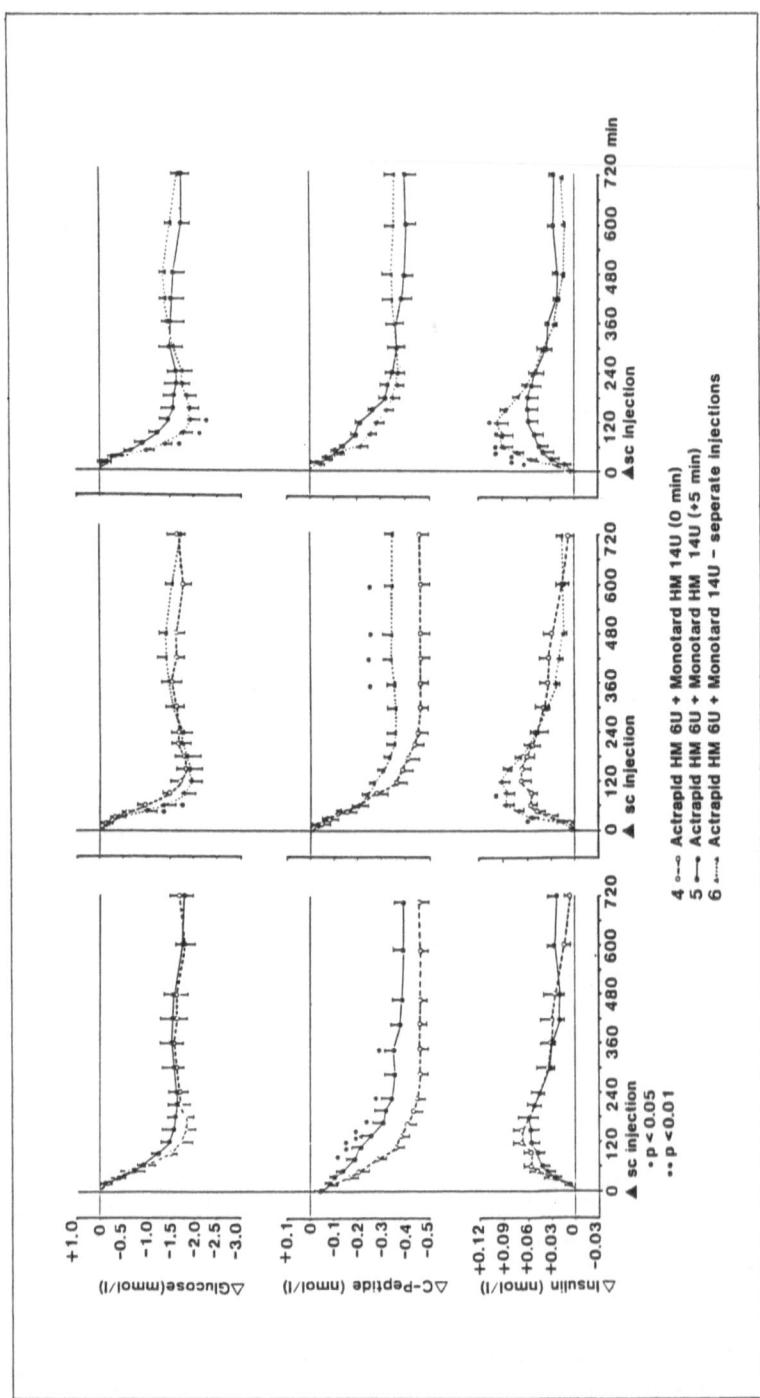

Figure 4.73 Comparison of effect of neutral, soluble (Actrapid HM: U–100) plus lente (Monotard HM: U–100) insulins admixed and injected immediately (4) and after 5 min (5) or administered by separate injections (6) on plasma glucose, C-peptide and insulin (IRI) concentrations in ten subjects. Insulins (Actrapid HM 6U, Monotard HM 14U) given subcutaneously (sc) at time 0. Results shown as means ± SE of Δ values

mmol/l was achieved at 120 min, followed by a slow recovery to within 1.7 ± 0.1 mmol/l of basal values at 720 min. With the admixtures of soluble and Lente insulin injected immediately and 5 min after preparation there was a slower hypoglycaemic response and lesser maximal reductions in glucose levels of 1.5 ± 0.2 and 1.6 ± 0.3 mmol/l at 150 and 210 min, respectively. The hypoglycaemic response was significantly greater ($p < 0.05$) with the separate injections at 45 to 60 min compared to the admixture injected immediately after preparation, and from 60 to 120 min ($p < 0.05$) when compared to the admixture allowed to stand for 5 min.

(b) Plasma C-peptide. After insulin administration the C-peptide levels fell relatively rapidly during the initial 180 to 240 min, with the levels remaining essentially unchanged thereafter. The reduction in C-peptide levels was significantly greater between 60 and 360 min ($p < 0.05$–0.01) with the soluble/Lente admixture injected immediately compared to the same admixture allowed to stand for 5 min and the separate injections between 360 and 600 min ($p < 0.05$). There was no difference in the plasma C-peptide levels between the separate injections and the admixture given 5 min after preparation although there was a tendency to a more delayed response with the latter regimen.

(c) Plasma insulin. The subcutaneous administration of soluble and Lente insulin by separate injections, admixed and given immediately or after 5 min, resulted in peak incremental insulin levels of 0.10 ± 0.02, 0.072 ± 0.01 and 0.061 ± 0.01 nmol/l, respectively, at 120 min. The insulin level was higher during the first 150 min with the separate injections of soluble and Lente insulin than with either of the two admixtures. The values were significantly higher with the separate injections at 30 and 90 min ($p < 0.05$) compared to the admixture given immediately, and from 30 to 120 min ($p < 0.05$–0.01) compared to the admixture given after 5 min. There was no difference between the two admixtures. From 180 min onwards the plasma insulin level was similar in the three comparative groups.

(iii) *Soluble insulin versus soluble plus Lente insulin admixtures and separate administration (Figure 4.74).* These comparisons were carried out to examine the early response (0 to 120 min) to subcutaneously injected soluble insulin when given alone (with diluting medium), together with Lente insulin but by separate injection, and following its admixture with Lente insulin and injected immediately or 5 min after preparation in the syringe. The individual comparisons are shown in Figure 4.74.

(a) Plasma glucose. The early hypoglycaemic response to soluble insulin diluted in its own medium was significantly greater at 45 and 60 min ($p < 0.05$) compared to the soluble plus Lente admixture injected immediately after preparation, and at 60 and 90 min ($p < 0.05$–0.01) compared to the admixture injected 5 min after preparation. There was no difference in the early hypoglycaemic response between the soluble insulin given alone compared to the soluble and Lente insulin given by separate simultaneous injections.

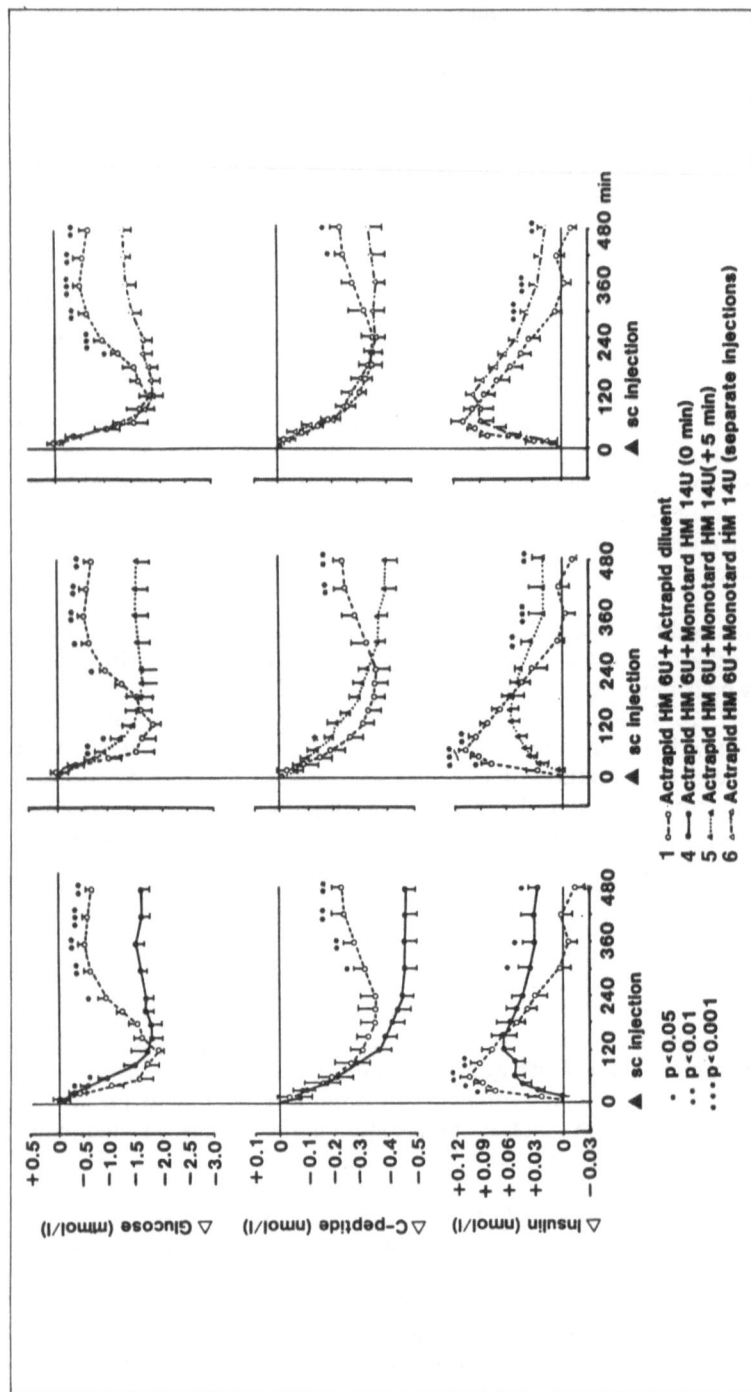

Figure 4.74 Comparison of effect of Actrapid HM (U–100) admixed with Actrapid diluent and injected immediately (1) with Actrapid HM (U–100) and Monotard HM (U–100) insulins, either admixed and given immediately (4) and after 5 min (5) or by separate injections (6) on plasma glucose, C-peptide and insulin (IRI) concentrations in ten subjects. Preparations given subcutaneously (sc) at time 0. Results shown as means of Δ values

(b) Plasma C-peptide. The fall in plasma C-peptide levels was the same when the soluble insulin was given by itself or by separate injection as part of the soluble plus Lente regimen. The early suppression of C-peptide levels was least with the soluble/Lente admixture allowed to stand for 5 min before injection, being significantly less than that observed with the soluble insulin plus its own diluting medium at 90 min ($p < 0.05$).

(c) Plasma insulin. Compared to the admixtures of soluble and Lente insulin administered immediately or 5 min after preparation, the injection of soluble insulin with its own diluent achieved significantly higher ($p < 0.05–0.01$) insulin levels between 30 and 90 min. There was no difference in the early incremental plasma insulin levels between the soluble insulin with its diluent compared to the separate injections of soluble and Lente insulins.

Peak insulin levels were, however, reached earlier at 60 min with the diluted soluble insulin compared to 120 min observed with the undiluted insulin as a part of the separate injections regimen.

4.3.3.3 Discussion

The results confirm the *in vitro* and *in vivo* findings of decreased solubility of the 'short-acting' insulin when admixed with 'intermediate-acting' Lente insulin (Berger et al, 1982; Galloway et al, 1982b; Grootendorst et al, 1983; Nolte et al, 1983; Heine et al, 1984a, b; Misawa et al, 1984). The goal of insulin treatment is to attain glycaemic control as close to physiological as possible, which requires insulin availability to mimic normal endogenous insulin secretion consisting of basal and meal-related secretory patterns. Twice-a-day mixtures of 'short-' and 'intermediate-acting' insulins are commonly used in an attempt to provide insulin with each meal and a basal supply as part of a multicomponent regimen (Skyler et al, 1982; Schade et al, 1983). Such regimens are based on the assumption that the constituent insulin preparations retain their individual physicochemical characteristics.

The results clearly demonstrate that when soluble insulin is admixed with Lente medium there is a marked reduction in insulin levels during the first 90 min after injection. Compared to the rapid increase in plasma insulin reaching peak levels at 60 min with soluble insulin diluted in its own medium, there was a slower rate of absorption resulting in a lower and delayed peak with the insulin plus Lente medium. These differences, however, were barely reflected in the hypoglycaemic response, although there was a tendency to an earlier and shorter-lived effect with the soluble insulin in its own medium. As there was no difference in the plasma insulin profiles between the admixtures of insulin and Lente medium, given immediately or after 5 min, the findings suggest an almost immediate precipitation of the dissolved insulin by the free zinc ions contained in the Lente medium.

Admixing soluble and Lente insulin resulted in a marked blunting of the early plasma insulin profile which occurred even when the admixture was injected almost immediately after preparation. Leaving the admixture to stand for a further 5 min prior to injection caused only a relatively small additional reduction in the resultant plasma insulin levels. Compared to the hypoglycaemic response observed with separate injections of soluble and Lente insulin, admixing the two insulins resulted in a reduced effect during the first 120 min after injection. Delaying the injection of the admixtures further reduced the early hypoglycaemic response.

Therefore, the results demonstrate that to retain the individual characteristics of soluble and Lente insulin when used together they should be administered by separate injection. When soluble and Lente insulin are admixed in a ratio of 3:7, precipitation appears to occur immediately, with only a small additional change when the admixture is left for a further 5 min before injection. Despite the rapid modification of the soluble insulin fraction about 50% is still preserved (Nolte et al, 1983). A lesser interaction is evident with a higher soluble to Lente ratio (Galloway et al, 1981a; Berger et al, 1982; Nolte et al, 1983) and also with the USP formulation (U–100) compared to the BP formulation (U–40) (Brange et al, 1985).

Whereas admixtures of soluble and isophane insulin are also physically unstable (Galloway et al, 1982b; Nolte et al, 1983) there is little or no loss of the early plasma insulin peak due primarily to the 'short-acting' insulin, even when such admixtures are allowed to stand for up to 2 days prior to administration (Heine et al, 1984a, b). This has not, however, been confirmed for the pre-mixed soluble/isophane insulin preparations.

It is important to be aware of the interaction of soluble and Lente insulin, which may necessitate an adjustment in the ratio of the soluble to Lente insulin. The influence of admixing on glycaemic control may be minimised by ensuring that the insulin mixing procedure is standardised, and the insulin is given 15–30min before the meal (Kinmonth and Baum, 1980; Lean et al, 1985). However, to retain the individual characteristics of the soluble and Lente insulins within the limitations of the day-to-day variation, they should not be mixed in the same syringe but administered by separate injections.

4.3.4 'Within' and 'between' subject variation

Introduction

One of the important features of subcutaneous insulin absorption is the 'within' and 'between' subject variation (Binder, 1969; Galloway et al, 1981a; Binder et al, 1984). Despite its obvious clinical relevance, relatively little attention has been paid to this important aspect of insulin absorption.

There is considerable systematic (non-random), as well as random 'within' subject variation in insulin absorption from a subcutaneous depot, when using ^{125}I-labelled insulin and examining the disappearance of radioactivity by external counting over the injection site (Nora et al, 1964; Binder et al, 1967). The systematic part of the 'within' subject variation using this method of assessing the absorption of insulin varies according to the site of injection and formulation of the insulin used (Binder et al, 1967; Binder, 1969; Kølendorf et al, 1978, 1983a; Hansen et al, 1979; Lauritzen et al, 1979; Kølendorf and Bojsen, 1982). The random 'within' subject coefficient of variation for insulin absorption (expressed as $T_{50\%}$) is approximately 30% for the purified insulins when measured on two consecutive days using this indirect technique (Kølendorf et al, 1978). In comparison, the 'between' subject coefficient of variation for the half-time of disappearance ($T_{50\%}$) of labelled insulin is up to 50% for all the insulins studied (Binder, 1969; Kølendorf et al, 1983a). Lauritzen et al (1979) observed that the daily absorption of the 'intermediate-acting' insulin (Lente, NPH) varied from 19 to 104% of the insulin dose. Galloway and co-workers (1981b) observed a 'within' and 'between' subject coefficient of variation in peak plasma insulin levels for soluble, NPH and Lente insulins of approximately 50 and 64%, 37 and 44%, and 36 and 28%, respectively. Such a variation could well contribute to the day-to-day variation in glycaemic control observed in insulin-treated diabetics (Molnar et al, 1972; Molnar and Reynolds, 1977). Changes in subcutaneous blood flow may account for the majority of the variability in insulin absorption (Nielsen and Larsen, 1973; Kølendorf et al, 1979). Differences in subcutaneous blood flow have also been described with varying thickness of adipose tissue (Larsen et al, 1966), a possible explanation for the delayed pattern of insulin absorption with increased adiposity (Birtwell et al, 1983).

It is therefore necessary to examine the 'within' and 'between' subject variation in both the absorption and response to subcutaneously administered insulin preparations.

Purpose of study

The main purpose of this study was to investigate the 'within' and 'between' subject variability in the plasma glucose, C-peptide and insulin concentrations following the subcutaneous injection in fasted healthy normal volunteer subjects of:

(i) neutral, soluble human insulin (Actrapid HM: U–100);
(ii) Lente human insulin (Monotard HM: U–100).

The study involved two separate groups of 12 volunteers for sections (i) and (ii), respectively. In each study the subjects received only the 'short-acting' or 'intermediate-acting' insulin preparation on two separate occasions 7 to 10 days apart.

All samples were assayed for glucose (glucose oxidase, Yellow Springs glucose analyser, Ohio, USA), insulin (IRI) (modification of Heding, 1972) and C-peptide (modification of Heding, 1975).

Statistical methods

The individual pairs of treatments were compared using the Student's t-test. The 'within' subject $SD_W = \sqrt{(\Sigma d^2/2n)}$, where Σd^2 is the sum of the squared differences between the pairs and n is the number of subjects. The 'between' subject SD_B was calculated as

$$SD_B = \sqrt{(SD_W^2/2 + \Sigma(x-\bar{x})^2/n-1)}$$

where $\Sigma (x-\bar{x})^2/n-1$ is the usual variance estimate calculated from the means ($\bar{x}$) of the pairs. The $SD^2w/2$ is added to account for the reduced 'within' subject variation of the mean of the pairs. The analyses were carried out on the absolute and Δ values, the latter derived by subtracting the mean pre-injection value of the -30 and 0 min samples from all subsequent levels for each study day. An estimate of the exogenous insulin level was determined according to the 'initial ratio method' described in study 4.2.1.1.

For each study the results obtained on the first and second study days were compared to check whether significant 'order of treatment' effects were present. In addition, the data were re-analysed after randomisation of the study days into two hypothetical 'treatment' groups, i.e. treatment 1 and 2 for the two categories of insulin, i.e. the 'short-' and 'intermediate-acting' insulins.

The two parts of the study dealing with the 'short-acting' neutral, soluble human insulin and 'intermediate-acting' Lente human insulin are presented separately in sections 4.3.4.1 and 4.3.4.2, respectively.

4.3.4.1 Soluble insulin (U-100)

Subjects, materials and methods

Twelve normal male subjects were recruited into the study, although one subject did not complete the study for unrelated reasons. The eleven volunteers who completed the study had a mean age of 28 years (range 20–35 years) and weight of 79 kg (range 61–85 kg).

The insulin preparation used was Actrapid HM (U–100), nitrogen content 0.537 mg/ml, potency 99.3 IU/ml (theoretical potency 185 IU/mg N). The subjects were studied on two separate occasions 7–10 days apart, i.e. Day 1 and 2, respectively.

After a 30 min basal period the insulin was injected at a dose level of 0.1 U/kg subcutaneously into the right or left side of the anterior abdominal wall. Samples were taken every 10 min during the first hour, and every 30 min up to 360 min post-injection.

Results

The results are presented as follows:

(i) Day 1 versus day 2,
(ii) 'Treatment 1' versus 'treatment 2'.

(i) *Day 1 versus day 2 (Figures 4.75–4.77).* The mean absolute and Δ plasma glucose, C-peptide and insulin levels are illustrated in Figures 4.75a and 4.75b, respectively. The mean difference between the response variables on the two study days with 95% confidence limits are shown in Figures 4.75c and 4.75d for the absolute and adjusted values, respectively.

After insulin administration on the first day, the plasma glucose fell from 5.1 ± 0.1 mmol/l to a nadir of 3.0 ± 0.2 mmol/l at 150 min. Thereafter, the glucose

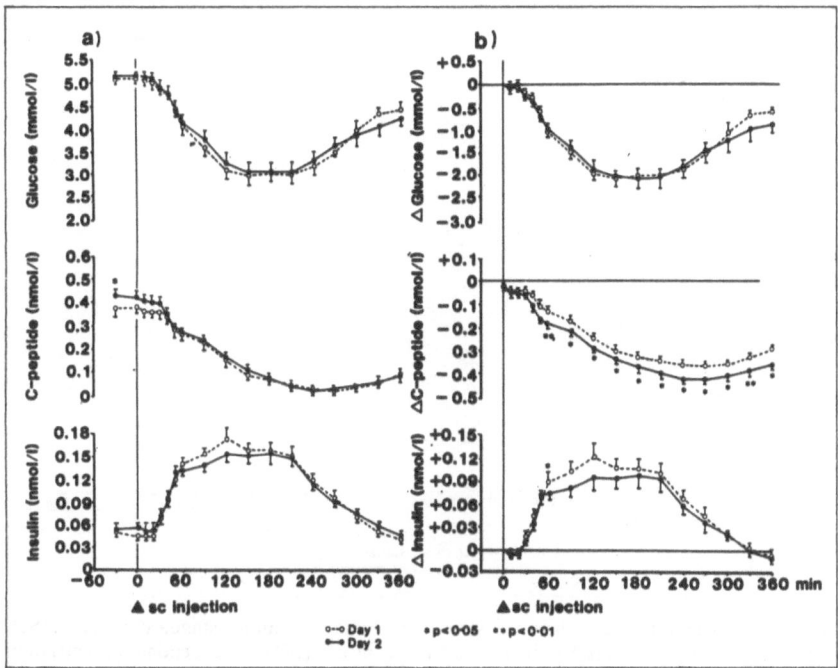

Figure 4.75a, b (a) Comparison of effect of neutral, soluble human insulin (Actrapid HM: U–100) on two separate days (day 1 and 2) on plasma glucose, C-peptide and insulin (IRI) concentrations (means ± SE) in eleven subjects. Insulin (0.10 U/kg) given subcutaneously (sc) at time 0. (b) Results shown as means ± SE of Δ values

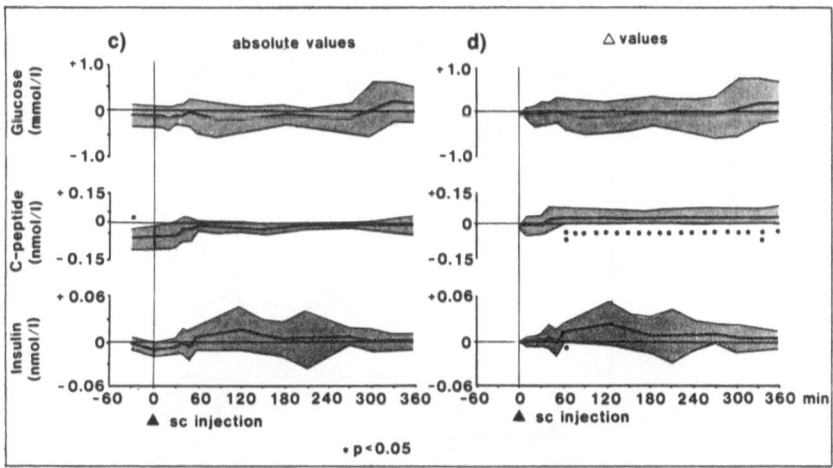

Figure 4.75c, d (c) Comparison of effect of neutral, soluble human insulin (Actrapid HM: U–100) on two separate days on plasma glucose, C-peptide and insulin (IRI) concentrations in eleven subjects. Insulin (0.10 U/kg) given subcutaneously (sc) at time 0. Results shown as means of differences (with 95% confidence limits) between responses on the two days. (d) Results shown as means of differences (with 95% confidence limits) between the Δ values on the two days

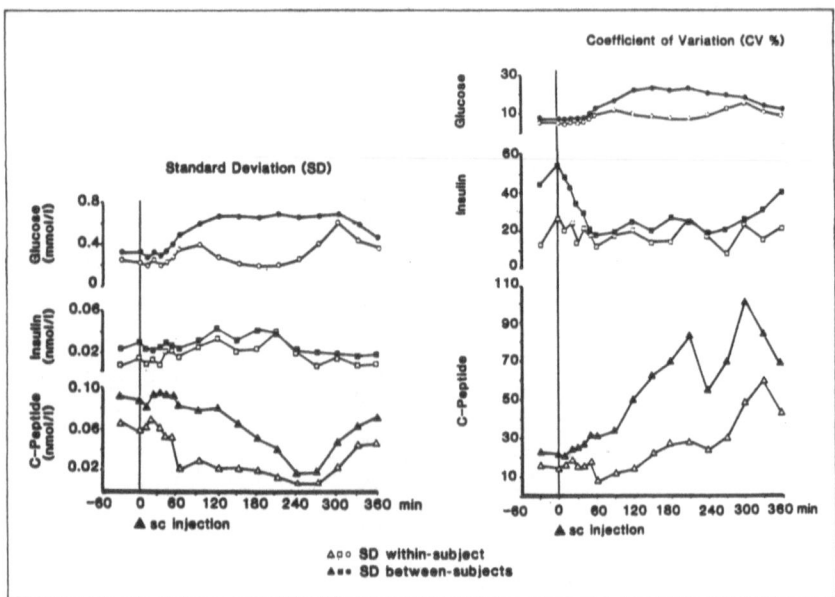

Figure 4.76 The 'within' and 'between' subject day-to-day variation – standard deviation (SD) and coefficient of variation (CV) – in plasma glucose, insulin (IRI) and C-peptide concentrations in eleven subjects. Insulin (Actrapid HM: U–100; 0.10 U/kg) given subcutaneously (sc) at time 0

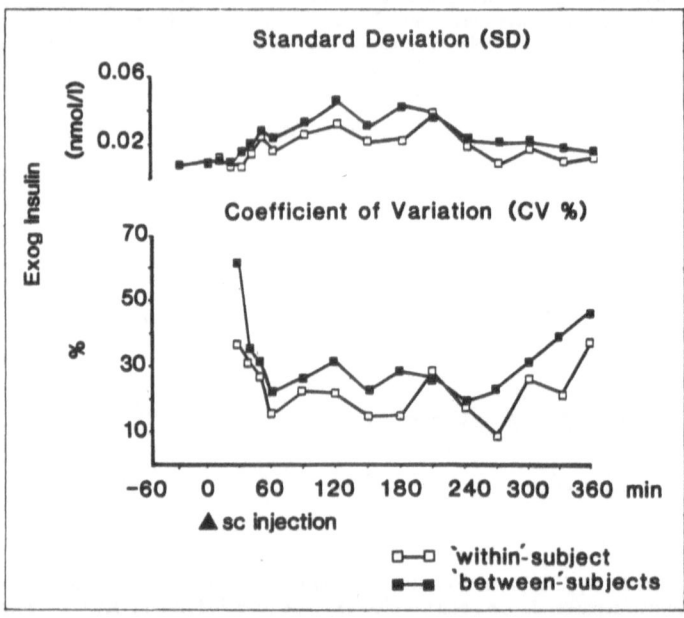

Figure 4.77 The 'within' and 'between' subject day-to-day variation – standard deviation (SD) and coefficient of variation (CV) – in the estimated ('initial ratio method') exogenous insulin concentrations. Insulin (Actrapid HM: U–100; 0.10 U/kg) given subcutaneously (sc) at time 0

slowly recovered to 4.5 ± 0.1 mmol/l by the end of the study period. In comparison on the second study day, the pre-injection glucose level was similar at 5.2 ± 0.1 mmol/l falling to 3.1 ± 0.12 nmol/l at 150 min and returning to 4.3 ± 0.2 mmol/l at 360 min. There was no significant difference in the hypoglycaemic response to the same insulin given on the two serial occasions.

The plasma insulin level increased from 0.048 ± 0.008 and 0.059 ± 0.01 nmol/l at time 0 min to reach peak levels of 0.18 ± 0.01 and 0.16 ± 0.01 nmol/l at 120 and 150 min on the first and second study days, respectively. The plasma insulin levels were not significantly different on the two study days for the absolute values. The incremental insulin values (Δ values), however, were significantly higher ($p < 0.05$) on the first day at 60 and 270 min.

The C-peptide concentrations fell from 0.39 ± 0.02 and 0.43 ± 0.03 nmol/l to the minimum level of 0.25 ± 0.01 and 0.27 ± 0.01 nmol/l at 270 min during study days 1 and 2, respectively. The absolute C-peptide levels differed between the two study days only for the first basal sample (–60 min), which was significantly higher ($p < 0.05$) on the second day. Consequently, when the Δ values were compared, the reduction in plasma C-peptide levels was significantly greater ($p < 0.05$–0.01) on the second day from 60 min onwards.

The 'within' and 'between' subject standard deviations for plasma glucose insulin and C-peptide are represented in Figures 4.76 and 4.77. The results demonstrate considerable 'between' subject variation in the basal 'fasting' insulin and C-peptide levels. After insulin a greater degree of heterogeneity, SD 'between' (SD_B) relative to SD 'within' subjects (SD_W) was observed in the hypoglycaemic response ('insulin sensitivity') compared to the plasma insulin profiles ('insulin pharmacokinetics'). This observation was reflected in the coefficient of variation estimates (Figures 4.76, 4.77).

(ii) 'Treatment 1' versus 'treatment 2' (Figure 4.78).   The mean absolute and Δ plasma glucose, C-peptide and insulin levels between the two hypothetical treatments ('treatments' 1 and 2) are shown in Figures 4.78a and 4.78b, respectively, with the mean difference plus 95% confidence limits included in Figures 4.78c and 4.78d, respectively.

The hypoglycaemic response was, as expected, almost identical for the two treatments, with the plasma glucose falling from 5.1 ± 0.1 mmol/l to 3.0 ± 0.2 and 3.1 ± 0.2 mmol/l on treatments 1 and 2, respectively, before recovering to 4.4 ± 0.2 mmol/l at the end of both treatment periods. Similarly there was no difference in the degree of C-peptide suppression between the treatments. The plasma insulin profiles were also similar for the two treatments.

Discussion

(i) Day 1 versus day 2

There was no difference in the hypoglycaemic response to neutral, soluble human insulin (U–100) at a dose level of 0.1 U/kg when administered to normal man on two sequential occasions 7–10 days apart. The suppression of C-peptide levels was apparently greater on the second day despite no difference in

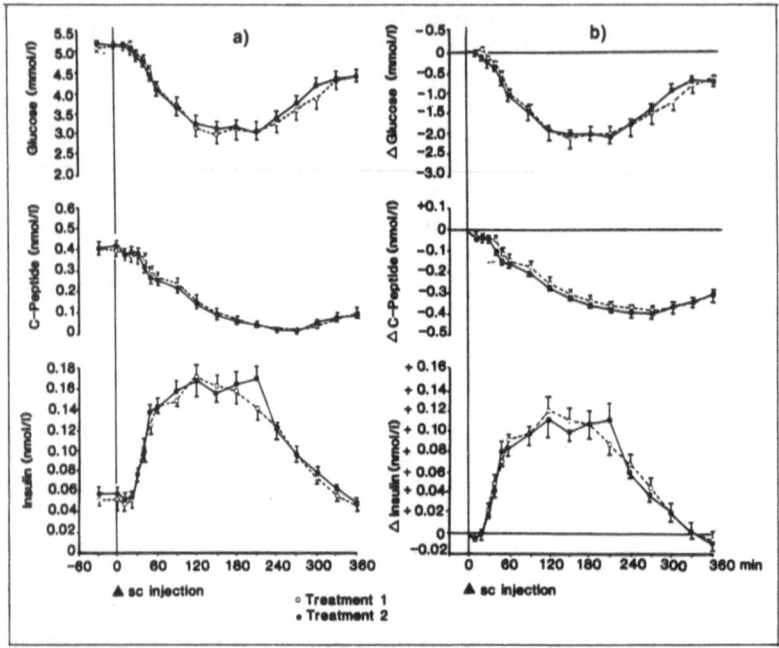

Figure 4.78a, b (a) Comparison of effect of hypothetical treatments 1 and 2 (Actrapid HM: U-100) on plasma glucose, C-peptide and insulin concentrations (means ± SE) in eleven subjects. Insulin (IRI) (0.10 U/kg) given subcutaneously (sc) at time 0. (b) Results shown as means ± SE of Δ values

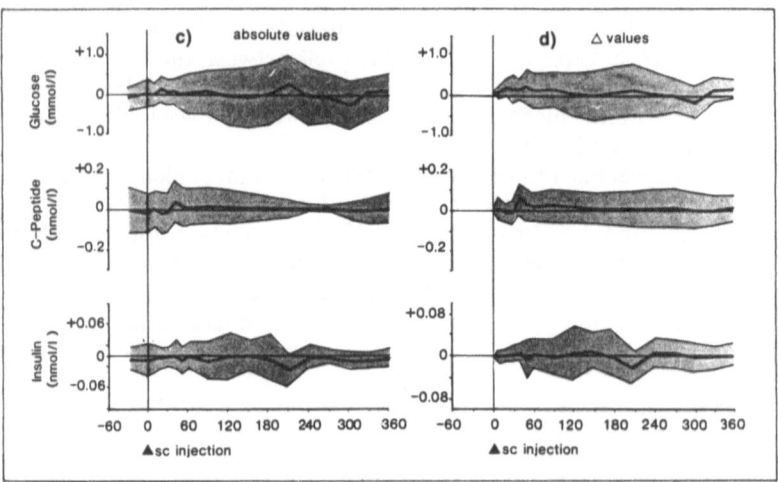

Figure 4.78c, d (c) Comparison of effect of hypothetical treatments 1 and 2 (Actrapid HM: U-100) on plasma glucose, C-peptide and insulin (IRI) concentrations in eleven subjects. Insulin (0.10 U/kg) given subcutaneously (sc) at time 0. Results shown as means of differences (with 95% confidence limits) between responses to the two 'treatments'. (d) Results shown as means of differences (with 95% confidence limits) between the Δ values with the two 'treatments'

the glucose responses and the higher incremental insulin levels on the first compared to the second study day. The significantly higher fasting C-peptide level on the second study day reflects a systematic change in the subject's basal insulin secretion from the first to the second experimental day, but a few random significant outcomes could also be expected.

The results demonstrate a greater 'between' than 'within' subject variability in the hypoglycaemic response, in contrast to the similar 'between' and 'within' subject variations in plasma insulin levels. This suggests a larger difference in 'insulin sensitivity' than 'insulin kinetics' between the subjects.

(ii) 'Treatment 1' versus 'treatment 2'

There was no statistically significant difference in the hypoglycaemic response, C-peptide and insulin levels between the study days when randomised into two hypothetical treatment groups, emphasising the importance of adopting a randomisation procedure when comparing insulin preparations of similar type.

4.3.4.2 Lente insulin (U-100)

Subjects, materials and methods

Twelve normal male subjects aged 20–40 years (mean 26 years) and weighing 60–92 kg (mean 74 kg) were included in the study. The insulin dose ranged from 18 to 28 U, i.e. 0.30 U/kg body weight. The insulin preparation used was Monotard HM (U–100), nitrogen content 0.531 mg/ml, potency 98.2 IU/ml (theoretical potency 185 IU/mgN). The volunteers were studied on two separate occasions 7–10 days apart, i.e. day 1 and 2, respectively. After a 1h basal period the insulin was injected at a dose of 0.30 U/kg subcutaneously into the left or right side of the anterior-abdominal wall mid-way between the umbilicus and anterior superior iliac spine. Venous blood samples were taken $\frac{1}{2}$-hourly during the basal period and for the first 3h after injection, then hourly up to 8h, 2-hourly up to 16h and, finally, 4-hourly up to 24h.

Results

The results are presented as follows:
(i)   Day 1 versus day 2,
(ii) 'Treatment 1' versus 'treatment 2'.

(i) *Day 1 versus day 2 (Figures 4.79–4.81).*   The mean absolute and Δ plasma glucose, C-peptide and insulin levels are shown in Figures 4.79a and 4.79b, respectively. Figures 4.79c and 4.79d represent the mean difference with 95% confidence limits between the two study days.

Following the subcutaneous insulin injection of the Lente insulin, there was a relatively slow fall in plasma glucose over the 24h study period from pre-injection levels of 5.1 ± 0.1 and 5.0 ± 0.1 mmol/l to 3.3 ± 0.1 and 3.3 ± 0.2

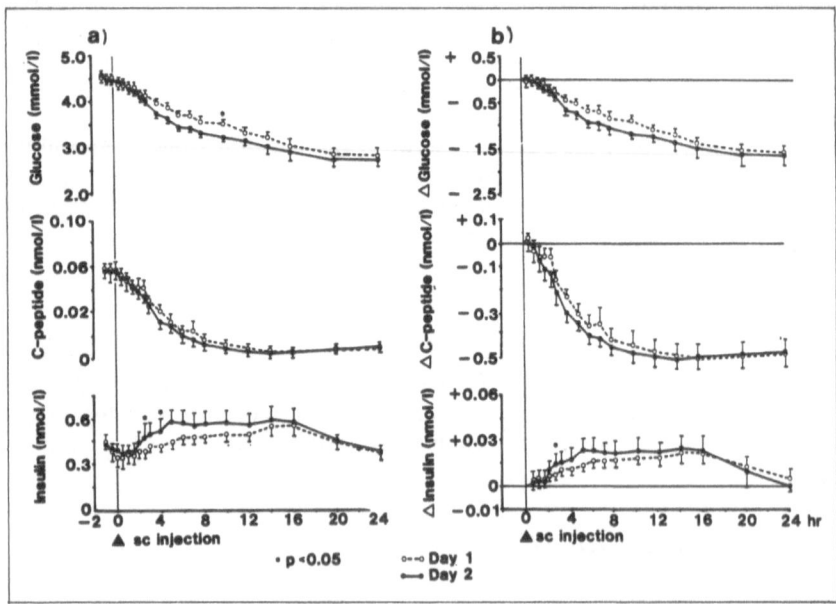

Figure 4.79a, b (a) Comparison of effect of human Monotard insulin (Monotard HM: U–100) on two separate days (day 1 and 2) on plasma glucose, C-peptide and insulin (IRI) concentrations (means ± SE) in twelve subjects. Insulin (0.30 U/kg) given subcutaneously (sc) at time 0. (b) Results shown as means ± SE of Δ values

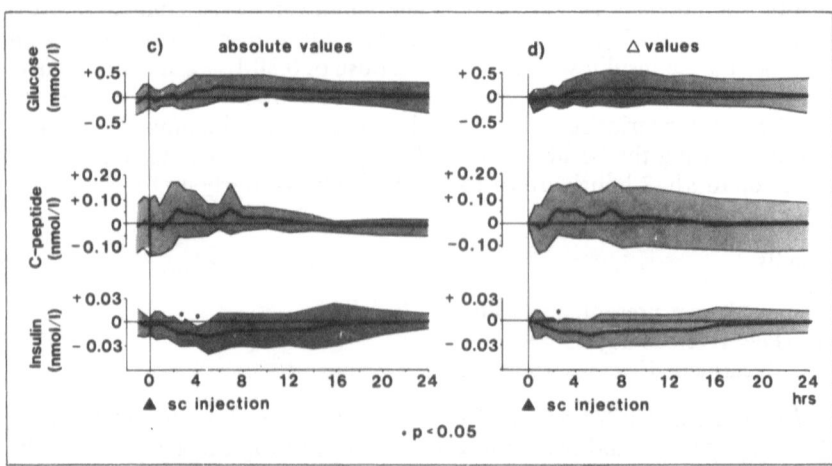

Figure 4.79c, d (c) Comparison of effect of human Monotard insulin (Monotard HM: U–100) on two separate days on plasma glucose, C-peptide and insulin (IRI) concentrations in twelve subjects. Insulin (0.30 U/kg) given subcutaneously (sc) at time 0. Results shown as means of differences (with 95% confidence limits) between responses on the two days. (d) Results shown as means of differences (with 95% confidence limits) between the Δ values on the two days

mmol/l for the first and second study days respectively. The plasma glucose level was significantly lower at 10 h ($p<0.05$) on day 2, which was not apparent for the Δ values.

During study days 1 and 2 the C-peptide fell from basal levels of 0.58 ± 0.05 and 0.59 ± 0.05 nmol/l to 0.07 ± 0.02 and 0.05 ± 0.02 nmol/l at 12 h, i.e. a fall to approximately 10% of pre-injection levels. Thereafter, the levels remained unchanged up to the end of the 24 h study period. There was no significant difference in the plasma C-peptide concentrations between the two study days, although the levels tended to be higher during the first 12 h on the first day in agreement with the glucose levels.

After injection, the plasma insulin increased from fasting levels of 0.046 ± 0.006 and 0.052 ± 0.006 nmol/l reaching similar peak levels of 0.075 ± 0.01 and 0.082 ± 0.01 nmol/l at 14 h. The insulin level was significantly higher ($p<0.05$) on the second study day at 2.5 and 5 h post-administration. For the incremental insulin levels the difference was significant at only one time point, i.e. 2.5 h ($p<0.05$). This difference was reflected in the C-peptide levels.

The 'within' and 'between' subject standard deviation (SD) and coefficient of variation (CV%) for each variable are shown in Figures 4.80 and 4.81. During the first 12 h the 'within' and 'between' subject coefficients of variation for

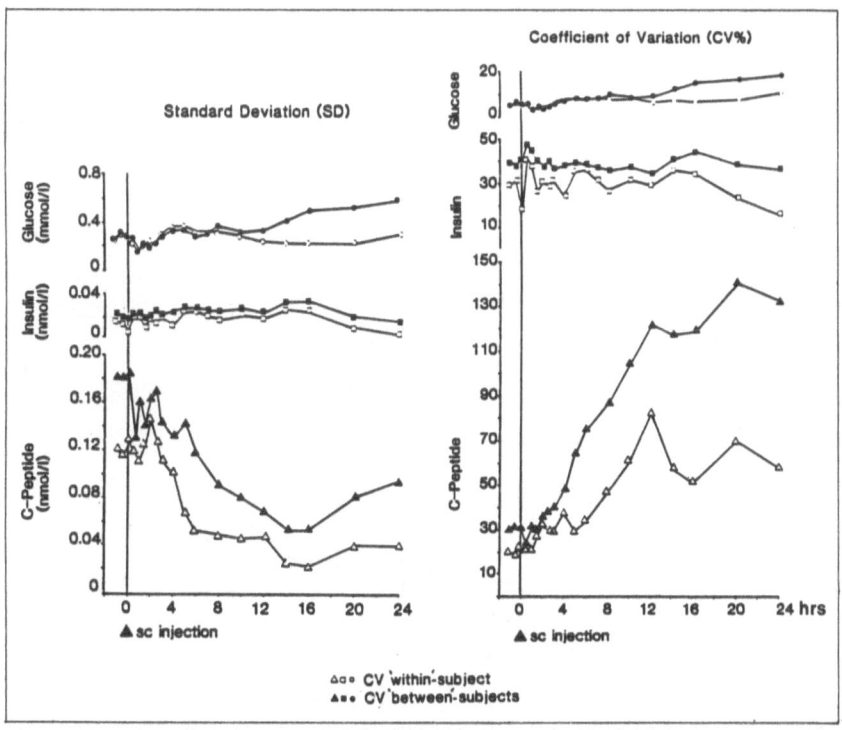

Figure 4.80 The 'within' and 'between' subject day-to-day variation – standard deviation (SD) and coefficient of variation (CV) – in plasma glucose, insulin (IRI) and C-peptide concentrations in twelve subjects. Insulin (Monotard HM: U–100; 0.30 U/kg) given subcutaneously (sc) at time 0

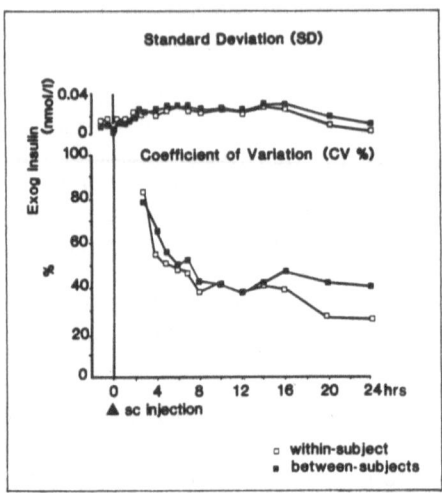

Figure 4.81 The 'within' and 'between' subject day-to-day variation – standard deviation (SD) and coefficient of variation (CV) – in the estimated ('initial ratio method') exogenous insulin concentrations. Insulin (Monotard HM: U–100; 0.30 U/kg) given subcutaneously (sc) at time 0

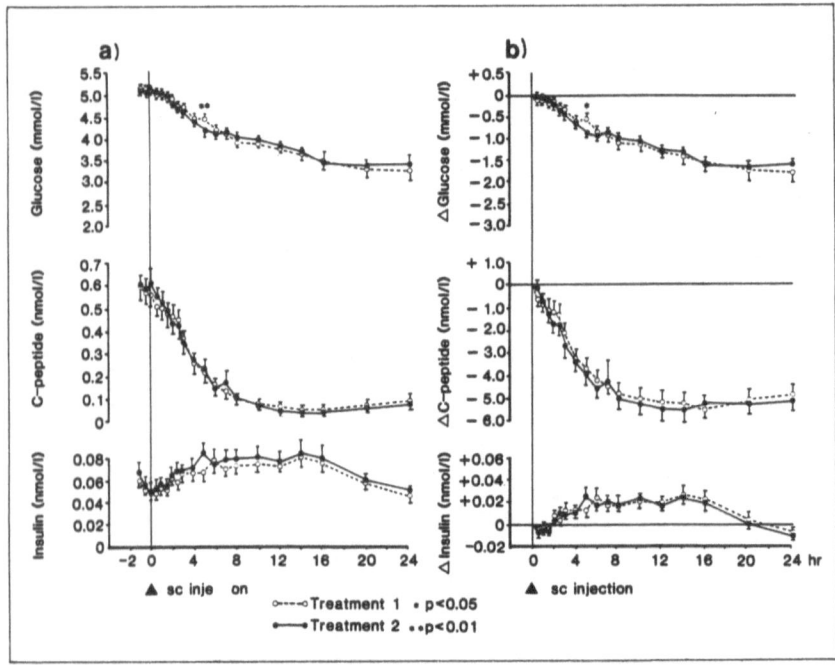

Figure 4.82a, b (a) Comparison of the effect of hypothetical treatments 1 and 2 (Monotard HM: U–100) on plasma glucose, C-peptide and insulin concentration (means ± SE) in twelve subjects. Insulin (0.30 U/kg) given subcutaneously (sc) at time 0. (b) Results shown as means ± SE of Δ values

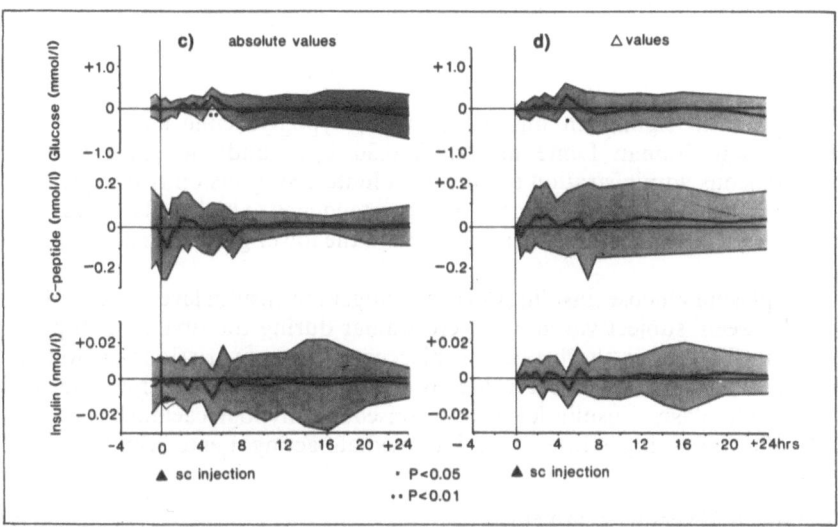

Figure 4.82c, d (c) Comparison of effect of hypothetical treatments 1 and 2 (Monotard HM: U–100) on plasma glucose, C-peptide and insulin (IRI) concentrations in twelve subjects. Insulin (0.30 U/kg) given subcutaneously (sc) at time 0. Results shown as means of differences (with 95% confidence limits) between responses to the two 'treatments'. (d) Results shown as means of differences (with 95% confidence limits) between the Δ values with the two 'treatments'

plasma glucose were both below 10%. Thereafter, the 'between' subject coefficient of variation increased to 20% by 24h relative to the 10% 'within' subject coefficient of variation (CV). During the first 16h the 'within' and 'between' subject coefficients of variation for plasma insulin were relatively stable at 30 and 40% respectively, becoming 20 and 40%, respectively at 24h. Similarly, there was little or no difference between the 'within' and 'between' subject coefficient of variation for the estimated exogenous insulin levels up to 14h, whereas at 24h the values were 26 and 41%, respectively (Figure 4.81). The 'within' and 'between' subject CV for C-peptide were below 40% up to 3h post-injection. Subsequently the 'within' and 'between' CV increased to 83 and 141% at 12 and 20h, respectively.

(ii) 'Treatment 1' versus 'treatment 2' (Figure 4.82). The mean absolute and Δ plasma glucose, C-peptide and insulin for the two 'treatments' 1 and 2 are shown in Figures 4.82a and 4.82b, respectively, with the mean differences (with 95% confidence limits) between the treatments represented in Figures 4.82c and 4.82d, respectively.

The hypoglycaemic response was, as expected, similar for the two treatments except at 5h when the glucose was significantly lower with treatment 2 ($p < 0.01$). There was no difference, however, in either the plasma C-peptide or insulin levels between the two treatment groups.

Discussion

Day 1 versus day 2

There was no significant difference in the hypoglycaemic and C-peptide responses to human Lente insulin at 0.30 U/kg body weight following subcutaneous administration to normal volunteer subjects on two sequential days 7–10 days apart. There was, however, a tendency to higher plasma insulin levels on the second study day as reflected in the lower glucose and C-peptide levels.

For plasma glucose, insulin (IRI) and exogenous insulin levels, the 'within' and 'between' subject variability were similar during the first 14–16 h post-injection. Thereafter, the 'between' subject coefficient of variation was twice as high as the 'within' subject value by 24 h. The results illustrate the less predictable plasma insulin levels and consequent hypoglycaemic effects 12–14 h following a single dose of the 'intermediate-acting' Lente insulin.

'Treatment 1' versus 'treatment 2'

Apart from a significantly lower glucose level with 'treatment 2' at one time-point only, i.e. 5 h ($p < 0.01$) there were no other differences in the hypoglycaemic and C-peptide responses and insulin levels between the two hypothetical treatments.

4.3.4.3   General discussion

The hypoglycaemic response to neutral, soluble human insulin (U–100) at a dose level of 0.10 U/kg body weight, did not differ either between the first and second sequential study days or between the study days when randomly allocated into two hypothetical treatment groups. In contrast, there were few significant 'order of treatment' effects for both the plasma C-peptide and insulin levels which could be due to random variation. The 'within' and 'between' subject variation indicates a greater degree of heterogeneity in the hypoglycaemic response relative to the plasma insulin profiles.

Differences were also observed between the first and second study days with the 'intermediate-acting' Lente human insulin (U–100). Higher plasma insulin levels were observed on the second day associated with a tendency towards lower glucose levels on the second compared to the first study day. However, when the study days were randomised into two comparative treatment groups, there were no differences to be found between the two hypothetical treatments. The 'within' and 'between' subject coefficient of variation for plasma glucose and insulin levels were similar up to 16 h after administration. Thereafter, there was a greater variability 'between' subjects for both parameters indicating a less predictable 'bioavailability' and hypoglycaemic response.

These results support the need for randomisation to remove any 'order' effects when comparing different treatments on different study days. In addition, for any comparative study it is important to ascertain both the 'within' and 'between' subject variability for each of the response variables.

5
Summary

Prior to the availability of insulin, the treatment of all diabetics was limited to an array of different diets, the use of herbal mixtures and the recommendation to exercise. The severe diabetic faced a shortened life, enduring intense starvation, with emaciation, intermittent and terminal infections.

The observation of von Mering and Minkowski (1889) that surgical removal of the pancreas from dogs induced a condition similar to diabetes mellitus in man, led to attempts to isolate the active principle produced by the islets by Langerhans in the pancreas. The search was rewarded with varying success by only a few of the 20 to 30 principal investigators at the beginning of this century (Blumenthal, 1898; Grey, 1905; De Witt, 1906; Rennie and Fraser, 1907; Zuelzer, 1908; Knowlton and Sterling, 1911; Scott, 1911; Murlin and Kramer, 1913; Clark, 1916; Kleiner, 1919; Paulesco, 1921; Banting and Best, 1921). In contrast to the other researchers who also succeeded in extracting insulin from pancreatic glands, the work of the two Canadians, Banting and Best, during 1921 and 1922, set into motion the extensive machinery needed to make insulin available for the treatment of diabetic patients world-wide (Banting and Best, 1922a, b).

Early in the era of insulin treatment, physicians confronted by the immunological side effects of animal pancreatic extracts (Joslin et al, 1922; Williams, 1922; Lawrence, 1925; Tuft, 1928) believed that the human, insulin protein must be different and that no patient should be sensitive to his own insulin (Karr et al, 1931; Lewis, 1937).

Until recently insulin has been produced almost exclusively from bovine and porcine pancreas, the general principles of the process remaining remarkably similar over the past 50 years (Romans et al, 1940; Schlichtkrull et al, 1975). The importance of insulin purity was soon recognised following the introduction of recrystallised insulin used successfully in treating insulin allergy due to unpurified insulins (Jorpes, 1949). Nevertheless, recrystallised insulin still contained several impurities (Harfenist and Craig, 1952; Mirsky and Kawamura, 1966; Steiner, 1967). The observation that almost all insulin-treated diabetics had circulating insulin binding antibodies (Berson et al, 1956; Berson and Yalow, 1964, 1966) further stimulated the development of additional purification procedures (Schlichtkrull et al, 1970, 1974; Root et al, 1972; Deckert et al, 1974; Chance et al, 1976; Jørgensen et al, 1982). The reduced immunogenicity of highly purified insulins offers numerous potential advantages to the insulin-treated patient (Bloom et al, 1979; Heding et al, 1980a; Kurtz and Nabarro, 1980; Home and Alberti, 1982). Insulin preparations with prolonged effect had been developed in an attempt to reduce the number of daily injections. Delaying the absorption of insulin after subcutaneous injection was achieved by complexing the insulin with globin: Globin insulin (Bauman, 1939; Reiner et al, 1939), surfen: Surfen insulin (Umber et al, 1938) protamine: Protamine, Protamine Zinc and Neutral Protamine Hagedorn insulin (Krayenbühl and Rosenburg, 1946) and excess zinc: Lente (Semilente, Lente, Ultralente) insulin (Hallas-Møller et al, 1952; 1954).

In 1960, crystalline human insulin was first prepared from cadaveric pancreas glands, allowing the determination of its amino acid composition and sequence which were shown to differ from other mammalian insulin.(Nicol and Smith, 1960). Porcine insulin differs from human insulin only at the C-terminal amino acid residue of the B-chain featuring alanine, instead of a threonine residue, with bovine insulin differing at two additional sites on the A-chain at positions 8 and 10. Soon after, human insulin extracted from human pancreas glands became available for limited clinical use such as skin testing in allergic patients (Kreines, 1965) and clinical–pharmacological studies (Ørskov and Christensen, 1969; Sönksen et al, 1973).

During the 1970s chemists tried to synthesize human insulin by various methods with varying success (reviewed by Geiger, 1976; Markussen, 1977). Total synthetis by Sieber and co-workers (1974) made available a small amount of human insulin sufficient only for a short-term study in diabetic patients demonstrating its biological efficacy and safety (Teuscher, 1979). Quantities sufficient for therapeutic use have relied on two techniques developed in parallel utilising either recombinant DNA technology (Goeddel et al, 1979; Chance et al, 1981c; Frank et al, 1981) or semi-synthesis from porcine insulin (Morihara et al, 1979; Gattner et al, 1980; Markussen, 1980). To differentiate between these, the British Pharmacopoeia designates the human insulins as 'emp' – enzymatically modified porcine, 'crb' – chain recombinant bacterial or 'prb' – proinsulin recombinant bacterial. In the following text the codes 'emp' and 'crb' have been replaced by the terms 'semi-synthetic' and 'biosynthetic'. Unfortunately, compendial definitions of insulin still differ from one pharmacopoeia to another, although it should not be too much to expect an international monograph for insulin and approved definitions for human insulin along the lines adopted by the British Pharmacopoeial Commission.

Since its first therapeutic use more than 60 years ago (Banting and Best, 1922b), insulin continues, and will continue, to be administered by subcutaneous injections in the majority of the insulin-requiring patient population for decades to come. Therefore, the bulk of the studies were centred on describing the plasma insulin profiles, metabolic and hormonal responses to the recently available 'semi-synthetic' human (emp) insulin preparations in normal man following subcutaneous administration (Table 5.1). These studies represent the first safety and efficacy evaluation of each of the above preparations in man after the pre-clinical toxicological and general pharmacological investigations (Gamst-Andersen et al, 1983; Jørgensen et al.

1983). They also included, for comparative purposes, equivalent pharma-ceutical formulations of porcine and/or bovine insulin and two formulations of 'biosynthetic' human insulin.

Table 5.1

Human insulin preparations (emp)	Timing category
Human Actrapid (Actrapid® HM)	'Short-acting'
Human Monotard (Monotard® HM)	'Intermediate-acting'
Human Protaphane (Protaphane® HM)	'Intermediate-acting'
Human Actraphane (Actraphane® HM)	'Biphasic'
Human Ultralente (Ultratard® HM)	'Long-acting'

The hormonal counterregulatory responses to hypoglycaemia induced by the subcutaneous and intravenous administration of neutral, soluble human ('semi-synthetic', 'biosynthetic') and porcine insulin were also examined.

In addition to evaluating the influence of *species* and *pharmaceutical formulation* on insulin absorption and biological response, other factors such as the *route of administration, site of subcutaneous injection,* the addition of an *'enzyme inhibitor', insulin concentration, admixing of insulins,* and the *'within' and 'between' subject variation* were also examined.

All the studies were conducted in normal volunteer subjects in accordance with internationally agreed guidelines for human experimentation (Helsinki Declaration, WHO, 1976). Well-established laboratory techniques were used for the measurement of metabolic and hormonal responses and the antibodies used in the insulin radioimmunoassay reacted identically with human, porcine and bovine insulin. Statistical analyses of the data involved a variety of methods including the Student's t-test and analysis of variance for paired comparisons, dose–response analysis utilising the parallel line models and new multivariate analyses for estimating the relative 'potency' and 'bioavailability' of the different species of insulin (Finney, 1978, Vølund, 1980).

All the statistical analyses were carried out by means of already available computer programs (Statistical Package for the Social Sciences) or specially developed APL computer programs. The findings will be summarised under the following headings:

Insulin species/pharmaceutical formulations

(a) 'short-acting' insulin preparations
(b) insulin preparations with prolonged effect
(c) additional factors that influence subcutaneous insulin absorption.

Up to the late 1970s insulin for therapeutic use consisted almost entirely of porcine and/or bovine insulin, derived from pancreas glands, a source still capable of satisfying requirements up to the end of the 20th century (WHO Expert Committee on Diabetes Mellitus, 1980). The advent of human insulin formulated into 'short-', 'intermediate-' and 'long-acting' preparations represents the latest achievement in the development of insulin preparations.

In view of the large numbers the last sample for each subject was screened for the presence of insulin antibodies. As the level was below 5 μg/l for all subjects, irrespective of type and number of studies, no further analyses were performed.

INSULIN SPECIES/PHARMACEUTICAL FORMULATIONS

(a) 'Short-acting' insulin preparations

The initial study confirmed the equivalent safety and efficacy of human insulin relative to its porcine counterpart following subcutaneous administration to man at a dose level of 6 U (Owens et al, 1981a). A continuous low-dose somatostatin infusion (100 μg/h) was used throughout the study to suppress endogenous insulin secretion (Alberti et al, 1973), so that the plasma insulin concentrations reflected more precisely the absorption and elimination characteristics of the insulins. The known influence of somatostatin on splanchnic blood flow (Felig and Wahren, 1976) and possibly on subcutaneous blood flow plus its potent inhibition of other hormones (Assan, 1976) prevented any firm physiological conclusions being drawn, although the comparative results remain valid. In this study both human and porcine insulins were well tolerated, and no local or systemic adverse effects were observed. No differences were found between the neutral, soluble human and porcine insulin in their effect on plasma glucose, insulin, C-peptide and blood intermediary metabolite concentrations.

In an otherwise identical follow-up study, but excluding somatostatin, again no difference was observed between human and porcine insulin. Comparison of the two studies demonstrated that somatostatin potentiates insulin-induced hypoglycaemia and delays, but does not prevent, recovery towards normoglycaemia. Somatostatin had little effect on plasma lactate or alanine concentrations, whereas a marked increase in both blood glycerol and 3-hydroxybutyrate levels was observed due to a state of accelerated lipolysis and ketogenesis resulting from insulin deficiency (Mahler et al, 1964).

Therefore 'long-acting' and more selective analogues of somatostatin could be useful as an adjunct to insulin therapy, potentiating its hypoglycaemic action, although extensive clinical studies would be necessary to ascertain any long-term benefits that may accrue from better counterregulatory hormone profiles (Hansen and Johansen, 1970; Gerich et al, 1975a).

Physicochemical differences between the three species of insulin used clinically form the basis of the high-performance liquid chromatographic (HPLC) techniques for the species analysis of insulins (Terabe et al, 1979; Kroeff and Chance, 1982). A preliminary study indicated that in man the hypoglycaemic effect of bovine insulin was delayed relative to human and porcine insulin despite the presence of similar plasma insulin profiles (Owens et al, 1984a). The data suggested a time-dependent variation in hypoglycaemic 'potency' between bovine and porcine insulin (Owens et al, 1984a) in part agreement with earlier results in the rabbit bioassay system (Vølund et al,

SUMMARY

1982), thereby bringing into question the validity of using the mixed species 4th International Standard (Bangham and Mussett, 1959) for the estimation of the biological 'potency' of the individual insulin species in such assay systems. Further 'human bioassay' studies were therefore conducted to compare the three species of insulin at three dose levels (0.05, 0.075 and 0.15 U/kg body weight) without the concomitant use of somatostatin. The results revealed significant time-dependent species differences in hypoglycaemic 'potency' between human, porcine and bovine insulins. Human insulin showed a quicker and less prolonged hypoglycaemic action relative to bovine insulin, whereas porcine insulin produced an intermediate response with a tendency to an overall lower 'potency' relative to human and bovine insulin. The relative 'bioavailaibilities' determined from the plasma insulin profiles showed rather small and insignificant differences, though largely in the same direction as the hypoglycaemic 'potencies', indicating that the species differences in the timing of hypoglycaemia exceed those due to absorption or 'bioavailability' differences. Relatively crude analyses of the intravenous kinetics of the three species of insulin from a separate study also indicate that there may be some species differences. There was a tendency towards a higher area under the insulin curve ($AUC_{0-240 min}$) with human relative to porcine insulin, and bovine relative to porcine insulin. The plasma clearance and, to some extent, the apparent volume of distribution were also less with bovine than human or porcine insulin. Others have observed little or no difference in the plasma or biological half-lives of 'biosynthetic' human and bovine insulin at the end of an intravenous infusion (Gray et al, 1984). Further studies are therefore necessary to explore the relative contribution of kinetic and tissue sensitivity differences between the three species of insulin to explain time-related variation in hypoglycaemic 'potency' of the three species of insulin following subcutaneous administration.

Comparison of the subcutaneous and intramuscular routes of administration of human insulin showed that the hypoglycaemic responses seen after subcutaneous injection into the abdomen and intramuscular injection into the thigh were similar, although tending to be of shorter duration after intramuscular injection (Owens et al, 1981d). In contrast, a rapid reduction of plasma glucose was seen after intravenous human insulin, reaching a nadir within 30 min as expected (Greenwood and Landon, 1966). After subcutaneous and intramuscular injections peak plasma insulin levels were achieved at 60 to 90 min, followed by a slightly more rapid clearance after intramuscular injection. Following intravenous administration, the maximum level was achieved at 2 min with a disappearance half-time ($T_{1/2}$) of approximately 5 min, in agreement with previous investigators using human (Sönksen et al, 1973), porcine or bovine pancreatic insulin (Burt and Davidson, 1974).

The elimination kinetics of intravenous human insulin during somatostatin infusion was described by a sum of two exponential functions indicating a rapid elimination component with $T_{1/2}$ in the range of 3 to 5 min. The volume of distribution was seen to be about 100 ml/kg with a plasma clearance rate of approximately 15 ml/min/kg in agreement with Tranberg and Dencker (1978). Somatostatin did not appear to influence the kinetics of intravenously administered human insulin, but markedly delayed the recovery of plasma glucose, as seen also in the subcutaneous studies.

Several investigators have observed a lesser hormonal counterregulatory response with human ('semi-synthetic', 'biosynthetic') than porcine insulin following subcutaneous and intravenous administration despite an equivalent degree of hypoglycaemia (Schlüter et al, 1981, 1982, 1983a, b; Rosak et al, 1982; Christensen et al, 1984). Therefore, in view of the proposed theoretical advantage of using human insulin, studies were conducted to examine the response to the two species of insulin after subcutaneous and intravenous bolus injection. The subcutaneous study illustrates the problem of trying to interpret such responses in a small group of subjects.

In this study human insulin achieved higher peak insulin levels, although there was no real difference in the hypoglycaemic response between the two insulins. There was, however, a trend towards an earlier glucagon response with human compared to porcine insulin but no difference between the growth hormone and cortisol levels. In view of the fact that variation in hypoglycaemia may bias the comparison of the hormonal counterregulatory responses to human and porcine insulin, these were compared after adjusting for differences in the hypoglycaemic response, i.e. rate of fall, minimum level and decrease of plasma glucose. None of these analyses showed any statistically significant differences between human and porcine insulin. Apart from a significant correlation between the minimum glucose and maximum glucagon levels, no other correlation could be established between the hypoglycaemic effects and counterregulatory responses. This is not surprising considering the size of the study, which limits the statistical power to detect any real difference. The demonstration of a difference in the glucagon, catecholamine, cortisol and growth hormone responses between subcutaneous human and porcine insulin by some (Schlüter et al, 1981, 1982; Petersen et al, 1982; Rosak et al, 1982) but not others (Ebihara et al, 1983; Landgraf-Leurs et al, 1984) may be partly related to the relatively small number of subjects included in the studies. The intravenous study involved 'semi-synthetic' and 'biosynthetic' human and porcine insulins given by bolus injection. No differences were observed in the hormonal counterregulatory response (glucagon, adrenaline, growth hormone and cortisol) between 'semi-synthetic' human and porcine insulin. The catecholamine response following the administration of 'biosynthetic' human insulin tended to be less than with the other two insulins, possibly related to its shorter hypoglycaemic effect. Pharmacokinetic analysis of the insulin data indicated that the reduced hypoglycaemic effect of the 'biosynthetic' human insulin may be associated with an increased plasma clearance rate compared to that of the other two insulins. In view of the sampling times, only the one-compartment model could be fitted consistently to the individual insulin curves, thus no firm conclusions about pharmacokinetic differences between the three insulins can be drawn.

Therefore, in conclusion, little or no clinically relevant difference exists between the neutral, soluble formulations of 'semi-synthetic' human and porcine insulin following subcutaneous or intravenous administration to normal man. Combining the results from several of the subcutaneous studies does, however, indicate a tendency to an earlier hypoglycaemic response with human relative to porcine insulin, when administered at a dose level of 6 U into the anterior abdominal wall. Whereas the insulin levels tended to be higher with human insulin between 30 and 60 min after injection, the difference does not reach statistical significance. There is, however, a time-dependent variation in 'potency' between the three species of insulin used clinically, human insulin possessing a relatively quicker and less prolonged hypoglycaemic action relative to bovine insulin, with porcine insulin occupying an intermediate position. The results from these subcutaneous studies with the 'short-acting' insulin preparatins tentatively indicate that species differences in the hypoglycaemic responses exceed those due to 'bioavailability' differences. The reverse also appears to be the case in some studies, emphasising the variability of the absorption process and state of 'insulin responsiveness' in fasting normal subjects. The studies do not indicate any real difference in the hormonal counterregulatory response betwen human and porcine insulin given either by the subcutaneous or intravenous route of administration.

(b) Insulin preparations with prolonged effect

In comparison to the 'short-acting' insulins, the preparations with a protracted action have a much slower absorption rate from the subcutaneous tissue resulting in lower but more prolonged insulin profiles. Therefore, methods were used to derive an approximate estimate of the prevailing exogenous insulin levels based on the ratio between insulin and C-peptide when no exogenous insulin is present, i.e. either during a control day (control day method) or for the basal (pre-insulin) period (initial ratio method). The C-peptide levels following insulin administration were utilised as an index of endogenous insulin secretion. Such methods have limitations as they are based on certain assumptions about constancy (in time) of insulin and C-peptide kinetics, including endogenous secretion in a constant ratio. The relationship can only be expected to hold approximately, deteriorating with rapid changes in endogenous insulin secretion (Polonsky and Rubenstein, 1984), thereby underestimating the exogenous insulin level during the early hypoglycaemic phase. The two methods agree very well for the exogenous insulin estimates for the studies involving 'short-' and intermediate-acting' insulins, although this constitutes no test of whether they are valid in that they estimate the exogenous insulin correctly. The comparative results between similar protracted insulin preparations should, however, remain valid. The relative hypoglycaemic 'potency' and 'bioavailability' of the test insulins were determined from the dose response analysis utilising the parallel line model (Finney, 1978) the response variables being measured over 3 or 4 h periods.

The hypoglycaemic 'potency' of 'semi-synthetic' human Lente insulin was greater than its porcine counterpart for the periods 3 to 7, 7 to 11 and 0 to 11 h after injection for the dose range of 0.1–0.30 U/kg body weight. There was a 40% greater 'bioavailability' of human insulin over the 11 h study period. This contrasts with the findings of Galloway et al (1982a), who showed no difference between 'biosynthetic' human and porcine Lente insulin preparations at 0.25 U/kg body weight, which may be due to a difference in the formulation of the 'semi-synthetic' and 'biosynthetic' human zinc insulin suspensions. The data also re-emphasise that small dosage changes of the 'intermediate-acting' Lente insulin are unlikely to have any clinical relevance in the majority of patients (Lauritzen et al, 1982; Hildebrandt et al, 1984b).

Comparing equivalent formulations of human and porcine NPH insulins at 0.15 and 0.30 U/kg body weight in a similar study, the 'bioavailability' of human insulin was also greater relative to porcine insulin with the difference reaching significance during the 7 to 11 h period after injection. The 'potency' difference between the two species of NPH insulin was in the same direction but did not reach statistical significance, whereas in the same study, the 'potency' of 'semi-synthetic' human insulin was greater than 'biosynthetic' human insulin for the 7 to 11 and 0 to 11 h study periods. These findings underline the influence of species and pharmaceutical formulations on the pharmacokinetics and hypoglycaemic response to NPH (Isophane) insulin preparations (Owens et al, 1984b).

Recent clinical studies also suggest a trend towards a relatively shorter duration of blood glucose lowering effect with 'biosynthetic' human NPH insulin, relative to porcine or bovine NPH insulin preparations (Clark et al, 1982; Galloway et al, 1982c, d, 1983).

Comparison of the 'intermediate-acting' Lente and NPH U–40 insulin preparations in the above studies demonstrates a clear tendency to an earlier hypoglycaemic response with NPH insulin at the 0.30 U/kg dose level. This difference reflected the quicker absorption of the NPH insulin. These findings were consistent for both the human and porcine 'intermediate-acting' insulin. Similar observations were made between human Lente and NPH U–100 insulin preparations in a 'within' subject comparative study over a 24 h period. NPH insulin achieved higher insulin levels during the first 3 h after injection associated with lower glucose levels during the first 5 h. Thereafter the trend was reversed, the insulin levels falling on NPH with no exogenous insulin detected at 22 h, whereas with Lente insulin the level was still about 30% of the peak values. While both NPH and Lente insulins are 'intermediate-acting' preparations (Bressler and Galloway, 1978) there are clear differences between them, especially during the first few hours after injection.

Much greater differences were observed between the new human Ultralente and the standard, commercially available, 'long-acting' bovine Ultralente (U–100) preparation. The onset of hypoglycaemia was evident at 5 and 10 h after injection of human and bovine insulin, respectively, with the hypoglycaemic response significantly greater with human insulin at 10 h and from 18 to 32 h. The estimated exogenous insulin level was significantly higher with human relative to bovine Ultralente between 4 and 22 h after administration.

These differences are likely to be clinically relevant when transferring patients from bovine to human Ultralente insulin, especially when associated with the lower antigenic and immunogenic properties of human insulin (Holman et al, 1984).

In conclusion, the differences between human and porcine insulin formulated either as Lente, Ultralente or NPH insulin are consistent in that human insulin tends to be 'more rapidly' absorbed with an earlier hypoglycaemic effect than its porcine counterpart. The largest difference, as expected, was between human and bovine Ultralente insulin (Owens et al, 1984c).

SUMMARY

The results from these studies can only be considered in the context of single-dose clinical–pharmacological studies in normal man. The data cannot therefore be directly extrapolated to diabetic patients. Attempts to characterise the timing of action of insulin preparations using animal models, normal subjects and diabetic patients, under standardised conditions – to arrive at idealised time–action curves – have limited clinical relevance (Schlichtkrull et al, 1975). Nevertheless, it is important to be able to compare the insulin preparations within each of the main categories of 'short-', 'intermediate-' and 'long-acting' insulins. This knowledge should form the basis for a rational approach to intensified conventional therapy in the insulin-requiring diabetic patient (Skyler et al, 1981; Schade et al, 1983).

(c) Additional factors that influence subcutaneous insulin absorption

Of the remaining factors known to influence subcutaneous insulin absorption, the effect of site of injection, the addition of a protease inhibitor to insulin, insulin concentration, mixing of insulin preparations and the 'within' and 'between' subject variation in the absorption and response to neutral, soluble 'semi-synthetic' human insulin have been examined. The studies confirm the more rapid absorption of insulin from the anterior abdominal wall relative to the thigh region, as previously documented for the other species of insulin (Binder, 1969; Koivisto and Felig, 1978; Galloway et al, 1981a; Berger et al, 1982). The reputed faster absorption of human compared to porcine insulin, when injected into the thigh (Sundermann et al, 1981), and the lack of a difference between the species when administered into the abdomen (Owens et al, 1981a), do not contradict a region difference in the absorption of human insulin.

The addition of aprotinin to human insulin was seen to increase insulin absorption within the first 30 to 60 min with an acceleration of the onset of hypoglycaemia, in agreement with earlier investigations (Berger et al, 1980; Linde and Gunnarsson, 1983). The response was very short-lived, consistent with an acute local hyperaemic effect of aprotinin (Williams et al, 1983). This possibility is supported by the similar time course of the local hyperaemic response and acceleration of insulin absorption seen with prostaglandin E_1 (Williams et al, 1984). The data do not support the hypothesis that inhibition of subcutaneous insulin degradation is the primary mechanism by which aprotinin enhances insulin absorption. The chronic use of subcutaneous aprotinin cannot be advocated, as it may lead to local and systemic immune damage.

The availability of insulin in different strengths has led to countless dosage errors (Watkins et al, 1967; Bloom et al, 1981). Whereas a change to 100-unit (U–100) insulin has been undertaken in many countries, most European countries still retain the 40-unit (U–40) insulin preparations. Studies were therefore conducted to compare the U–40 and U–100 strengths of soluble, Lente and NPH insulins. Absorption of U–40 neutral, soluble human insulin was clearly more rapid than the U–100 formulation, consistent with a quicker decrease in plasma glucose and C-peptide levels. Five to six hours later there was a trend towards higher insulin and lower glucose values with the U–100 insulin.

The 'within' subject variability was higher with the U–40 than the U–100 insulin preparation. Previous studies have not found a difference between U–40 and U–100 soluble insulin (Galloway et al, 1981a; Lauritzen et al, 1984). There appears to be less of a difference between the U–40 and U–100 strengths of the 'intermediate-acting' insulin preparations. This question as it relates to the Lente and NPH insulin preparation needs further evaluation as the comparisons were carried out between subjects from separate studies. Whilst supporting the need to adopt a single strength of insulin (Bloom et al, 1981), the lower concentration of U–40 would appear to be more appropriate, due to the quicker absorption of the U–40 'short-acting' insulin preparation, with its possible therapeutic benefits (Berger et al, 1982). The magnitude of the difference suggests, however, that it is of little clinical relevance. Therefore, the diabetic patients are best served by a change to U–100 insulin to avoid unnecessary and life-threatening dosage errors (Bloom et al, 1981).

In an attempt to achieve glycaemic control as close to physiological as possible, multi-component insulin regimens have been used to provide both mean and basal insulin requirements (Skyler et al, 1982). The most popular regimen has been the 'split-and-mixed' regimen, involving twice-daily injection of combinations of 'short-' and 'intermediate-acting' NPH or Lente insulins (Oakley et al, 1966; Skyler et al, 1981; Schade et al, 1983).

Mixing of 'short-' and 'intermediate-acting' insulins in the majority of instances is made on the unsupported assumption that the constituent insulins retain their individual characteristics. It has been known for some time that mixtures of soluble and Lente, and soluble and NPH, insulins are unstable, resulting in the loss of the soluble insulin fraction, the extent of which is dependent upon the ratio of the two insulins and the time allowed for interaction (Nolte et al, 1983; Galloway et al, 1982b). Two studies were therefore conducted to examine the influence of mixing soluble insulin with NPH and Lente insulin. The results of the studies confirm a greater loss of soluble insulin when admixed with Lente relative to NPH insulin (Berger et al, 1982; Heine et al, 1984a, b; Heine et al, 1985). There was little or no difference in the plasma insulin profile between the separate injection of soluble and NPH insulins compared to admixtures of the two insulins given immediately or 30 min after preparation. There was, however, blunting of the early insulin peak with the pre-mixed insulin prepared with soluble and NPH insulin, in a ratio of 30:70. Mixing soluble and Lente insulin, even when injected immediately after preparation, indicated a significant loss of the soluble fraction, resulting in lower plasma insulin levels and a reduced hypoglycaemic response during the first 90 min after injection, when compared to the two preparations given simulatenously by separate injection. The difference between the soluble/NPH and soluble/Lente admixtures is reflected in the higher post-prandial glucose levels observed with soluble and Lente insulin in insulin-treated diabetics (Heine et al, 1985). A similar interaction occurs with soluble and Ultralente insulin mixtures (Mulhauser et al, 1985). Therefore, when it is considered necessary to retain the individual characteristics of the soluble and insulin zinc suspensions, they should be administered by separate injections. However, for the majority of patients, twice-a-day mixtures of soluble and Lente insulin achieve 'satisfactory' glycaemic control with the appropriate ratio of soluble and Lente insulin (Birtwell et al, 1984). It must be noted also that the pre-mixed soluble and NPH insulin preparations are not equivalent to the constituent insulins admixed in the same ratio and injected up to 30 min after preparation. The concept of intensified conventional insulin therapy requires a flexible approach exploiting the properties of the individual insulin preparations, with the insulin regimens designed to meet each individual patient's requirements.

It is of importance, in the evaluation and use of insulin, to be aware of the 'within' and 'between' subject variation in subcutaneous insulin absorption (Binder et al, 1984). This facet of insulin absorption was examined for both the neutral, soluble and Lente, U–100, human insulin preparations, with the subjects undergoing two study days 1 week apart. The results indicate an order effect between the first and second study days, which was greater for the 'intermediate-acting' insulin. However, when randomly allocating the study days to two hypothetical treatment days, no differences were observed, which emphasises the need to employ a randomised design or randomised block design for the comparison of different insulins in the 'human bioassay system'. This procedure was adopted in all the studies for comparing different species and formulations of insulin, and when evaluating the influence of a number of factors on subcutaneous insulin absorption using the newly available 'semi-synthetic' human insulin preparations.

The studies outlined above indicate the many factors that may affect the quality of insulin treatment. Primarily the influence of species and pharmaceutical formulation were examined. Other factors such as concentrations, dose, site of administration, local vasodilation at site of injection and mixing of 'short-' and 'intermediate-acting' insulin are important. The 'within' and 'between' subject day-to-day variation in the insulin absorption and hypoglycaemia following subcutaneous administration demonstrates the dominating influence of the state of insulin responsiveness. Whereas alterations in the species and formulation of insulin and the adoption of insulin regimens based on small doses of soluble insulin to improve reproducibility are intended to improve the quality of insulin treatment, the insulin responsiveness of the patient will remain the ultimate constraint.

Therefore, in conclusion, human insulin, a product of the ongoing evolution in insulin treatment, represents the realisation of the wishes of physicians and chemists alike to make available homologous insulin for the treatment of diabetes mellitus in man. Producing insulin identical to human pancreatic insulin either by the enzymatic conversion of porcine insulin or by employing recombinant DNA technology, are undisputed technological achievements. The availability of human insulin also provides the basic material for future generations of insulin preparations. The contribution of human insulin to the evolution of insulin treatment compared to the major advances achieved earlier by the modification and purification of insulin, remains to be established.

Acknowledgements

The studies were commenced during August 1979 and continued up to December 1984. The work would not have been possible without the support of many with whom I have been associated in the course of the investigations. As only a few can be mentioned I offer my sincere gratitude to all who have helped.

All the clinical studies were conducted in the Diabetes and Metabolism Investigations Unit in the Department of Medicine, University of Wales College of Medicine (UWCM), Cardiff. I am indebted to Professor R. Hall and Dr T. M. Hayes for their encouragement and advice, and for the excellent facilities.

It is a pleasure to express my sincere thanks to all my colleagues in Diabetes Research and Development, Novo Research Institute (NRI), Copenhagen. My special thanks go to Dr Lise G. Heding for her invaluable advice and encouragement throughout these studies and for making available to me both at NRI and UWCM the necessary reagents, laboratory and computing facilities to perform the radioimmunoassays and analyse the results. The assistance and guidance of Aage Vølund and Birgit Jensen in developing APL computer programs for statistically analysing the large volume of data, was indispensable. Other colleagues who have helped me include: Clive Burge, Kathleen Larsen, Drs J. Schlichtkrull, Jan Markussen, Klavs Jørgensen, Jens Brange, Ivan Jensen and Bente Tronier, also Frank Petersen, Bente Hansen, Lisbet Pedersen, Marianne Heiden, Lena Jensen, Kirsten Vilhelmsen, Richter Friis, Bent Wier, Inger Marie Krogh and Else Jørgensen.

I am indebted to my colleagues at the Department of Medicine and University of Wales College of Medicine during the past 5 years, including Drs M. Keston Jones, John Birtwell, Ian Jones, Robert Ryder, Jiten Vora and Jameel Atiea. The task of performing the innumerable radioimmunoassays at UHW was undertaken by Steve Luzio. My thanks also go to Sheila Williams and Christopher Davies for their technical assistance in the laboratory and Investigations Unit. I would also like to acknowledge the additional support given by Professor George Alberti and Dr Philip Home, Newcastle; Professor Gordon Reeves, Nottingham; Professor Steven Bloom, London; Dr Ulrich Keller, Basle; Professor George Elder and Dr Stewart Woodhead, Cardiff.

Thanks are also due to the nursing staff of the Diabetes and Metabolism

ACKNOWLEDGEMENTS

Unit during the past 5 years – Alison Rochester, Margaret Abouharb, Rosemary Williams, and Anne Griffiths-Jones, to C. J. Borthwick for assisting with the literature research, to Angela Evans and Linda Webb for secretarial work, to Dr Ralph Marshall and his staff of the Department of Medical Illustration, especially Adrian Shaw and Janice Sharp for the artwork.

I wish to record my appreciation to all the volunteer subjects who so willingly co-operated in these studies.

Finally, I would also like to credit Dr Guy Dodson, York, for the X-ray diffraction photographs of human and porcine insulins, The British Library, London, for the photographic copy of the map of Thebes by Edward Lane (Frontispiece), and the Wellcome Institute Library, London, for the print of a page from G. Ebers (ed.), *Papyros Ebers*, 2 vols Leipzig: W. Englemann, 1875, Vol 1. Tafel XXXIX.

Bibliography

Abel, J. J. Crystalline insulin. Proc. Natl. Acad. Sci. (Wash.) 1926; 12: 132–136.

Abel, J. J., Geiling, E. M. K., Rouiller, C. A., Bell, F. K., Wintersteiner, O. Crystalline insulin. J. Pharmacol. Exp. Ther. 1927; 31: 65–85.

Adeniyi-Jones, R. O. C., Jones, R. H., Barnes, D. G., Gerlis, L. S., Sönksen, P. H. Porcine and human insulin (Novo): a comparison of their metabolism and hypoglycaemic activity in normal man. Diabetes Care 1983; 6 (Suppl. 1): 9–12.

Agarwal, R. C. A new least-squares refinement technique based on the fast Fourier transform algorithm. Acta Crystallographica 1978; Sect. A34: 791–809.

Åkerblom, H. K., Mäkela, A. L. Insulin antibodies in the serum of diabetic children treated from the diagnosis of the disease with highly purified insulins. Acta Paediatr. Scand. 1977; 270 (Suppl.): 69–79.

Akre, P. R., Kirtley, W. R., Galloway, J. A. Comparative hypoglycaemic response of diabetic subjects to human insulin or structurally similar insulins of animal source. Diabetes 1964; 13: 135–143.

Alberti, K. G. M. M., Christensen, N. J., Christensen, S. E., et al. Inhibition of insulin secretion by somatostatin. Lancet 1973; ii: 1299–1301.

Alberti, K. G. M. M. and Nattrass, M. Highly purified insulins. Diabetologia 1978; 15: 77–80.

Alberti, K. G. M. M., Home, P. D. Monitoring of insulin therapy in insulin dependent diabetes mellitus. In: Skyler, J. S. (ed.), Insulin Update, 1982. Princeton: Excerpta Medica, 1982: 175–184.

Albisser, A. M., Leibel, B. S., Ewart, T. G., Davidovac, Z., Botz, C. K., Zingg, W. An artificial endocrine pancreas. Diabetes 1974; 23: 389–396.

Alford, F. P., Bloom, S. R., Nabarro, J. D. N. et al. Glucagon control of fasting glucose in man. Lancet 1974; ii: 974–977.

Alford, F. P., Bloom, S. R., Nabarro, J. D. N. Glucagon levels in normal and diabetic subjects: use of a specific immunoabsorbent for glucagon radio-immunoassay. Diabetologia 1977; 13: 1–6.

Allen, F. M. Studies concerning glycosuria and diabetes. Cambridge, Mass: Harvard University Press, 1913.

Allen, F. M., Stillman, E., Fritz, R. Total dietary regulation in the treatment of diabetes. New York, Rockefeller Institute for Medical Research 1919, Monograph No. 11: 1–78.

American Diabetes Association special report. U–100: a new era in diabetes mellitus therapy. Diabetes 1972a; 21: 832.

American Diabetes Association. Preventing insulin dosage errors. JAMA 1972b; 222: 140.

Andersen, O. O. Insulin antibody formation. I. The influence of age, sex, infections, insulin dosage and regulation of diabetes. Acta Endocrinol. (Copenh.) 1972; 71: 126–140.

Andersen, O. O. Insulin antibody formation. II. The influence of species difference and method of administration. Acta Endocrinol. (Copenh.) 1973; 72: 33–45.

Andersen, O. O., Egeberg, J. The clinical significance of insulin antibodies. Acta Paediatr. Scand. 1977; 270 (Suppl.): 63–68.

Andersen, O. O. Insulin antibodies and late diabetic complications. Irvine, J. (ed.), Immunology of Diabetes. Edinburgh: Teviot Scientific Publications, 1980: 319–324.

Andreani, D., Iavicoli, M., Colletti, A., Menzinger, G., Maltavello, C. Esperienze nel trattamento del diabete con le insuline de tipo mono-componente (MC) e monospecie (MS). Folia Endocrinol. (Roma) 1972; 25: 516–539.

Andreani, D. Some aspects of treatment with monocomponent (MC) and monospecies (MS) insulins. Excerpta Medica Int. Congress Series 1973; 316: 68–75.

Andreani, D., Iavicoli, M., Tamburrano, G., Menzinger, G. Comparative trials with monocomponent (MC) and monospecies (MS) pork insulins in the treatment of diabetes mellitus. Horm. Metab. Res. 1974; 6: 447–454.

Aretaeus, The Cappadocian. The extant works. Ed. and trans. by Adams, F. London, 1856.

Arias, P., Kerner, W., Navascués, I., Schäfauer, G., Pfeiffer, E. F. Semisynthetic human insulin and purified pork insulin do not differ in their biological potency. Klin. Wochenschr. 1984; 62: 1145–1150.

Arimura, A., Sato, H., DuPont, A., et al. Somatostatin: abundance of immunoreactive hormone in rat stomach and pancreas. Science 1975; 189: 1007–1008.

Arnozan and Vaillard. Contribution à l'étude du pancreas du lapin; lésions provoquées par la ligature du canal de Wirsung. Arch. de Physiol. Horm. et Path., Paris, 1884; 3: 287.

Arquilla, E. R., Thiene, P., Brugman, T., Ruess, W., Sugiyama, R. Effects of zinc ion on the conformation of antigenic determinants on insulin. Biochem. J. 1978; 175: 289–297.

Asplin, C. M., Hartog, M., Goldie, D. J. Change of insulin dosage, circulating free and bound insulin and insulin antibodies on transferring diabetics from conventional to highly purified porcine insulin. Diabetologia 1978; 14: 99–105.

Assan, R. La somatostatine: une nouvelle hormone. Diabète Metab. 1976; 2: 135–146.

Baker, E. N., Dodson, E. J. Crystallographic refinement of the structure of actinidin at 1.7 Å resolution by fast Fourier least-squares methods. Acta Crystallographica 1980; Sect. A36: 559–572.

Baker, R. S., Schmidtke, J. R., Ross, J. W., Smith, W. C. Preliminary studies on the immunogenicity and amount of *Escherichia coli* polypeptides in biosynthetic human insulin produced by recombinant DNA technology. Lancet 1981; ii: 1139–1142.

Ball, E. G., Jungas, R. L. Studies on the metabolism of adipose tissue XIII. The effect of anaerobic conditions and dietary regime on the response to insulin and epinephrine. Biochemistry 1963; 2: 586–592.

Bangham, D. R., Mussett, M. V. The Fourth International Standard for Insulin. Bull. Wld. Hlth. Org. 1959; 20: 1209–1220.

Banting, F. G., Best, C. H. The internal secretion of the pancreas. J. Lab. Clin. Med. 1922a; 7: 251–256.

Banting, F. G., Best, C. H. Pancreatic extracts. J. Lab. Clin. Med. 1922b; 7: 464–472.

Banting, F. G., Best, C. H., Collip, J. B., Macleod, J. J. R. The preparation of pancreatic extracts containing insulin. I. The preparation of the earlier extracts. Trans. Roy. Soc. Can. 1922a; 16: Section V, 1–2.

Banting, F. G., Best, C. H., Collip, J. B., Campbell, W. R., Fletcher, A. A. Pancreatic extracts in the treatment of diabetes mellitus: Preliminary report. Can. Med. Assoc. J. 1922b; 12: 141–146.

Banting, F. G., Best, C. H., Collip, J. B., Macleod, J. J. R., Noble, E. C. The effect of pancreatic extract (insulin) on normal rabbits. Am. J. Physiol. 1922c; 62: 162–176.

Banting, F. G., Campbell, W. R., Fletcher, A. A. Further experience with insulin in the treatment of diabetes mellitus. Br. Med. J. 1923; i: 8–12.

Banting, F. G. Diabetes and Insulin. Nobel Prize Lecture, Stockholm, 1925. Can. Med. Assoc. J. 1926; 16: 221–232.

Banting, F. G. The history of insulin. Edin. Med. J. 1929; 36: 1–18.

Banting, F. G., Frank, W. R., Gairns, S. Experimental insulin and metrazole shock. VII. Anti-insulin activity of insulin-treated patients. Am. J. Psychiatry 1938; 95: 553–556.

Barach, J. H. The history of the disease. In: Diabetes and its treatment. New York: OUP, 1949: 3–20.

Barron, Moses. The relation of the islets of Langerhans to diabetes with special reference to cases of pancreatic lithiasis. Surg. Gynecol. Obstet. 1920; 31: 437–448.

Barros D'Sa, A. A. J., Bloom, S. R., Baron, J. H. Direct inhibition of gastric acid by growth hormone release inhibiting hormone in dogs. Lancet 1975; i: 886–887.

Baum, C. K., Tudor, R., Landon, J. A simple competitive protein binding assay for plasma cortisol. Clin. Chim. Acta 1974; 55: 147–154.

Bauman, L. Clinical experience with globin insulin. Proc. Soc. Exp. Biol. Med. (N.Y.) 1939; 40: 170–171.

Bauman, W. A., Yalow, R. S. Differential diagnosis between endogenous and exogenous insulin-induced refractory hypoglycemia in a non-diabetic patient. N. Engl. J. Med. 1980; 303: 198–199.

Beecher, H. K., Krogh, A. Microscopic observation of the absorption of insulin and protamine insulinate. Nature 1936; 137: 458.

Bellmann, O., Hartmann, E. Influence of pregnancy on the kinetics of insulin. Am. J. Obstet. Gynecol. 1975; 122: 829–833.

Berger, M., Halban, P. A., Assal, J. P., Offord, R. E., Vranić, M., Renold, A. E. Pharmacokinetics of subcutaneously injected tritiated insulin: effects of exercise. Diabetes 1979; 28: 53–57.

Berger, M., Cüppers, H. J., Halban, P. A., Offord, R. E. The effect of aprotinin on the absorption of subcutaneously injected regular insulin in normal subjects. Diabetes 1980; 29: 81–83.

Berger, M., Cüppers, H. J., Hegner, H., Jörgens, V., Berchtold, P. Absorption kinetics and biologic effects of subcutaneously injected insulin preparations. Diabetes Care 1982; 5: 77–91.

Bernard, C. De l'origine du sucré dans l'economie animale. C.R. Soc. Biol. (Paris) 1849; 1: 121–133.

Bernard, C. Nouvelles recherches experimentales sur les phenomenes glycogenique due foie. C.R. Soc. Biol. (Paris) 1857; 9: 1.

Bernard, C. Leçons sur le diabete et la glycogenese animale, Paris, 1877.

Berson, S. A., Yalow, R. S., Bauman, A., Rothschild, M. A., Newerly, K. Insulin-I^{131} metabolism in human subjects: demonstration of insulin binding globulin in the circulation of insulin-treated subjects. J. Clin. Invest. 1956; 35: 170–190.

Berson, S. A., Yalow, R. S. Species specificity of human anti-beef, pork insulin serum. J. Clin. Invest. 1959; 38: 2017–2025.

Berson, S. A., Yalow, R. S. Insulin inhibitors and insulin resistance. N.Y. State J. Med. 1960; 60: 3658–3665.

Berson, S. A., Yalow, R. S. The present status of insulin antagonists in plasma. Diabetes 1964; 13: 247–259.

Berson, S. A., Yalow, R. S. Insulin in blood and insulin antibodies. Am. J. Med. 1966; 40: 676–690.

Best, C. H. The prolongation of insulin action. Symposium on hormones (Sigma X1 Lect.) 1937; 362–377.

Best, C. H. The first clinical use of insulin. Diabetes 1956; 5: 65–67.

Best, C. H. The internal secretion of the pancreas. Can. Med. Assoc. J. 1962; 87: 1046–1051.

Best, C. H. Nineteen hundred and twenty one in Toronto. Diabetes 1972; 21 (Suppl. 2): 385–395.

Beyer, J., Weber, Th., Schultz, G., Hassinger, W., Westerburg, A., Cordes, V. Comparison of biosynthetic human insulin and pork insulin during rest, food ingestion and physical work in insulin dependent diabetic subjects using a glucose controlled insulin infusion system. Diabetes Care 1981; 4: 189–192.

Biemond, M. E. F., Sipman, W. A., Olivié, J. Quantitative determination of polypeptides by gradient elution high-pressure liquid chromatography. J. Liq. Chromatogr. 1979; 2: 1407–1435.

Biemond, M. E. F., Sipman, W. A., Olivié, J. Quantitative determination of insulin by gradiant elution HPLC. In: Brandenburg, D., Wollmer A. (eds.), Proceedings 2nd International Insulin Symposium, Aachen. Berlin, New York: Walter de Gruyter, 1980: 201–206.

Binder, C., Nielsen, Aa, Jørgensen, K. The absorption of an acid and a neutral insulin solution after subcutaneous injection into different regions in diabetic patients. Scand. J. Clin. Lab. Invest. 1967; 19: 156–163.

Binder, C., Absorption of injected insulin. A clinical pharmacological study. *Thesis.* Copenhagen: Munksgaard, 1969.

Binder, C., Lauritzen, T., Faber, O., Pramming, S. Insulin pharmacokinetics. Diabetes Care 1984; 7: 188–199.

Birtwell, A. J., Owens, D. R., Luzio, S., Jones, I. R., Hayes, T. M., Vølund, Aa. Subcutaneous adiposity influences the absorption of radio-labelled Actrapid insulin. (Abstract). Diabetologia 1983; 25: 141.

Birtwell, A. J., Owens, D. R., Jones. I. R., et al. Comparison of highly purified semi-synthetic insulin and highly purified porcine insulin in the treatment of Type I diabetes: an interim report of a multi-centre randomised single blind study. Diabète Metab. 1984; 10: 295–298.

Bischoff, F., Jemtegaard, L. M. Divided dosage of insulin. Am. J. Physiol. 1937; 119: 149.

Blatherwick, N. R., Ewing, M. E., Bradshaw, P. J. Some effects of zinc and iron salts on the hypoglycaemic action of insulin in rats. Am. J. Physiol. 1938; 121: 44.

Blauth, C., Sönksen, P., Tomkins, C., et al. The hypoglycaemic action of somatostatin in the anaesthetised dog. Clin. Endocrinol. 1977; 6: 17–25.

Bliss, M. Banting's, Best's and Collip's accounts of the discovery of insulin. Bull. Hist. Med. 1982a; 56: 554–568.

Bliss, M. The discovery of insulin. Toronto: McClelland & Stewart, 1982b.

Bloom, A., Keen, H., Watkins, P. J. A change to 100-unit insulin dosage will reduce errors. Br. Med. J. 1981; 283: 33–34.

Bloom, S., Mortimer, C., Thorner, M., et al. Inhibition of gastrin and gastric acid secretion by growth-hormone release-inhibiting hormone. Lancet 1974; ii: 1106–1109.

Bloom, S. R., Adrian, T. E., Mitchell, S. J., Barnes, A. J., Kohner, E. M. Dirty insulin – a stimulant to autoimmunity (Abstract). Diabetologia 1976; 12: 381.

Bloom, S. R., West, A. M., Polak, J. M., Barnes, A. J., Adrian, T. E. Hormonal contaminants of insulin. In: Bloom, S. R. (ed.), Gut hormones. Edinburgh, London, New York: Churchill Livingstone, 1978: 318–322.

Bloom, S. R., Barnes, A. J., Adrian, T. E., Polak, J. M. Autoimmunity in diabetics induced by hormonal contaminants of insulin. Lancet 1979; i: 14–17.

Blundell, T. L., Johnson, L. N. Protein crystallography. New York: Academic Press, 1976: 404–419.

Bodanszky, M., and Fried, J. Process for preparing human insulin. U. S. Patent 3276961, 1966.

Boden, G., Soeldner, J. S. A sensitive double antibody radioimmunoassay for human growth hormone (HGH). Levels of serum HGH following rapid tolbutamide infusion. Diabetologia 1976; 3: 413–421.

Boden, G., Reichard, G. A. Jr., Hoeldtke, R. D., Rezvani, I., Owen, O. E. Severe insulin-induced hypoglycemia associated with deficiencies in the release of counterregulatory hormones. N. Engl. J. Med. 1981; 305: 1200–1205.

Bolli, G., Feoc. P. D., Compangnucci, P., et al. Abnormal counterregulation in insulin-dependent diabetes mellitus. Interaction of anti-insulin antibodies and impaired glucagon and epinephrine secretion. Diabetes 1983; 32: 134–141.

Bollinger, R. E., Morris, J. H., McKnight, F. G., Diederich, D. A. Disappearance of ^{131}I-labelled insulin from plasma as a guide to management of diabetes. N. Engl. J. Med. 1964; 270: 767–770.

Bonnici, F. Making the change to U–100 insulins. A patient education guide. S. Afr. Med. J. 1983; 64: 201–203.

Bottermann, P., Gyaram, H., Wahl, K., Ermler, R., Lebender, A. Pharmacokinetics of biosynthetic human insulin and characteristics of its effect. Diabetes Care 1981; 4: 168–169.

Bottermann, P., Gyaram, H., Wahl, K., Ermler, R., Lebender, A. Insulin concentrations and time-action profiles of three different intermediate-acting insulin preparations in non-diabetic volunteers under glucose-controlled infusion technique. Diabetes Care 1982; 5 (Suppl. 2): 43–52.

Bouchardat, A. De la glycosurie ou diabète sucré; son traitement hygiénique. Paris: Germer-Bailliere, 1875.

Brange, J., Skelbaek-Pedersen, B., Langkjær, L. et al. Galenics of insulin preparations. In: Berger, M. (ed.) Subcutaneous insulin therapy. Berlin – Heidelberg: Springer-Verlag, 1985.

Brearly, B. F., Mackie, J. British standard insulin syringe (Letter). Br. Med. J. 1978; i: 713.

Bressler, R., Galloway, J. A. Insulin treatment of diabetes mellitus. Med. Clin. N. Am. 1971; 55: 861–876.

Bressler, R., Galloway, J. A. The insulins: Pharmacology and uses. Drug Therapy 1978; March: 43–61.

British Pharmacopoeia; Biological assay of insulin Cambridge University Press, 1980: A141–A142.

Brogard, J. M., Blickle, J. F., Pinget, M., Stahl, A., Dorner, M. Biosynthetic human insulin: pharmacokinetics and effects in healthy human volunteers. Int. J. Clin. Pharmacol. Ther. Toxicol. 1983; 21: 575–580.

Brogard, J. M., Blickle, J. F., Stahl, A., Pinget, M., Dorner, M. Insulin humaine biosynthetique. La Presse Medicale 1984; 13: 265–268.

Brown, H., Sanger, F., Kital, R. The structure of pig and sheep insulins. Biochem. J. 1955; 60: 556–565.

Brownlee, M. Insulin treatment of diabetes. Hosp. Pract. 1979; 14: 85–94.

Brownlee, M., Cahill, G. F. Diabetic control and vascular complications. Atherosclerosis Rev. 1979; 4: 29–70.

Brownstein, M., Arimura, A., Sato, H., et al. The regional distribution of somatostatin in the rat brain. Endocrinology 1975; 96: 1456–1461.

Brunfeldt, K., Deckert, T. The antigenic properties of pig insulin. Acta Endocrinol. (Copenh.) 1964; 47: 353–366.

Brunfeldt, K., Deckert, T. Antibodies in the pig against pig insulin. Acta Endocrinol. (Copenh.) 1966; 47: 367–370.

Brunfeldt, K., Deckert, T., Thomsen, J. Human crystalline insulin from non-diabetic and diabetic patients. Acta Endocrinol. 1969; 60: 543–549.

Bruni, B., Ricci, C., Giolitti, A., Osenda, M., D'Alberto, M., Turco, G. L. Insulin antibody production studied quantitatively with a modified radio-immunoassay technique and with radioimmunoelectrophoresis in patients treated with monocomponent (MC) insulin. J. Nucl. Biol. Med. 1973; 17: 123.

Bruni, B., Bruni, K. B., Gamba, S., Giolitti, A., Rittatore, R., Turco, G. L. Long-term clinical trial with porcine monocomponent Lente insulin (Monotard). Panminerva Med. 1977; 19: 247–254.

Brunner, J. C. Experimenta Nova Circa Pancreas. Amsterdam (Amstelaedami), 1682.

Burday, S. Z., Fine, P. H., Schalch, D. S. Growth hormone secretion in response to arginine infusion in normal and diabetic subjects. Relationship to blood glucose levels. J. Lab. Clin. Med. 1968; 71: 897–911.

Burgess, N., Campbell, J. M. H., Osman, A. A., Payne, W. W., Poulton, E. P. Early experiences with insulin in the treatment of diabetes mellitus. Lancet, 1923; ii: 777.

Burgus, R., Ling, N., Butcher, M., et al. Primary structure of somatostatin, a hypothalamic peptide that inhibits the secretion of pituitary growth hormone. Proc. Natl. Acad. Sci. USA 1973; 79: 684–688.

Burrow, G. N., Hazlett, B. E., Phillips, M. J. A case of diabetes mellitus. N. Engl. J. Med. 1982; 306: 340–343.

Burt, R. L., Davidson, I. W. F. Insulin half-life and utilisation in normal pregnancy. Obstet. Gynecol. 1974; 43: 161–170.

Cahill, G. F. Jr. Physiology of insulin in man. Diabetes 1971; 20: 785–799.

Cahill, G. F. Jr., Etzwiler, D. D., Freinkel, N. 'Control' and diabetes. N. Engl. J. Med. 1976; 294: 1004–1005.

Camerini-Davalos, R. A., Velasco, C., Glasser, M., Bloodworth, J. M. B. Jr. Drug-induced reversal of early diabetic microangiopathy. N. Engl. J. Med. 1983; 309: 1551–1556.

Campbell, W. R., Fletcher, A. A., Kerr, R. B. Protamine insulin in treatment of diabetes mellitus. Am. J. Med. Sci. 1936; 192: 589–600.

Carpenter, F. H. Partition column chromatography of insulin in z-butanol-aqueous acid systems. Arch. Biochem. Biophys. 1958; 78: 539–545.

Carpenter, F. H. Relationship of structure to biological activity of insulin as revealed by degradative studies. Am. J. Med. 1966; 40: 750–758.

Cartwright, B. J., Owens, C., Kassimi, F., Baksi, A. K. A study of clinical aspects of the change to U-100 insulin. Abstract of paper presented at the British Diabetic Association Spring Meeting, York, 1983.

Castillo, M., Nemery, A., Verdin, E., Lefebvre, P. J., Luyckx, A. S. Circadian profiles of blood glucose and plasma free insulin during treatment with semi-synthetic and bio-synthetic human insulin, and comparison with conventional monocomponent preparations. Eur. J. Clin. Pharmacol. 1983; 25: 767–771.

Cawley, T. A singular case of diabetes, consisting entirely in the quality of the urine; with an enquiry into the different theories of that disease. London Med. J. 1788; 9: 286–308.

Celsus, A. C. De Medicina (with an English translation by Spencer, W. G.) Harvard University Press, 1960.

Champion, M. C., Shepherd, G. A. A., Rodger, N. W., Dupre, J. Continuous subcutaneous insulin infusion in the management of diabetes mellitus. Diabetes 1980; 29: 206–212.

Chan, S. J., Kwok, S. C. M., Steiner, D. F. The biosynthesis of insulin: some genetic and evolutionary aspects. Diabetes Care 1981; 4: 4–10.

Chance, R. E., Ellis, R. M., Bromer, W. W. Porcine proinsulin: characterisation and amino acid sequence. Science 1968; 161: 165–167.

Chance, R. E. Amino acid sequences of proinsulin and intermediates. Diabetes 1972; 21 (Suppl. 2): 461–467.

Chance, R. E., Root, M. A., Galloway, J. A. The immunogenicity of insulin preparations. Acta Endocrinol. (Copenh.) 1976; 83 (Suppl. 205): 185–196.

Chance, R. E., Hoffman, J. A., Kroeff, E. P., et al. The production of human insulin using recombinant DNA technology and a new chain combination procedure. In: Rich, D. H., Gross, E. (eds.), Peptides: Synthesis–Structure–Function. Proceedings of the Seventh American Peptide Symposium, Rockford II, Pierce Chemical Co., 1981a: 721–728.

Chance, R. E., Kroeff, E. P., Hoffman, J. A., Frank, B. H. Chemical, physical and biological properties of biosynthetic human insulin. Diabetes Care 1981b; 4: 147–154.

Chance, R. E., Kroeff, E. P., Hoffman, J. A. Chemical, physical and biological properties of recombinant human insulin. In: Gueriguian, J. L. (ed.), Insulins, Growth Hormone and Recombinant DNA Technology. New York: Raven Press, 1981c: 71–86.

Chang, J., Brauer, D., Wittman-Leibold, B. Microsequence analysis of peptides and proteins using 4-N, N-dimethylaminoazobenzene 4-isothiocyanate/phenylisothiocyanate double coupling methods. FEBS Lett. 1978; 93: 205–214.

Charles, W. A., Szekeres, A., Staten, M., Worcester, B., Walsh, K. M. Comparison of porcine insulin and human insulin (Novo) using the glucose-controlled insulin infusion system, glucose-insulin dose-response curves and the out-patient effectiveness of human insulin (Novo) in insulin-dependent diabetes. Diabetes Care 1983; 6 (Suppl. 1): 29–34.

Chawdhury, S. A., Dodson, E. J., Dodson, G. G., et al. The crystal structure of two zinc human insulins. In: Gueriguian, J. L., Bransome, E. D., Outschoorn, A. S. (eds.), Hormone drugs. Proceedings of the FDA-USP Workshop on Drug and Reference Standards for Insulins, Somatotropins and Thyroid-axis Hormones, Bethesda, Maryland. Rockville: USP Convention Inc., 1982: 106–115.

Chawdhury, S. A., Dodson, E. J., Dodson, G. G., et al. The crystal structure in three non-pancreatic human insulins. Diabetologia 1983; 25: 460–464.

Chevreul, M. E. Note sur le sucre de diabétes. Ann. Chim. Paris 1815; 95: 319–320.

Chideckel, E. W., Palmer, J., Koerker, D. J., Ensinck, J., Davidson, M. B., Goodner, C. J. Somatostatin blockade of acute and chronic stimuli of the endocrine pancreas and the consequences of this blockade on glucose homeostasis. J. Clin. Invest. 1975; 55: 754–762.

Chideckel, E. W., Goodner, C. J., Koerker, D. J., Johnson, D. G., Ensinck, J. E. Role of glucagon in mediating metabolic effects of epinephrine. Am. J. Physiol. 1977; 232: 464–470.

Chisholm, D. J., Kraegen, E. W., Hewett, M. J., Lazarus, L. Comparison of potency of porcine insulin with semisynthetic human insulin at three dose levels using the euglycaemic clamp. Horm. Metab. Res. 1983; 15: 415–418.

Christensen, N. J., Christensen, S. E., Hansen, Aa. P., Lundbaek, K. The effect of somatostatin on plasma noradrenaline and plasma adrenaline concentrations during exercise and hypoglycemia. Metabolism 1975; 24: 1267–1272.

Christensen, S. E., Hansen, Aa. P., Iversen, J., et al. Somatostatin as a tool in studies of basal carbohydrate and lipid metabolism in man. Modifications of glucagon and insulin release. Scand. J. Clin. Lab. Invest. 1974; 34: 321–325.

Christensen, S. E., Schmitz, O., Hansen, Aa. P., Jensen, I., Heding, L. G. A double-blind study of the efficacy of neutral human and porcine insulin in Type I diabetes using a glucose-controlled insulin infusion system. Metabolism 1984; 33: 864–868.

Christy, M., Deckert, T., Nerup, J. Immunity and autoimmunity in diabetes mellitus. Clin. Endocrinol. Metab. 1977; 6: 305–332.

Clark, A. J. L., Adeniyi-Jones, R. O., Knight, G., et al. Biosynthetic human insulin in the treatment of diabetes. Lancet 1982; ii: 354–357.

Clausen, V. Kliniske Undersøgelser over Insulinresorptionens Paavirkelighed af Adrenalin, Pituitrin og Ephetonin. Monograph, Copenhagen, 1934.

Colagiuri, S., Kotowicz, M. A., Steinbeck, A. W., Kidson, W. Metabolic profiles in diabetic subjects treated with human insulin (Novo) and porcine insulin. Diabetes Care 1983; 6 (Suppl. 1): 49–52.

Cole, R. D., The chromatography of insulin in urea containing buffer. J. Biol. Chem. 1960; 235: 2294–2299.

Collip, J. B. The preparation of pancreatic extracts containing insulin. II. The preparation of the extracts as used in the first clinical cases. Trans. Roy. Soc. Can. 1922; 16 (Section V): 2–3.

Collip, J. B. The original method as used for the isolation of insulin in semipure form for the treatment of the first clinical cases. J. Biol. Chem. 1923; 55: 40–41.

Colwell, A. R., Izzo, J. L., Stryker, W. A. Intermediate action of mixtures of soluble insulin and protamine zinc insulin. Arch. Intern. Med. 1942; 69: 931–951.

Colwell, A. R. Protamine insulin mixtures in treatment of diabetes mellitus. N.Y. State J. Med. 1947; 47: 1103–1110.

Colwell, A. R. Fifty years of diabetes in perspective. Diabetes 1968; 17: 599–610.

Crea, R., Kraszewski, A., Hirose, T., Itakura, K. Chemical synthesis of genes for human insulin. Proc. Natl. Acad. Sci. USA 1978; 75: 5765–5769.

Cryer, P. E. Glucose counterregulation in man. Diabetes 1981; 30: 261–264.

Cryer, P. E., Gerich, J. E. Relevance of glucose counterregulatory systems to patients with diabetes: critical roles of glucagon and epinephrine. Diabetes Care 1983; 6: 95–99.

Cüppers, H. J. Pharmacokinetics of subcutaneously injected insulin. Thesis, Düsseldorf University, Medical Faculty, 1981.

Czyzyk, A., Lawecki, J., Rogala, H., Miedzinska, E., Popik-Hankiewicz, A.

Serum levels of insulin-binding antibodies in diabetic patients treated with monocomponent insulin. Diabetologia 1974; 10: 233–236.

Damgaard, U., Markussen, J. Analysis of insulins and related compounds by HPLC. Horm. Metab. Res. 1979; 11: 580–581.

Da Prada, M., Zürcher, G. Simultaneous radioenzymatic determination of plasma and tissue adrenaline, noradrenaline and dopamine within the femtomole range. Life Science 1976; 19: 1161–1174.

Debodo, R. C. R., Altszuler, A. Insulin hypersensitivity and physiological insulin antagonism. Physiol. Rev. 1958; 38: 389–423.

Deckert, T. Insulin antibodies. Thesis, Copenhagen University, 1964.

Deckert, T., Grundahl, E. The antigenicity of pig insulin. Diabetologia 1970; 6: 15–20.

Deckert, T., Andersen, O. O., Grundahl, E., Kerp, L. Iso-immunization of man by recrystallised human insulin. Diabetologia 1972; 8: 358–361.

Deckert, T., Andersen, O. O., Poulsen, J. E. The clinical significance of highly purified pig insulin preparations. Diabetologia 1974; 10: 703–708.

Deckert, T., Lorup, B. Regulation of brittle diabetes by a pre-planned insulin infusion programme. Diabetologia 1976; 12: 573–579.

Deckert, T. Intermediate-acting insulin preparations: NPH and Lente. Diabetes Care 1980; 3: 623–626.

Del Guercio, M., de Natale, B., Gargantini, L., et al. Effect of somatostatin on blood sugar, plasma growth hormone and glucagon levels in diabetic children. Diabetes 1976; 25: 550–553.

De Meyer, J. Action de la secretion interne du pancreas sur differents organes et en particulier su la secretion renale. Arch. di Fisiol. 1909; 7: 96–99.

De Pirro, R., Fusco, A., Spallone, L., Mignatia, R., Lauro, R. Insulin antibodies prevent insulin receptor interactions. Diabetologia 1980; 19: 118–122.

Devane, G., Siler, T., Yen, S. Acute suppression of insulin and glucose levels by synthetic somatostatin in normal human subjects. J. Clin. Endocrinol. Metab. 1974; 38: 913–915.

Devlin, J. G., Parameswaran, V. Immunologic response to monocomponent insulin in newly diagnosed diabetic patients. J. Irish Med. Assoc. 1975; 68: 301–305.

Devlin, J. G., Parameswaran, V. Characterisation of antibody response to monocomponent insulin. J. Irish Med. Assoc. 1978; 71: 256–260.

De Witt, L. M. Morphology and physiology of areas of Langerhans in some vertebrates. J. Exp. Med. 1906; 8: 193–239.

Diem, P., Teuscher, A. Immunologische Untersuchungen mit vollsynthetischem humanen Insulin bei Patienten mit Diabetes Mellitus. Schweiz Med. Wochenschr. 1979; 109: 1814–1816.

Dinner, A., Lorenz, L. High performance liquid chromatographic determination of bovine insulin. Anal. Chem. 1979; 51: 1872–1873.

Dixon, K., Exon, P. D., Malins, J. M. Insulin antibodies and the control of diabetes. Q. J. Med. 1975; 176: 543–553.

Dobson, M. Experiments and observations on the urine in diabetes. J. Phys. of London, 1776; 5: 298–316.

Doi, K., Morita, S., Yoshida, Y., Baba, S. Comparison of biosynthetic human insulin and pork insulin in noninsulin-dependent diabetic subjects during insulin clamp studies using a glucose controlled insulin infusion system. In: Sakamoto, N., Alberti, K. G. M. M. (eds.), Current and Future Therapies with Insulin. Excerpta Medica International Congress Series, Amsterdam–Oxford–Princeton, 1983, 607: 230–234.

Dörzbach, V. E., Müller, R. Die Insulintherapie: Die Insulinpräparate. In: Pfeiffer, E. F. Handbook of diabetes mellitus. Pathophysiology and clinical considerations. Vol. II. München: J. F. Lehmanns Verlag, 1971: 1087–1111.

Eaton, R. P., Allen, R. C., Schade, D. S., Erickson, K. M., Standefer, J. Prehepatic insulin production in man: kinetic analysis using peripheral connecting peptide behaviour. J. Clin. Endocrinol. Metab. 1980; 51: 520–528.

Ebihara, A., Kondo, K., Ohashi, K., Kosaka, K., Kuzuya, T., Tarui, S. Clinical pharmacology of human insulin of recombinant DNA origin in healthy volunteers. Diabetes Care 1982; 5 (Suppl. 2): 35–38.

Ebihara, A., Kondo, K., Ohashi, K., Kosaka, K., Kuzuya, T., Matsuda, A. Comparative clinical pharmacology of human insulin (Novo) and porcine insulin in normal subjects. Diabetes Care 1983; 6 (Suppl. l): 17–22.

Ellenberg, M., Rifkin, H. Clinical diabetes mellitus. New York: McGraw-Hill Book Company Inc., 1962.

Erwald, R., Hed, R., Nygren, A., Röjdmark, S., Weichel, K. Comparison of the effect of intraportal and intravenous infusion of insulin on blood glucose and free fatty acids in peripheral venous blood of man. Acta Med. Scand. 1974; 195: 351–357.

European Pharmacopoeia 1975; 75–77.

Evans, D. R., Smith, C. S. Hazards of monocomponent insulin. Br. Med. J. 1976; l: 1146 (Corres.).

Faber, O. K., Lauritzen, T., Binder, C., Mouridsen, H. T., Vølund, Aa. Insulin Monotard og Insulin Novo Lente Sammenligning af absorption og klinisk effekt. Ugeskr. Læg. 1975; 137: 2510–2514.

Faber, O. K., Binder, C., Markussen, J., et al. Characterization of seven C-peptide antisera. Diabetes 1978; 27 (Suppl. l): 170–177.

Falholt, K. Determination of insulin-specific IgE in serum of diabetic patients by solid-phase radioimmunoassay. Diabetologia 1982; 22: 254–257.

Fankhauser, E. Neuere Aspekte der Insulintherapie. Schweiz Med. Wochenschr. 1969; 99: 414–420.

Federlin, K., Laube, H., Velcovsky, H. G. Biologic and immunologic in vivo and in vitro studies with biosynthetic human insulin. Diabetes Care 1981; 4: 170–174.

Fehling, H. C. Von Quantitative Bestimmung des Zuckers in Harn. Arch. Physiol. Heilk. 1848, 7: 64–73.

Feldman, J. M., Plonk, J. W., Bivens, C. H. The role of cortisol and growth hormone in the counterregulation of insulin-induced hypoglycemia. Horm. Metab. Res. 1975; 7: 378–381.

Felig, P., Wahren, J. Somatostatin and diabetes: suppression of glucose absorption rather than stimulation of glucose disposal. Metabolism 1976; 25 (Suppl. l): 1509–1511.

Finney, D. J. Statistical method in biological assay, 3rd edn. Charles Griffin, 1978.

Fitz-Patrick, D., Patel, Y. C. Antibodies of insulin, pancreatic polypeptide, glucagon and somatostatin in insulin-treated diabetics. J. Clin. Endocrinol. Metab. 1981; 52: 948–952.

Forsham, P. H., Diabetes mellitus: a rational plan for management. Postgrad. Med. 1982; 71: 139–144; 148–154.

Foster, D. W. Studies in the ketosis of fasting. J. Clin. Invest. 1967; 46: 1283–1296.

Foster, K. J., Alberti, K. G. M. M., Hinks, L., et al. Blood intermediary metabolite and insulin concentrations after an overnight fast: reference ranges for adults and interrelations. Clin. Chem. 1978; 24: 1568–1572.

Francis, A. J., Home, P. D., Hanning, I., Alberti, K. G. M. M., Tunbridge, W. M. G. Intermediate acting insulin given at bedtime: effect on blood glucose concentrations before and after breakfast. Br. Med. J. 1983; 286: 1173–1176.

Frank, L. L. Diabetes mellitus in the text of old Hindu medicine (Charaka, Susruta, Vagbhata). Am. J. Gastroenterol. 1957; 27: 76–95.

Frank, B. H., Pettee, J. M., Zimmermann, R. E., Burck, P. J. The production of human proinsulin and its transformation to human insulin and C-peptide. In: Rich, D. H., Gross, E. (eds.), Peptides: Synthesis–Structure–Function. Proceedings of the Seventh American Peptide Symposium, Rockford. Pierce Chemical Co., 1981; 729–738.

Freidenberg, G. R., White, N., Cataland, S., O'Dorisio, T. M., Sotos, J. F., Santiago, J. V. Effectiveness of aprotinin (Trasylol) in protease-mediated insulin resistance. Diabetes 1980; 29 (Suppl. 2): 23A.

Freidenberg, G. R., White, N., Cataland, S., O'Dorisio, T. M., Sotos, J. F., Santiago, J. V. Diabetes responsive to intravenous but not subcutaneous insulin: effectiveness of aprotinin. N. Engl. J. Med. 1981; 305: 363–368.

Frost, D. P., Srivastava, M. C., Jones, R. H., Nabarro, J. D. N., Sönksen, P. H. The kinetics of insulin metabolism in diabetes mellitus. Postgrad. Med. J. 1973; 49 (Dec. Suppl.): 949–954.

Fukumoto, Y., Ichihara, K., Nonaka, K., Tarui, S. Comparison of diurnal serum insulin levels during short term treatments with sulphonylurea and with insulin in non-insulin dependent diabetics. Horm. Met. Res. 1982; 14: 1–4.

Galloway, J. A., Bressler, R. Insulin treatment in diabetes. Med. Clin. North. Am. 1978; 62: 663–680.

Galloway, J. A., Spradlin, C. T., Nelson, R. L., Wentworth, S. M., Davidson, J. A., Swarner, J. L. Factors influencing the absorption, serum insulin concentration, and blood glucose responses after injections of regular insulin and various insulin mixtures. Diabetes Care 1981a; 4: 366–376.

Galloway, J. A., Spradlin, C. T., Root, M. A., Fineberg, S. E. The plasma glucose response of normal fasting subjects to neutral regular and NPH biosynthetic human and purified pork insulins. Diabetes Care 1981b; 4: 183–188.

Galloway, J. A., Root, M. A., Bergstrom, R., et al. Clinical pharmacologic studies with human insulin (recombinant DNA). Diabetes Care 1982a; 5 (Suppl. 2): 13–22.

Galloway, J. A., Spradlin, C. T., Jackson, R. L., Otto, D. C., Bechtel, L. D. Mixtures of intermediate-acting insulin (NPH and lente) with regular insulin: An update. In: Skyler, J. S. (ed.), Insulin Update: 1982. Princeton: Excerpta Medica 1982b: 111–119.

Galloway, J. A., Peck, F. B., Fineberg, S. E., et al. The U. S. 'New patient' and 'transfer' studies. Diabetes Care 1982c; 5 (Suppl. 2): 135–139.

Galloway, J. A., Fineberg, S. E., Fineberg, N. S., Goldman, J. Effect of purity and beef content on complications of insulin therapy. In: Gueriguian, J. L., Bransome, E. D., Outschoorn, A. S. (eds), Hormone drugs. Proceedings of the FDA-USP Workshop on Drug and Reference Standards for Insulins, Somatotropins and Thyroid-axis Hormones, Bethesda, Maryland. USP Convention Inc., 1982d: 244–253.

Galloway, J. A., Root, M. A. The use of biosynthetic human insulin in man. From gene to protein. Translation into biotechnology. In: Ahmad, F., Schultz, J., Smith, E. E., Wheland, W. J. (eds), Proceedings of Miami Winter symposium, 1982. New York, London. Academic Press, 1982: 391–417.

Galloway, J. A., Fineberg, S. E., Root, M. A., Spradlin, T. C. Human insulin (rDNA): a summary of clinical studies in the USA. In: Sakamoto, N., Alberti, K. G. M. M. (eds), Current and future therapies with insulin. Excerpta Medica Int. Congress Series, 1983; 607: 80–89.

Gamst-Andersen, H., Hjortkjaer, R. K., Lorenzen, F. H., Ashby, R. Preclinical studies on human insulin I. Acute and subacute toxicity studies. Acta Pharmacol. Toxicol. 1983; 52: 261–267.

Garber, A. J., Cryer, P. E., Santiago, J. V., Haymond, M. W., Pagliara, A. S., Kipnis, D. M. The role of adrenergic mechanisms in the substrate and hormonal response to insulin-induced hypoglycemia in man. J. Clin. Invest. 1976; 58: 7–15.

Garrison, F. H. An introduction to the history of medicine, 4th edn. Philadelphia: W. B. Saunders, 1929: 261.

Gattner, H–G., Danho, W., Naithani, V. K. Enzyme-catalysed semisynthesis with insulin derivatives. In: Brandenburg, D., Wollmer, A. (eds), Proceedings 2nd International Insulin Symposium, Aachen. Berlin, New York: Walter de Gruyther, 1980: 117–123.

Geiger, R. Chemie des Insulins. Chemiker Zeitung 1976; 100: 111–129.

Gerich, J. E., Langlois, M., Noacco, C., Karam, J. H., Forsham, P. H. Lack of glucagon response to hypoglycemia in diabetes: evidence for an intrinsic pancreatic alpha cell defect. Science 1973; 182: 171–173.

Gerich, J. E., Lorenzi, M., Schneider, V., et al. Effects of somatostatin on plasma glucose and glucagon levels in human diabetes mellitus: pathophysiologic and therapeutic implications. N. Engl. J. Med. 1974a; 291: 544–547.

Gerich, J. E., Lorenzi, M., Schneider, V., et al. Inhibition of pancreatic glucagon responses to arginine by somatostatin in normal man and in insulin-dependent diabetics. Diabetes 1974b; 23: 876–880.

Gerich, J. E., Lorenzi, M., Karam, J. H., et al. Abnormal pancreatic glucagon secretion and postprandial hyperglycaemia in diabetes mellitus. JAMA 1975a; 234: 159–165.

Gerich, J. E., Lorenzi, M., Bier, D., et al. Prevention of human diabetic ketoacidosis by somatostatin: evidence for an essential role of glucagon. N. Engl. J. Med. 1975b; 292: 985–989.

Gerich, J. E., Lovinger, R., Grodsky, G. M. Inhibition by somatostatin of glucagon and insulin release from the perfused rat pancreas in response to arginine, isoproterenol and theophylline: evidence for a preferential effect on glucagon secretion. Endocrinology 1975c; 96: 749–754.

Gerich, J. E., Schultz, T., Tsalikian, E., et al. Clinical evaluation of somatostatin as a potential adjunct to insulin in the management of diabetes mellitus. Diabetologia 1977; 13: 537–544.

Gerich, J. E., Davis, J., Lorenzi, M., et al. Hormonal mechanisms of recovery from insulin-induced hypoglycaemia in man. Am. J. Physiol. 1979a; 236: E380–385.

Gerich, J. E., David, J., Lorenzi, M., et al. Mechanisms of recovery from hypoglycaemia in man. I. Interaction of glucagon and epinephrine. Am. J. Physiol. 1979b; 236: 209–215.

Gerich, J. E. Somatostatin and diabetes. Am. J. Med. 1980; 70(3): 619–626.

Gerlis, L. S., Adeniyi-Jones, R., Jones, R. H., Sönksen, P. H., Barnes, G. D. The metabolism and distribution of human monocomponent insulin in man. Minerva Endocrinologica 1982; 7 (Suppl. l): 49–54.

Gerritzen, F. The duration of the action of different insulins. Br. Med. J. 1952; i: 249–250.

Gilbert, W., Villa-Komaroff, L. Useful proteins from recombinant bacteria. Sci. Am. 1980; 242: 74–94.

Ginsberg, S., Block, M. B., Mako, M. E., Rubenstein, A. H. Serum insulin levels following administration of exogenous insulin. J. Clin. Endocrinol. Metab. 1973; 36: 1175–1179.

Giustina, G., Peracchi, M., Reschini, E., et al. Dose-response study of the inhibiting effect of somatostatin on growth hormone and insulin secretion in normal subjects and acromegalic patients. Metabolism 1975; 24: 807–815.

Goeddel, D. V., Kleid, D. G., Bolivar, F., et al. Expression in Escherichia coli of chemically synthesized genes for human insulin. Proc. Natl. Acad. Sci. USA 1979; 76: 106–110.

Gomez-Pan, A., Reed, J. D., Albinus, M. et al. Direct inhibition of gastric acid and pepsin secretion by growth hormone release-inhibiting hormone in cats. Lancet 1975; i: 888–890.

Gonen, B., Goldman, J., Baldwin, D., et al. Metabolic control in diabetic patients. Effect of insulin-secretory reserve (measured by plasma C-peptide levels) and circulating insulin antibodies. Diabetes 1979; 28: 749–753.

Gray, R. S., Cowan, P., Duncan, L. J. P., Clarke, B. F. A comparison of the biological actions and pharmacokinetics of intravenously infused highly purified beef and biosynthetic human insulins in normal man. Diabète Metab. 1984; 10: 188–193.

Greene, S. A., Smith, M. A., Cartwright, B., Baum, J. D. Comparison of human versus porcine insulin in treatment of diabetes in children. Br. Med. J. 1983; 287: 1578–1579.

Greenwood, F. C., Landon, J. Assessment of hypothalamic pituitary function in endocrine disease. J. Clin. Pathol. 1966; 19: 284–292.

Griffin, N. K., Spanos, A., Jenkins, P. A., Turner, R. C., Werther, G., Baum, J. D. 24-hour metabolic profiles in diabetic children. Arch. Dis. Child. 1980; 55: 112–117.

Grootendorst, B. C., Jonkers, J. R., Kruit, I. The miscibility of short acting insulins with depot insulins: an in vitro study. Pharm. Weekbl. 1983; 118: 746–751.

Guerra, S. M. O., Kitabchi, A. E. Comparison of the effectiveness of various routes of insulin injection: insulin levels and glucose response in normal subjects. J. Clin. Endocrinol. Metab. 1976; 42: 869–874.

Guillemin, R., Gerich, J. Somatostatin: physiological and clinical significance. Ann. Rev. Med. 1976; 27: 379–388.

Gunnarsson, R., Arner, P., Heding, L., Linde, B., Östman, J. Aprotinin reduced insulin resistance caused by excessive degradation in subcutaneous tissue (Abstract). Diabetologia 1980; 19: 279.

Gwinup, G., Elias, A. N. The poor man's insulin 'pump'. Postgrad. Med. 1982; 72: 113–118.

Haft, D. E., Miller, L. L. Alloxan diabetes and demonstrated direct action of insulin on metabolism of isolated perfused rat liver. Am. J. Physiol. 1958; 192: 33–42.

Hagedorn, H. C., Jensen, B. N., Krarup, N. B., Woodstrup, I. Protamine insulinate. JAMA 1936; 106: 177–180.

Hagedorn, H. C. The absorption of protamine insulin. Rep. Steno Hospital (Copenh.) 1946; 1: 25–28.

Hales, C. N., Randall, P. J. Immunoassay of insulin with insulin antibody precipitate. Biochem. J. 1963; 88: 137–146.

Hall, R., Schally, A., Evered, D., et al. Action of growth-hormone-release inhibitory hormone in healthy men and in acromegaly. Lancet 1973; ii: 581–584.

Hall, R., Anderson, J., Smart, G. A., Besser, M. Fundamentals of clinical endocrinology. 2nd edn. London: Pitman, 1974.

Hallas-Møller, K., Hey, A. Iso-insulin Novo: Et nyt protraheret virkende insulinpraeparat (A new insulin preparation with prolonged action). Ugeskr. Laeg. 1944; 23: 265.

Hallas-Møller, K., Jersild, M., Petersen, K., Schlichtkrull, J. Crystalline and amorphous insulin-zinc compounds with prolonged action (Danish). Ugeskr. Laeg. 1951; 113: 1761–1767.

Hallas-Møller, K., Jersild, M., Petersen, K., Schlichtkrull, J. Zinc insulin preparations for single daily injections. JAMA 1952; 150: 1667–1671.

Hallas-Møller, K., Jersild, M., Petersen, K., Schlichtkrull, J. The Lente insulins. Insulin zinc suspensions. Dan. Med. Bull. 1954; 1: 132–142.

Hallas-Møller, K. Clinical, biological and physiological background of the new insulin-zinc suspensions. Lancet 1954; ii: 1029–1034.

Hallas-Møller, K. The Lente insulins. Diabetes 1956; 5: 7–14.

Hansen, Aa. P., Johansen, K. Diurnal patterns of blood glucose, serum free fatty acids, insulin, glucagon and growth hormone in normals and juvenile diabetics. Diabetologia 1970; 6: 27–33.

Hansen, Aa. P., Ørskov, H., Seyer-Hansen, K., et al. Some action of growth hormone release inhibiting factor. Br. Med. J. 1973; iii: 523–524.

Hansen, Aa. P., Lundbaek, K. Somatostatin: a review of its effects especially in human beings. Diabète Metab. 1976; 2: 203–218.

Hansen, Aa. P., Ledet, T., Lundbaek, K. Growth hormone and diabetes. In: Brownlee, M. (ed.), Handbook of Diabetes Mellitus, Vol. 4. New York: John Wiley, 1981: 231–275.

Hansen, B., Linde, S., Kølendorf, K., Jensen, F. Absorption of protamine-insulin in diabetic patients. I. Preparation and characterisation of protamine-^{125}I-insulin. Horm. Metab. Res. 1979; 11: 85–90.

Hansen, B., Welinder, B., Nielsen, J. H. Physico-chemical properties of insulin. In; Gueriguian, J. L., Bransome, E. D., Outschoorn, A. S. (eds), Hormone Drugs. Proceedings of the FDA–USP Workshop on Drug and Reference Standards for Insulin, Somatotropins and Thyroid-axis Hormones, Bethesda, Maryland. Rockville: USP Convention Inc., 1982: 72–83.

Harano, Y., Ohgaku, S., Hidaka, H., et al. Glucose, insulin and somatostatin infusion for the determination of insulin sensitivity. J. Clin. Endocrinol. Metab. 1977; 45: 1124–1127.

Harfenist, E. J., Craig, L. C. Countercurrent distribution studies with insulin. J. Am. Chem. Soc. 1952; 74: 3083–3087.

Harris, J. I., Sanger, F., Naughton, M. A. Species differences in insulin. Arch. Biochem. Biophys. 1956; 65: 427–438.

Heding, L. G. Radioimmunological determination of pancreatic and gut glucagon in plasma. Diabetologia, 1971; 7: 10–19.

Heding, L. G. Determination of total serum insulin (IRI) in insulin treated diabetic patients. Diabetologia 1972; 8: 260–266.

Heding, L. G., Larsen, U. D., Markussen, J., Jørgensen, K. H., Hallund, O. Radioimmunoassays for human, pork and ox C-peptide and related substances. Horm. Metab. Res. 1974; 5(Suppl.1): 40–44.

Heding, L. G. Radioimmunological determination of human C-peptide in serum. Diabetologia 1975; 11: 541–548.

Heding, L. G., Larsson, Y., Ludvigsson, J. The immunogenicity of insulin preparations. Antibody levels before and after transfer to highly purified porcine insulin. Diabetologia 1980a, 19: 511–515.

Heding, L. G., Persson, B., Stangenberg, M. B-cell function in newborn infants of diabetic mothers. Diabetologia 1980b; 19: 427–432.

Heding, L. G. Human Insulin. Facts and perspectives. Acta Med. Scand. 1983; Suppl. 671: 107–115.

Heine, R. J., Bilo, H. J. G., Fonk, T. van der., Veen, E. A. van der., Meer, J. Insulin absorption kinetics and action profiles after the administration of regular and intermediate acting insulin mixtures (NPH and lente). Diabetes 1984a; 33 (Suppl. l): 39A.

Heine, R. J., Bilo, H. J. G., Fonk, T. van der., Veen, E. A. van der., Meer, J. Absorption kinetics and action profiles of mixtures of short- and intermediate-acting insulins. Diabetologia 1984b; 27: 558–562.

Heine, R. J., Bilo, H. J. G., Sikkenk, A. C. van der., Veen, E. A. van der. Mixing short- and intermediate-acting insulins in the syringe: effect on postprandial blood glucose concentrations in type I diabetes. Br. Med. J. 1985; 209: 204–205.

Heiskell, C. L., Florsheim, W. H., Meister, L. Electrophoretic distribution of allergenic and hormonal fractions of commercial insulins. Diabetes 1959; 8: 388–391.

Henschen, F. On the term 'diabetes' in the works of Aretaeus and Galen. Med. Hist. 1969; 13: 190–192.

Hildebrandt, P., Birch, K., Sestoft, L., Nielsen, S. L. Non-linear relationship between subcutaneous blood flow and insulin absorption. (Abstract). Diabetologia 1982; 23: 174.

Hildebrandt, P., Birch, K., Nielsen, S. L., Sestoft, L. Absorption on infused insulin: kinetics and relation to subcutaneous blood flow (Abstract). Diabetologia 1983a; 25: 164.

Hildebrandt, P., Sestoft, L., Nielsen, S. L. The absorption of subcutaneously injected short-acting soluble insulin: influence of injection technique and concentration. Diabetes Care 1983b; 6: 459–462.

Hildebrandt, P., Birch, K., Sestoft, L., Vølund, Aa. Subcutaneous absorption of insulin Monotard. Acta Endocrinol. 1983c; 257: 25 (Abstract).

Hildebrandt, P., Birch, K., Sestoft, L., Vølund, Aa. Dose-dependent subcutaneous absorption of porcine, bovine and human NPH insulins. Acta Med. Scand. 1984a; 215: 69–73.

Hildebrandt, P., Vølund, Aa., Kühl, C., Berger, A. Subcutaneous absorption of human and bovine Ultratard insulins. Diabetologia 1984b; 27: 287–288A.

Hildebrandt, P., Birch, K., Sestoft, L., Vølund, Aa. Human Monotard insulin dose-dependent subcutaneous absorption. Diabetes Research 1984c; 1: 183–185.

Hilsted, J., Madsbad, S., Krarup, T., et al. Hormonal, metabolic and cardiovascular responses to hypoglycaemia in diabetic autonomic neuropathy. Diabetes 1981; 30: 626–633.

Hirsh, A. Handbook of geographical and historical pathology. (Translation by Charles Creighton), 3 vols. London: 1883–1886.

Ho, L. S., Jawadi, M. H. Biological activity of premixing short acting (SA) and intermediate acting (IA) insulins. Diabetes 1984; 33 (Suppl. l): 102A.

Hoeldtke, R. D., Boden, G., Shuman, C. R., Owen, O. E. Reduced epinephrine secretion and hypoglycaemia unawareness in diabetic autonomic neuropathy. Ann. Intern. Med. 1982; 96: 459–462.

Holman, R. R., Turner, R. C. Diabetes: the quest for basal normoglycaemia. Lancet 1977; i: 469–474.

Holman, R. R., Dornan, T. L., Mayon-White, V., et al. Prevention of deterioration of renal and sensory-nerve function by more intensive management of insulin-dependent diabetic patients: a two-year randomised prospective study. Lancet 1983; i: 204–208.

Holman, R. R., Steemson, J., Darling, P., Reeves, W. G., Turner, R. C. Human Ultralente insulin. Br. Med. J. 1984; 288: 665–668.

Homandberg, G. A., Mattis, J. A., Laskowski, M. Synthesis of peptide bond by proteinases. Addition of organic cosolvents shifts peptide bond equilibria toward synthesis. Biochemistry 1978; 17: 5220–5227.

Home, P. D., Alberti, K. G. M. M. The new insulins, their characteristics and clinical indications, Drugs 1982; 24: 401–413.

Home, P. D., Massi-Benedetti, M., Shepherd, G. A. A., Hanning, I., Alberti, K. G. M. M., Owens, D. R. A comparison of the activity and disposal of semi-synthetic human insulin and porcine insulin in normal man by the glucose clamp technique. Diabetologia 1982a; 22: 41–45.

Home, P. D., Alberti, K. G. M. M., Owens, D. R. Some observations on insulin absorption and pharmacokinetics. In: Skyler, J. S. (ed.), Insulin Update: 1982. Princeton: Excerpta Medica, 1982b: 120–124.

Home, P. D., Capaldo, B., Burrin, J. M., Worth, R., Alberti, K. G. M. M. A crossover comparison of continuous subcutaneous insulin infusion (CSII) against multiple insulin injections in insulin-dependent diabetic subjects: improved control with CSII. Diabetes Care 1982c; 5: 466–471.

Home, P. D., Hanning, I., Capaldo, B., Alberti, K. G. M. M. Bioavailability of highly purified bovine Ultralente insulin. Diabetes Care 1983; 6: 210.

Home, P. D., Mann, N. P., Hutchinson, A. S., et al. A fifteen-month double-blind cross-over study of the efficacy and antigenicity of human and pork insulins. Diabetic Medicine 1984; 1: 93–98.

Horwitz, D. L., Rubenstein, A. H., Reynolds, C., Molnar, D., Yamaihara, N. Prolonged suppression of insulin release by insulin-induced hypoglycaemia: demonstration by C-peptide assay. Horm. Metab. Res. 1975; 7: 449–452.

Hosker, J. P., Turner, R. C. Insulin treatment of newly-presenting ketotic diabetic patients into the honeymoon period. Lancet 1982; ii: 633–635.

Hulst, S. G. Th. Treatment of insulin-induced lipoatrophy. Diabetes 1976; 25: 1052–1054.

Hurn, B. A. L., Farrant, P. C., Young, B. A., Grahame, A. Insulin-binding antibody and hormone dosage in non-resistant diabetes. Postgrad. Med. J. 1969; 45 (Suppl.): 819–824.

IDF Special Committee. Report to the special committee set up to present a written summary of work leading up to the discovery of insulin. IDF Bull. 1971; XVI: 29–49.

International Pharmacopoeia 1967; 797–799.

Irsigler, K., Kritz, H., Hagmüller, G., et al. Long-term continuous intraperitoneal insulin infusion with an implanted remote-controlled infusion device. Diabetes 1981; 30: 1072–1075.

Ishihara, Y., Saito, T., Ito, Y., Fujino, M. Structure of sperm- and sei-whale insulins and their breakdown by whale pepsin. Nature 1958; 181: 1468–1469.

Iversen, J. Inhibition of pancreatic glucagon release by somatostatin: In vitro. Scand. J. Clin. Lab. Invest. 1974; 33: 125–129.

Izzo, J. L., Gabiga, A. M., Hoffmaster, J. Pharmacologic and clinical studies on two new types of long-acting insulins with special reference to zinc insulin preparations (Novo): Preliminary report. Diabetes 1953; 2: 358–364.

Jackson, R. L., Storvick, W. O., Hollinden, C. S. et al. Neutral regular insulin. Diabetes 1972; 21: 235–245.

Jackson, J. G. L. Insulin 1922–1982. IDF Bull. 1982; 27: 9–13.

Jiang, Guo-Yan. Diabetes mellitus in China, past and present. In: Clinico-genetic genesis of diabetes mellitus. Proceedings of an International Symposium on clinico-genetic genesis of diabetes mellitus, Kobe, Japan. Amsterdam: Excerpta Medica, 1982: 27–33.

Johansen, K., Hansen, Aa. P. Diurnal serum growth hormone levels in poorly and well-controlled juvenile diabetics. Diabetes 1971; 20: 239–245.

Johnson, I. S. Authenticity and purity of human insulin (recombinant DNA). Diabetes Care 1982; 5 (Suppl. 2): 4–12.

Jørgensen, K. D., Hallund, O., Heding L. G., et al. Estimation of insulin purity in the light of developments in analytical methods. In: Gueriguian, J. L., Bransome, E. D., Outschoorn A. S. (eds), Hormone Drugs. Proceedings of the FDA-USP Workshop on Drug and Reference Standards for Insulins, Somatropins and Thyroid-axis Hormones, Bethesda, Maryland. Rockville: USP Convention Inc., 1982: 139–147.

Jørgensen, K. H., Brange, J., Hallund, O., Pingel, M. A method for the preparation of essentially pure insulin. In: Rodriguez, R. R., Eblin, F. J. G., Henderson, I., Assan, R. (eds), VII Congress of the International Diabetes Federation. Amsterdam: Excerpta Medica Int. Congress Series, 1970; 209: Abstract 334: p 149.

Jørgensen, K. H., Wolffbrandt, K. H., Weis, J. U. Preclinical studies on human insulin II. General pharmacological studies. Acta Pharmacol. Toxicol. (Copenh.). 1983; 52: 268–272.

Jorpes, J. E. Recrystallised insulin for diabetic patients with insulin allergy. Arch. Intern. Med. 1949; 83: 363–371.

Joslin, E. P. The treatment of diabetes mellitus. Philadelphia: Lea & Febiger, 1916.

Joslin, E. P., Gray, H., Root, H. F. Insulin in hospital and home. J. Metab. Res. 1922; 2: 651–699.

Joslin, E. P. The treatment of diabetes mellitus, 8th edn. Philadelphia: Lea & Febiger, 1946.

Joslin, E. P., Root, H. F., White, P., Marble, A. The treatment of diabetes mellitus, 10th edn. Philadelphia: Lea & Febiger, 1959.

Kamimura. Über die Bedeutung der Langerhanschem Inseln für den Kohlen-hydratstoffwechsel. Mitt. Med. Fak. d.k. Univ. zu Tokyo, 1917; 17: 95.

Karr, W. G., Kreidler, W. A., Scull, C. W., Petty, O. H. Certain immunologic studies in insulin sensitivity. Am. J. Med. Sci. 1931; 181: 293–296.

Kasama, T., Iwata, Y., Okubo, T., Sakaguchi, Y., Sugiura, M. Determination of purity and identification of animal sources of insulin in various insulin preparations. Jpn. J. Pharmacol. 1980; 30: 293–300.

Keck, K. Ir-gene control of immunogenicity of insulin and A-chain loop as a carrier determinant. Nature 1975; 254: 78–79.

Keck, K. Ir-gene control of carrier recognition: III. Cooperative recognition of two or more carrier determinants of insulins of different species. Eur. J. Immunol. 1977; 7: 811–816.

Keen, H., Glynne, A., Pickup, J. C., et al. Human insulin produced by recombinant DNA technology: safety and hypoglycaemic potency in healthy men. Lancet 1980; ii: 398–401.

Kemmer, F. W., Sonnenberg, G., Cüppers, H. J., Berger, M. Absorption kinetics of semi-synthetic human insulin and biosynthetic (recombinant DNA) human insulin. Diabetes Care 1982; 5 (Suppl. 2): 23–28.

Kemmler, W., Peterson, J. D., Steiner, D. F. Studies on the conversion of proinsulin to insulin. I. Conversion in vitro with trypsin and carboxypeptidase B. J. Biol. Chem. 1971; 246: 6786–6791.

Kern, R. A., Langner, P. H. Protamine and allergy: nature of local reactions after injections of protamine zinc insulin; induction of sensitivity to insulin by injections of protamine zinc insulin. JAMA 1939; 113: 198–200.

Kimmel, J. R., Pollock, H. G. Studies of human insulin from non-diabetic and diabetic pancreas. Diabetes 1967; 16: 687–694.

King, L. S. Empiricism, rationalism and diabetes. JAMA 1964; 187: 521.

Kinmonth, A. L., Baum, J. D. Timing of pre-breakfast insulin injection and postprandial metabolic control in diabetic children. Br. Med. J. 1980; 280: 604–606.

Kirkbride, M. E. The islands of Langerhans after ligation of the pancreatic ducts. J. Exp. Med. 1912; 15: 101–105.

Klaff, L. J., Vinik, A. I., Berelowitz, M., Jackson, W. P. U. Circulating antibodies in diabetics treated with conventional and purified insulin. S. Afr. Med. J. 1978; 54: 149–153.

Klier, M., Kerner, W., Torres, A. A., Pfeiffer, E. F. Comparison of the biologic activity of biosynthetic human insulin and natural pork insulin in juvenile onset diabetic subjects assessed by the glucose controlled insulin infusion system. Diabetes Care 1981; 4 (Suppl. 2): 193–195.

Koivisto, V. A., Felig, P., Effects of leg exercise on insulin absorption in diabetic patients. N. Engl. J. Med. 1978; 298: 79–83.

Koivisto, V. A. Sauna-induced acceleration in insulin absorption from subcutaneous injection site. Br. Med. J. 1980; 280: 1411–1413.

Koivisto, V. A., Felig, P. Alterations in insulin absorption and in blood glucose control associated with varying insulin injection sites in diabetic patients. Ann. Intern. Med. 1980; 92: 59–61.

Koivisto, V. A., Fortney, S., Hendler, R., Felig, P. A rise in ambient temperature augments insulin absorption in diabetic patients. Metabolism 1981; 30: 402–405.

Kølendorf, K., Aaby, P., Westergaard, S., Deckert, T. Absorption, effectiveness and side effects of highly purified porcine NPH-insulin preparations (Leo). Eur. J. Clin. Pharmacol. 1978; 14: 117–124.

Kølendorf, K., Bojsen, J., Nielsen, S. L. Adipose tissue blood flow and insulin disappearance from subcutaneous tissue. Clin. Pharmacol. Ther. 1979; 25: 598–604.

Kølendorf, K., Bojsen, J. Kinetics of subcutaneous NPH insulin in diabetics. Clin. Pharmacol. Ther. 1982; 31: 494–500.

Kølendorf, K., Bojsen, J., Deckert, T. Clinical factors influencing the absorption of ^{125}I-NPH insulin in diabetic patients. Horm. Metab. Res. 1983a; 15: 274–278.

Kølendorf, K., Bojsen, J., Deckert, T. Absorption and miscibility of regular porcine insulin after subcutaneous injection of insulin-treated diabetic patients. Diabetes Care 1983b; 6: 6–9.

Korp, W., Levett, R. E. Erfahrungen mit Monokomponenten-Insulin. Wien Klin. Wochenschr. 1973; 85: 326–330.

Kraegen, E. W., Campbell, L. V., Chia, Y. O., Meler, H., Lazarus, L. Control of blood glucose in diabetics using an artificial pancreas. Aust. NZ. J. Med. 1977; 7: 280–286.

Krayenbühl, C., Rosenberg, T. Crystalline protamine insulin. Rep. Steno. Hosp. (Copenh.). 1946; 1: 60–73.

Kreines, K. The use of various insulins in insulin allergy. Arch. Intern. Med. (Chicago) 1965; 116: 167–171.

Kroeff, E. P., Chance, R. E. Applications of high performance liquid chromatography for analysis of insulins. In: Gueriguian, J. L., Bransome, E. D., Outschoorn A. S. (eds), Hormone Drugs, Proceedings of the FDA–USP Workshop on Drug and Reference Standards for Insulins, Somatotropins and Thyroid-axis Hormones, Bethesda, Maryland. Rockville: USP Convention Inc., 1982: 148–162.

Kronheim, S., Berelowitz, M., Pimstone, B. A radioimmunoassay for growth hormone release-inhibiting hormone: Method and quantitative tissue distribution. Clin. Endocrinol. 1976; 5: 619–630.

Kruse, V. Effect of insulin-binding antibodies on free insulin in plasma and tissue after subcutaneous injection. A model study. In: Keck, Erb (ed.), Basic and clinical aspects of immunity to insulin. Berlin, New York: Walter de Gruyter & Co, 1981.

Kumar, D., Miller, L. V. Pork insulin resistance treated with dealaninated insulin (Abstract). Diabetes 1970; 19: 392.

Kumar, D. Immunoreactivity of insulin antibodies in insulin treated diabetics. Significance of the beta-chain carboxyterminal amino-acid (B30) of insulin. Diabetes 1979; 28: 994–1000.

Kung, Y., Du Yu-Cang., Haung Wei-teh., Chen Chan-chin., et al. Total synthesis of crystalline insulin. Scientia Sinica 1966; 15: 544–561.

Kurtz, A. B., Mustaffa, B. E., Daggett, P. R., Nabarro, J. D. N. Effect of insulin antibodies on free and total plasma insulin. Lancet 1977; ii: 56–58.

Kurtz, A. B., Matthews, J. A., Nabarro, J. D. N. Insulin-binding antibody: Reaction differences with bovine and porcine insulins. Diabetologia 1978; 15: 19–22.

Kurtz, A. B., Nabarro, J. D. N. Circulating insulin-binding antibodies. Diabetologia 1980; 19: 329–334.

Kurtz, A. B., Matthews, J. A., Mustaffa, B. E., Daggett, P. R., Nabarro, J. D. N. Decrease of antibodies to insulin, proinsulin and contaminating hormones after changing treatment from conventional beef to purified pork insulin. Diabetologia 1980; 8: 147–150.

Kurtz, A. B., Gray, R. S., Markanday, S., Nabarro, J. D. N. Circulating IgG antibody to protamine in patients treated with protamine-insulins. Diabetologia 1983; 25: 322–324.

Küssmaul, A. Zur Lehre vom Diabetes Mellitus. Dtsch. Arch. Klin. Med. Leipzig 1874; 14: 1–46.

Laguesse, E. G. Sur la formation des ilôts de Langerhans dans le pancreas. C.R. Soc. Biol. (Paris) 1893; 45: 819–820.

Landgraf-Leurs, M. M. C., Brügelmann, I., Kammerer, S., Lorenz, R., Landgraf, R. Counterregulatory hormone release after human and porcine insulin in healthy subjects and patients with pituitary disorders. Klin. Wochenschr. 1984; 62: 659–668.

Langdon, N., Hyland, K., Yudkin, J. S. Comparison of glucose control using U-80 and U-100 strength insulin. Diabetic Med. 1984; 1: 243.

Langerhans, P. Beiträge zur mikroskopischen Anatomie der Bauch-speicheldrüse Thesis. Berlin 1869.

Larsen, O. A., Lassen, N. A., Quaade, F. Blood flow through human adipose tissue determined with radioactive xenon. Acta Physiol. Scand. 1966; 66: 337–345.

Laube, H., Velcovsky, H. G., Federlin, K. Semisynthetisches Humaninsulin vergleichende Untersuchung über Stoffwechseleffekte beim Menschen. (Abstract). Aktuel. Endokrin. 1981a; 2: 102.

Laube, H., Velcovsky, H. G., Federlin, K. Comparative studies of semisynthetic and recombinant human insulins (Abstract). Diabetologia 1981b; 21: 296.

Laube, H., Velcovsky, H. G., Mäser, E., Federlin, K. Vergleichende Untersuchung zur Wirkung von unterschiedlichen Humaninsulinen bei gesunden Probanden. In: Petersen, K-G., Schlüter, K. J., Kerp, L. (eds), Proceedings of 1st International Symposium 'Neue Insuline'. Freiburg: Freiburger Graphische Betreibe, 1982: 61–65.

Lauritzen, T., Faber, O. K., Binder, C. Variation in ^{125}I-insulin absorption and blood glucose concentration. Diabetologia 1979; 17: 291–295.

Lauritzen, T., Binder, C., Falser, O. K. Importance of insulin absorption, subcutaneous blood flow, residual beta-cell function in insulin therapy. Acta Pediatr. Scand. 1980; Suppl. 283: 81–85.

Lauritzen, T., Pramming, S., Gale, E. A. M., Deckert, T., Binder, C. Absorption of isophane (NPH) insulin and its clinical implications. Br. Med. J. 1982; 285: 159–162.

Lauritzen, T., Frost-Larsen, K., Larsen, H. W., et al. Continuous subcutaneous insulin (Letter). Lancet 1983a; i: 1445–1446.

Lauritzen, T., Frost-Larsen, K., Larsen, H. W., et al. Effect of 1 year of near-normal blood glucose levels on retinopathy in insulin-dependent diabetics. Lancet 1983b; i: 200–204.

Lauritzen, T., Thorsteinsson, B., Pramming, S., Sørensen, L., Binder, C. Subcutaneous absorption of U-40 and U-100 insulin. Horm. Metab. Res. 1984; 16: 611–612.

Lavaux, J. P., Ooms, H. A., Christiansen, A. H. Insulin antibodies in insulin-treated patients; a clinical trial with highly purified insulins. Excerpta Medica Int. Congress Series 1973; 316: 40–46.

Lawrence, R. D. Local insulin reactions. Lancet 1925; i: 1125–1126.

Lawrence, R. D., Archer, N. Zinc protamine insulin. A clinical trial of the new preparation. Br. Med. J. 1937; i: 487–491.

League of Nations. The biological standardisation of insulin. Reports on the preparation of the international standard and definition of the unit. League of Nations 111. Health Organisation Report 1926; 7: 5–71.

League of Nations. The new international insulin standard and redefinition of the existing unit in terms thereof. Q. Bull. Hlth. Org. League of Nations 1936; 5: 584–658.

Leake, C. D. The Chief Egyptian Medical Papyri. In: The Old Egyptian Medical Papyri. Lawrence, Kansas: University of Kansas Press, 1952: 7–17.

Lean, M. E. J., Ng. L. L., Tennison, B. R. Interval between insulin injection and eating in relation to blood glucose control in adult diabetics. Br. Med. J. 1985; 290: 105–108.

Leslie, D. Generalised allergic reactions to monocomponent insulin. Br. Med. J. 1977; ii: 736–737.

Lewis, J. H. The antigenic properties of insulin. JAMA 1937; 108: 1336–1338.

Leyton, O. The administration of insulin in suspension. Lancet, 1929; i: 756.

Liljenquist, J., Mueller, G., Cherrington, A., et al. Evidence for an important role of glucagon in the regulation of hepatic glucose production in normal man. J. Clin. Invest. 1977; 59: 369–374.

Lind, S., Bell, S., Gilmore, E., Huisjes, H. J., Schally, A. V. Insulin disappearance rate in pregnant and non-pregnant women, and in non-pregnant women given GHRIH. Eur. J. Clin. Invest. 1977; 7: 47–51.

Linde, B., Gunnarsson, R. Effects of aprotinin on insulin absorption and subcutaneous blood flow in insulin-treated diabetic patients (Abstract). Diabetologia 1983; 25: 175.

Lins, P., Efendič, S. Hyperglycaemia induced by somatostatin in normal subjects. Horm. Metab. Res. 1976; 8: 497–498.

Lloyd, B., Burrin, J., Smythe, P., Alberti, K. G. M. M. Enzymic fluorimetric continuous-flow assays for blood glucose, lactate, pyruvate, alanine, glycerol and 3-hydroxybutyrate. Clin. Chem. 1978; 24: 1724–1729.

Lloyd, L. F., Corran, P. H. Analysis of insulin preparations by reversed phase high performance liquid chromatography. J. Chromatogr. 1982; 240: 445–454.

Lockwood, D. H., Prout, T. E. Antigenicity of heterologous and homologous insulin. Metabolism 1965; 14: 530–538.

Logie, A. W., Stowers, J. M. Hazards of monocomponent insulins. Br. Med. J. 1976; i: 879–880.

Lowell, F. C. Immunologic studies in insulin resistance: the presence of a neutralising factor in the blood exhibiting some characteristics of an antibody. J. Clin. Invest. 1944; 23: 225–240.

Ludvigsson, J., Heding, L. G. C-peptide in children with juvenile diabetes. Diabetologia 1976; 12: 627–630.

Luft, R., Efendič, S., Hökfelt, T. Somatostatin – both hormone and neurotransmitter. Diabetologia 1978; 14: 1–13.

Lundbæk, K., Christensen, N. J., Jensen, V. A., et al. Diabetes, diabetic angiopathy and growth hormone. Lancet 1970; ii: 131–133.

Lundbæk, K., Christensen, N. J., Jensen, V. A., et al. The pathogenesis of diabetic angiopathy and growth hormone. Dan. Med. Bull. 1971; 18: 1–7.

Lunetta, M., Leonardi, R., Rapisarda, S., Palermo, F., Mughini, L. Aprotinin administered together with insulin has no effect on blood glucose levels in Type I diabetics. IRCS. Med. Sci. 1984; 12: 23.

Maberly, G. F., Wait, G. A., Kilpatrick, J. A., et al. Evidence for insulin degradation by muscle and fat tissue in an insulin resistant diabetic patient. Diabetologia 1982; 23: 333–336.

MacCullum, W. G. On the relation of the islands of Langerhans to glycosuria. Bull. Johns Hopkins Hosp., Baltimore 1909; 20: 265–268.

Macleod, J. J. R. Pancreatic extract and diabetes. Can. Med. Assoc. J. 1922; 12: 423–425.

Macleod, J. J. R. History of the researches leading to the discovery of insulin. Bull. Hist. Med. 1978; 52: 295–312.

McKinlay, I., Farquhar, J. W. Use of 100 units/ml insulin in treatment of diabetic children. Arch. Dis. Child. 1976; 51: 796–798.

Mahler, R., Stafford, W. S., Tarraut, M. E., Ashmore, J. The effect of insulin on lipolysis. Diabetes 1964; 13: 297–302.

Malins, J. M. Insulins and diabetes. Prescriber's J. 1970; 10: 25–30.

Malone, J. I., Root, A. W. Plasma free insulin concentrations: Keystone to effective management of diabetes mellitus in children. J. Pediatr. 1981; 99: 862–867.

Mann, N. P., Johnston, D. I., Reeves, W. G., Murphy, M. A. Human insulin and porcine insulin in the treatment of diabetic children: Comparison of metabolic control and insulin antibody production. Br. Med. J. 1983; 287: 1580–1582.

Marble, A. Insulin in the treatment of diabetes. In: Marble, A., White, P., Bradley, R. F., Krall, L. P. (eds). Joslin's Diabetes Mellitus, 11th edn. Philadelphia: Lea & Febiger 1971; 287–301.

Märki, F., Albrecht, W. Biological activity of synthetic human insulin. Diabetologia 1977; 13: 293–295.

Markussen, J. Synthetic paths to insulin. Acta Paed. Scand. 1977; Suppl. 270: 121–126.

Markussen, J. Process for preparing insulin esters; United Kingdom Patent Application GB 2069502 A, 1980.

Markussen, J., Jørgensen, K., Thim, L., et al. Human monocomponent insulin: chemistry and characteristics of human insulin (Novo) (Abstract). Diabetologia 1981; 21: 302.

Markussen, J. Human monocomponent Insulin aus Schweine-Rohinsulin. In: Petersen, K-G., Schlüter, K. J., Kerp, L. (eds), Proceedings 1st International Symposium 'Neue Insuline', Freiburg: Freiburger Graphische Betriebe 1982a: 38–44.

Markussen J. The advent of human insulin in diabetes therapy. Medicographia 1982b; 4: 39–44.

Markussen, J., Damgaard, U., Jørgensen, K. H., et al. Production of human monocomponent insulin. In: Gueriguian, J. L., Bransome, E. D., Outschoorn, A. S. (eds), Hormone Drugs. Proceedings of the FDA-USP Workshop on Drug and Reference Standards for Insulins, Somatotropins and Thyroid-axis Hormones, Bethesda, Maryland. Rockville: USP Convention Inc., 1982, 116–126.

Markussen, J., Schaumburg, K. Reaction mechanism in trypsin-catalysed synthesis of human insulin studies by [17]O-nuclear magnetic resonance spectroscopy. (Abstract). Diabetologia 1982; 23: 185.

Markussen, J., Damgaard, V., Jørgensen, K. H., Sørensen, E., Thim, L.

Human monocomponent insulin – chemistry and characteristics. Acta Med. Scand. 1983a; Suppl. 671: 99–105.

Markussen, J., Damgaard, U., Pingel, M., Snel, L., Sørensen, A. R. Sørensen, E. Chemistry and characteristics of human monocomponent insulin. In: Sakamoto, N., Alberti, K. G. M. M. (eds). Current and future therapies with insulin. Excerpta Medica Int. Congress Series, 1983b; 607: 71–79.

Markussen, J., Damgaard, U., Pingel, M., Snel, L., Sørensen, A. R. Sørensen, E. Human insulin (Novo): Chemistry and characteristics. Diabetes Care 1983c; 6 (Suppl. l): 4–8.

Markussen, J. Production of human insulin. In: Nattrass, M., Santiago, J. V. (eds), Recent advances in diabetes. Edinburgh, London, New York: Churchill Livingstone, 1984: 45–53.

Martin, R. I. R., Stocks, A. E., Pearson, M. J. Significance of disappearance rate of injected insulin (Letter). Lancet 1967; i: 619–620.

Massi-Benedetti, M., Burrin, J. M., Capaldo, B., Alberti, K. G. M. M. A comparative study of the activity of biosynthetic human insulin and pork insulin using the glucose clamp technique in normal subjects. Diabetes Care 1981; 4: 163–167.

Mauer, S. M., Fish, A. J., Blau, E. B., Michael, A. F. The glomerular mesangium. I. Kinetic studies of macromolecular uptake in normal and nephrotic rats. J. Clin. Invest. 1972; 51: 1092–1101.

Maxwell, L. C., Bischoff, F. Augmentation of the physiologic response to insulin. Am. J. Physiol. 1935; 112: 172.

Mayer, A. M. Frederick Banting and the discovery of insulin. Charles Best, a brilliant assistant. Diabetes Forecast 1982; 35: 44–48.

Medvei, V. C. A history of endocrinology. MTP Press, Lancaster, Boston, The Hague, 1982.

Meienhofer, J., Shinabel, E., Bremer, H. et al. Synthese der Insulinketten und ihre Kombination zu insulinaktiven Präparaten. Z. Naturforsch 1963; 18b: 1120–1121.

Meissner, C., Thum, C., Beischer, W., et al. Antidiabetic action of somatostatin – assessed by the artificial pancreas. Diabetes 1975; 24: 988–996.

Mering, J. von, Minkowski, O. Diabetes Mellitus nach Pankreasextirpation. Arch. Exp. Pathol. Pharmakol. Leipzig 1890; 26: 371–387.

Metropolitan Life Insurance Company. Statistics Bulletin. New York 1960; 41: 6 (Feb.), 1 (Mar.).

Miles, A. A., Mussett, M. C., Perry, W. L. M. Third international standard for insulin. Bull. Wld. Hlth. Org. 1952; 7: 445–459.

Miller, W. L., Baxter, J. D. Recombinant DNA – a new source of insulin. Diabetologia 1980; 18: 431–436.

Mirouze, J., Orsetti, A., Schmouker, Y., Carty, E., Almes, N. Diabète sucré. Son traitment par les insulins purifiées monocomposées. Nouv. Presse Med. 1973; 2: 1981–1985.

Mirouze, J., Selam, J. L., Pham, T. C., Cavadore, D. Evaluation of exogenous insulin homeostasis by the artificial pancreas in insulin-dependent diabetes. Diabetologia 1977; 13: 273–278.

Mirouze, J., Selam, J. L., Pham, T. C., Mendoza, E., Orsetti, A. Sustained insulin-induced remissions of juvenile diabetes by means of an external artificial pancreas. Diabetologia 1978; 14: 223–227.

Mirouze, J., Selam, J. L., Pham, T. C., Chenon, D. Programming of an open-loop system for intravenous insulin infusion in insulin-dependent diabetes. Acta Diabetol. Lat. 1980; 17: 103–109.

Mirouze, J., Selam, J. L., Pham, T. C., Chenon, D. The outcome of juvenile ketotic diabetes following remissions induced by the artificial pancreas: a four year follow-up. Horm. Met. Res. 1982a; Suppl. Series Vol. 12: 238–240.

Mirouze, J., Monnier, L., Richard, J. L., Gancel, A., Soua, K. B. Comparative study of NPH human insulin (recombinant DNA) and pork insulin in diabetic subjects: preliminary report. Diabetes Care 1982b; 5 (Suppl. 2): 60–62.

Mirouze, J. Insulin treatment: A non-stop revolution. Diabetologia 1983; 25: 209–221.

Mirouze, J., Selam, J. L. Clinical experience in human diabetics with portable and implantable insulin minipumps. Life Support Systems 1983; 2: 39–50.

Mirouze, J., Benghernaout, O., Pham, T. C., Richard, J. L., Bringer, J. Comparative analysis of soluble porcine and human insulin (Novo) using the artificial pancreas. Diabetes Care 1983; 6 (Suppl. l): 40–42.

Mirsky, I. A., Jinks, R., Perisutti, G. The isolation and crystallisation of human insulin. J. Clin. Invest. 1963; 42: 1869–1872.

Mirsky, I. A., Kawamura, K. Heterogeneity of crystalline insulin. Endocrinology 1966; 78: 1115–1119.

Misawa, K., Nakayama, H., Aoki, S., et al. Decreased solubility of short-acting human insulins when mixed with intermediate-acting human insulins. J. Jpn. Diab. Soc. 1984; 27: 959–962.

Misbin, R. I., Almira, E. C., Cleman, M. W. Insulin degradation in serum of a patient with apparent insulin resistance. J. Clin. Endocrinol. Metab. 1981; 52: 177–180.

Miyasita, S. An historical analysis of Chinese drugs in the treatment of hormonal diseases, goitre and diabetes mellitus. Am. J. Chinese Med. 1980; 8: 17–25.

Mizuno, N., Ogawa, T., Ishida, M., Okada, K., Shigeaki, B. Pancreatic polypeptide binding antibodies in insulin treated diabetics. J. Jpn. Diab. Soc. 1980; 23: 219–226.

Molnar, G. D., Taylor, W. F., Langworthy, A. L. Plasma immunoreactive insulin patterns in insulin-treated diabetics. Mayo Clin. Proc. 1972; 47: 709–719.

Molnar, G. D., Reynolds, C. Diurnal glucose variability and hormonal regulation. Horm. Metab. Res. 1977; (Suppl. 7): 148–157.

Moore, E. W., Mitchell, M. L., Chalmers, T. C. Variability in absorption of insulin – I^{131} in normal and diabetic subjects after subcutaneous and intramuscular injection. J. Clin. Invest. 1959; 38: 1222–1227.

Morihara, K., Oka, T., Tsuzuki, H. Semi-synthesis of human insulin by trypsin-catalysed replacement of Ala-B30 by Thr in porcine insulin. Nature 1979; 280: 412–413.

Mortimer, C. H., Carr, D., Lind, T., et al. Effects of growth-hormone-release inhibiting hormone on circulating glucagon, insulin and growth hormone in normal, diabetic, acromegalic and hypopituitary patients. Lancet 1974; i: 697–701.

Mühlhauser, I., Broermann, C., Tsotsalas, M., Berger, M. Miscibility of human and bovine Ultralente insulin with soluble insulin. Br. Med. J. 1985; 289: 1656–1657.

Müller, R., Berger, W., Wick, H., Keller, U. Comparison of the effect of semisynthetic human insulin and porcine insulin on glucose kinetics, plasma free fatty acid and amino acid levels in man. Horm. Metab. Res. 1984; 16: 271–274.

Müller, W. A., Taillens, C., Lereret, S., Berger, M., Philippe, J., Halban, P. A., Offord, R. E. Resistance against subcutaneous insulin successfully managed with aprotinin (Letter). Lancet 1980; i: 1245–1246.

Munkgaard Rasmussen, S., Heding, L. G., Parbst, E., Vølund, Aa. Serum IRI in insulin-treated diabetics during a 24-hour period. Diabetologia 1975; 11: 151–158.

Mustaffa, B. E., Daggett, P. R., Nabarro, J. D. N. Insulin binding capacity in patients changed from conventional to highly purified insulins. An indicator of likely response. Diabetologia 1977; 13: 311–315.

Nabarro, J. D. N., Mustaffa, B. E., Morris, D. V., Walport, M. J., Kurtz, A. B. Insulin deficient diabetes. Contrasts with other endocrine deficiencies. Diabetologia 1979; 16: 5–12.

Nakagawa, S., Suda, N., Kudo, M., Kawasaki, M. A new type of hypoglycaemia in a newborn infant. Diabetologia 1973; 9: 367–375.

Nathan, D. M., Lou, P., Avruch, J. Intensified conventional and insulin pump therapies in adult Type I diabetes. A crossover study. Ann. Intern. Med. 1982; 97: 31–36.

Naunyn, B. Der Diabetes Mellitus. Wien: Alfred Hölder, 1898.

Naunyn, B. Der Diabetes Mellitus. Berlin-Wien: Die Deutsche Klinik 3, 1903.

Navalesi, R., Pilo, A., Ferrannini, E. Kinetic analysis of plasma insulin disappearance in non-ketotic diabetic patients and in normal subjects. J. Clin. Invest. 1978; 61: 197–208.

Nelson, W. E., Vaughane, M. Textbook of pediatrics. 9th edn. Philadelphia: W. B. Saunders, 1969.

Neubauer, H. P., Schöne, H. H. The immunogenicity of different insulins in several animal species. Diabetes 1978; 27: 8–15.

Nicol, D. S. H. W., Smith, L. F. Amino-acid sequence of human insulin. Nature 1960; 187: 483–485.

Nielsen, S. L., Larsen, O. A. Relationship of subcutaneous adipose tissue blood flow to thickness of subcutaneous tissue and total body fat mass. Scand. J. Clin. Lab. Invest. 1973; 31: 383–388.

Nolte, M. S., Ajoste, D., Forsham, P. H. Reduced solubility of rapid-acting insulins when mixed with longer acting insulins (Abstract). Diabetes 1982; 31 (Suppl. 2): 71A.

Nolte, M. S., Poon, V., Grodsky, G. M., Forsham, P. H., Karam, J. H. Reduced solubility of short-acting soluble insulins when mixed with longer-acting insulins. Diabetes 1983; 32: 1177–1181.

Nora, J. J., Smith, D. W., Cameron, J. R. The route of insulin administration in the management of diabetes mellitus. J. Paediatr. 1964; 64: 547–551.

Nosadini, R., Noy, G., Kurtz, A. B., Alberti, K. G. M. M. Differential response to infusions of highly purified and conventional bovine and porcine insulins. Diabetes 1981; 30: 650–655.

Oakley, N. W. Effect of 'fractionated' insulins on total plasma insulin binding capacity and insulin requirements in severe diabetes. Lancet 1976; i: 994–996.

Oakley, W. G., Hill, D., Oakley, N. W. Combined use of regular and crystalline protamine (NPH) insulins in the treatment of severe diabetes. Diabetes 1966; 15: 219–222.

Oakley, W. G., Pyke, D. A., Taylor, K. W. Clinical diabetes and its biochemical basis. Oxford: Blackwell Scientific Publications, 1968.

Obermeier, R., Geiger, R. A new semi-synthesis of human insulin. Hoppe-Seyler's Z. Physiol. Chem. 1976; 357: 759–767.

Offord, R. E., Philippe, J., Davis, J. G., Halban, P. A., Berger, M. Inhibition of degradation of insulin by opthalmic acid and by a bovine pancreatic protease inhibitor. Biochem. J. 1979; 182: 249–251.

Opie, E. L. The relation of diabetes mellitus to lesions of the pancreas. J. Exp. Med. 1901; 5: 527–540.

Orci, L., Baetens, D., Dubois, M. P. et al. Evidence for the D-cell of the pancreas secreting somatostatin. Horm. Metab. Res. 1975; 7: 400–402.

Ørskov, H., Christensen, N. J. Disappearance rate of exogenous human insulin. (Letter). Lancet 1966; ii: 701.

Ørskov, H., Christensen, N. J. Plasma disappearance rate of injected human insulin in juvenile diabetic, maturity-onset diabetic and non-diabetic subjects. Diabetes 1969; 18: 653–659.

Owen, O. E., Reichard, G. A. Jr. Ketone body metabolism in normal, obese and diabetic subjects. Isr. J. Med. Sci. 1975; 11: 560–570.

Owens, D. R., Wragg, K. G., Biggs, P. I., Luzio, S., Kimber, G., Davies, C. Comparison of the metabolic response to a glucose tolerance test and a standardised test meal and the response to serial test meals in normal healthy subjects. Diabetes Care 1979; 2: 409–413.

Owens, D. R., Jones, M. K., Hayes, T. M., et al. Human insulin: Study of safety and efficacy in man. Br. Med. J. 1981a; 282: 1264–1266.

Owens, D. R., Wragg, K. G., Biggs, P. I., Luzio, S., Davies, C. J., Jones, M. K. The reproducibility of serial meal and oral glucose tolerance tests in normal subjects. Diabète Metab. 1981b; 7: 25–33.

Owens, D. R., Jones, M. K., Rochester, A. J., et al. Comparative responses in normal man to subcutaneous human, porcine and bovine soluble insulin. (Abstract). Diabetologia 1981c; 21: 311.

Owens, D. R., Jones, M. K., Hayes, T. M., et al. Comparative study of subcutaneous, intramuscular and intravenous administration of human insulin. Lancet 1981d; ii: 118–122.

Owens, D. R., Jones, M. K., Birtwell, A. J., et al. A study of the comparative safety and efficacy of neutral soluble human (semi-synthetic) and porcine monocomponent insulin in non-diabetic subjects. Diabète Metab. 1982; 8: 155–158.

Owens, D. R., Heding, L. G., Birtwell, A. J., Jones, I. R., Home, P. D., Luzio, S. Clinical studies with 'semi-synthetic' human insulin. In: Sakamoto, N., Alberti, K. G. M. M (eds), current and future therapies with insulin. Excerpta Medica Int. Congress Series, 1983a; 607: 90–97.

Owens, D. R., Jones, M. K., Birtwell, A. J., Jones, I. R., Hayes, T. M., Heding, L. G. The clinical pharmacology of human insulin (Novo) in normal subjects. Diabetes Care 1983b; 6 (Suppl. l): 13–16.

Owens, D. R., Jones, M. K., Birtwell, A. J., Burge, C. T. R., Jones, I. R., Heyburn, T. M., Heding, L. G. Pharmacokinetics of subcutaneously administered human, porcine and bovine neutral soluble insulin to normal man. Horm. Metabol. Res. 1984a; 16: 195–199.

Owens, D. R., Jones, I. R., Birtwell, A. J., et al. Study of porcine and human isophane (NPH) insulins in normal subjects. Diabetologia 1984b; 26: 261–265.

Owens, D. R., Jones, I. R., Birtwell, A. J., et al. Pharmacokinetics of bovine and human Ultralente insulin. (Abstract) Diabetic Medicine 1984c; l: 154.

Paley, R. G. Analysis of accessory factors in causation of dermal reactions to insulin. J. Pharm. Pharmacol. 1950; 2: 304–310.

Palmer, J. P., Ensinck, J. W. Stimulation of glucagon secretion by ethanol-induced hypoglycaemia in man. Diabetes 1975; 24: 295–300.

Papaspyros, N. S. The history of diabetes mellitus, 2nd edn. Stuttgart: Georg Thieme Verlag, 1964.

Parr, J. H. Transfer to U–100 insulin. The metabolic control and experience of patients. Br. J. Pharm. Pract. 1983; 5: 14–18.

Patel, Y. C., Reichlin, S. Somatostatin in hypothalamus, extra hypothalamic brain and peripheral tissues of the rat. Endocrinology 1978; 102: 523–530.

Paulesco, N. C. Action de l'extrait pancréatique injecté dans le sang chez un animal diabétique. C.R. Soc. Biol. (Paris) 1921a; 85: 555.

Paulesco, N. C. Influence de la quantité de pancréas amplogée pour préparer l'extrait injecté dans le sang chez un animal diabétique. C.R. Soc. Biol. (Paris) 1921b; 85: 558.

Paulesco, N. C. Action de l'extrait pancreatique injecté dans le sang chez un animal diabétique. C.R. Soc. Biol. (Paris) 1921c; 85: 559.

Paulesco, N. C. Recherches sur le rôle du pancréas dans l'assimilation nutritive. Arch. Int. Physiol. 1921d; 17: 85–109.

Paulesco, N. C. Quelques réactions chimiques et physiques appliquées à l'extrait aqueux du pancréas pour le débarrasser des substances protéiques en excès. Arch. Int. Physiol. 1923a; 21: 71–85.

Paulesco, N. C. Divers procédés pour entroduire l'extrait pancréatique dans l'organisme d'un animal diabetique. Arch. Int. Physiol. 1923b; 21: 215–238.

Paulesco, N. C. Traitement du diabète. La Presse Médicale 1924; 32: 202–204.

Peck, F. B., Schechter, J. S. The newer insulin mixtures. Proc. Am. Diab. Assoc. 1944; 4: 57.

Peck, F. B. Insulin mixtures and modifications. Proc. Am. Diab. Assoc. 1946; 6: 275–300.

Pedersen, H. D. Absorption af ^{125}I-mærket protamin-insulin fra subcutis.

English abstract: (Absorption of NPH insulin labelled with ^{125}-I from subcutaneous tissue). Ugeskr. Laeg. 1978; 140: 1760–1764.

Peracchi, M., Reschini, E., Cantalamessa, L., Giustina, G., Cavagnini, F., Pinto, M., Bulgheroni, P. Effect of somatostatin on blood glucose, plasma growth hormone, insulin and free fatty acids in normal subjects and acromegalic patients. Metabolism 1974; 23: 1009–1015.

Petersen, K-G., Schlüter, K. J., Kerp. L. Less pronounced changes in serum potassium and epinephrine during hypoglycaemia induced by human insulin (recombinant DNA). Diabetes Care 1982; 5 (Suppl. 2): 90–92.

Pfeiffer, E. F., Thum, C. H., Clemens, A. H. The artificial beta cell: a continuous control of blood sugar by external regulation of insulin infusion (glucose controlled insulin infusion system). Horm. Metab. Res. 1974; 487 (Suppl. 6): 339–342.

Phelps, R. L., Freinkel, N., Rubenstein, A. H., et al. Carbohydrate metabolism in pregnancy. XV. Plasma C-peptide during intravenous glucose tolerance in neonates from normal and insulin treated diabetic mothers. J. Clin. Endocrinol. Metab. 1978; 46: 61–68.

Phillips, M., Simpson, R. W., Holman, R. R., Turner, R. C. A simple and rational twice daily insulin regime. Distinction between basal and meal insulin requirements. Q. J. Med. 1979; 191: 493–506.

Pickup, J. C., Keen, H., Parsons, J. A., Alberti, K. G. M. M. Continuous subcutaneous insulin infusion: an approach to achieving normoglycaemia. Br. Med. J. 1978; i: 204–207.

Pickup, J. C., White, M. C., Keen, H., Parsons, J. A., Alberti, K. G. M. M. Long-term continuous subcutaneous insulin infusion in diabetics at home. Lancet 1979; ii: 870–873.

Pickup, J. C., Keen, H., Viberti, G. C. Continuous subcutaneous insulin infusion in the treatment of diabetes mellitus. Diabetes Care 1980a; 3: 290–300.

Pickup, J. C., Bilous, R. W., Keen, H., Aprotinin and insulin resistance. (Letter). Lancet 1980b; ii: 93–94.

Pickup, J. C., Bilous, R. W., Viberti, G. C., et al. Plasma insulin and C-peptide after subcutaneous and intravenous administration of human insulin (recombinant DNA) and purified porcine insulin in healthy men. Diabetes Care 1982; 5 (Suppl. 2): 29–34.

Pimstone, B., Berelowitz, M. Somatostatin – paracrine and neuromodulator peptide in gut and nervous system. S. Afr. Med. J. 1978; 53: 7–9.

Pingel, M., Vølund, Aa., Sørensen, E., Sørensen, A. R. Assessment of insulin potency by chemical and biological methods. In: Gueriguian, J. L., Bransome, E. D., Outschoorn, A. S. (eds), Hormone drugs. Proceedings of the FDA-USP Workshop on Drug and Reference Standards for Insulins, Somatropins and Thyroid-axis Hormones, Bethesda, Maryland. Rockville: USP Convention Inc., 1982: 19–21.

Pingel, M., Vølund Aa., Sørensen, E., Collins, J. E., Dieter, C. T. Biological potency of porcine, bovine and human insulins in the rabbit bioassay system. Diabetologia 1985; 28: 862–869.

Pirart, J. Diabetes mellitus and its degenerative complications: a prospective study of 4,400 patients observed between 1947 and 1973. Diabète Metab. 1977; 3: 97–107, 173–182, 245–256.

Polak, J. M., Pearse, A. G., Grimelius, L. et al. Growth-hormone release-inhibiting hormone in gastrointestinal and pancreatic D-cells. Lancet 1975; i: 1220–1222.

Polonsky, K. S., Bergenstal, R., Pous, G., Schneider, M., Jaspan, J. B., Rubenstein, A. Relation of counterregulatory responses to hypoglycemia in Type I diabetics. N. Engl. J. Med. 1982; 307: 1106–1112.

Polonsky, K. S., Rubenstein, A. H. C-peptide as a measure of the secretion and hepatic extraction of insulin. Diabetes 1984; 33: 486–494.

Popp, D. A., Shah, S. D., Cryer, P. E. The role of epinephrine-mediated B-adrenergic mechanisms in hypoglycemic glucose counterregulation and post-hypoglycemic hyperglycemia in insulin-dependent diabetes mellitus. J. Clin. Invest. 1982; 69: 315–326.

Poulsen, J. E. Features of the history of diabetology. Copenhagen: Munksgaard, 1982.

Poulsen, J. S. D., Smith, M., Deckert, M., Deckert, T. Comparison of intraperitoneal and intravenous insulin infusion. Acta Endocrinol. (Copenh.). 1980; 95: 500–504.

Raptis, S., Karaiskos, C., Enzmann, F., et al. Biologic activities of biosynthetic human insulin in healthy volunteers and insulin-dependent diabetic patients monitored by the artificial endocrine pancreas. Diabetes Care 1981; 4: 155–162.

Raskin, P., Unger, R. Hyperglucagonemia and its suppression: Importance in the metabolic control of diabetes. N. Engl. J. Med. 1978; 299: 433–436.

Raskin, P., Pietri, A. O., Unger, R., Shannon, W. A. Jr. The effect of diabetic control on the width of skeletal-muscle capillary basement membrane in patients with Type I diabetes mellitus. N. Engl. J. Med. 1983; 309: 1546–1550.

Reed, J. A. 'Aretaeus, the Cappadocian'. Diabetes 1954; 3: 419–421.

Reeves, M. L., Seigler, D. E., Ryan E. A., Skyler, J. S. Glycaemic control in insulin-dependent diabetes mellitus: Comparison of outpatient intensified conventional therapy with continuous subcutaneous insulin infusion. Am. J. Med. 1982; 72: 673–680.

Reeves, W. G. Immunology of diabetes and insulin therapy. In: Thompson R. A. (ed.), Recent advances in clinical immunology. Edinburgh, London, New York: Churchill Livingstone, 1980: 183–220.

Reeves, W. G., Allen, B. R., Tattersall, R. B. Insulin-induced lipoatrophy: evidence for an immune pathogenesis. Br. Med. J. 1980; 280: 1500–1503.

Reeves, W. G., Kelly, U. An immunochemical method for the quantitation of insulin antibodies. J. Immunol. Meth. 1980; 34: 329–338.

Reeves, W. G., Kelly, U. Insulin antibodies induced by bovine insulin therapy. Clin. Exp. Immunol. 1982; 50: 163–170.

Reeves, W. G., Gelsthorpe, K., Van der Minne, P., Torenssma, R., Tattersall, R. B. HLA phenotype and insulin antibody production. Clin. Exp. Immunol. 1984a; 57: 443–448.

Reeves, W. G., Barr, D., Douglas, C. A., et al. Factors governing the human immune response to injected insulin. Diabetologia 1984b; 26: 266–271.

Reiner, L., Searle, D. S., Lang, E. H. On the hypoglycaemic activity of globin insulin. J. Pharmacol. Exp. Ther. 1939; 67: 330–340.

Reisner, C., Moul, D. J., Cudworth, A. G. Generalised urticaria precipitated by change to highly purified porcine insulin (Letter). Br. Med. J. 1978; ii: 56.

Renner, R., Vocke, K., Hepp, K. D. Search for the most practical regular NPH mixtures for Type I diabetic patients. Diabetes Care 1982; 5 (Suppl. 2): 53–56.

Renold, A. E., Winegrad, A. I., Martin, D. B. Diabète sucré et tissu adipeux. Helv. Med. Acta 1957; 24: 322–327.

Renold, A. E., Steinke, J., Soeldner, J. S., Antoniades, H. N., Smith, R. E. Immunological response to the prolonged administration of heterologous homologous insulin in cattle. J. Clin. Invest. 1966; 45: 702–713.

Richard, J.-L., Rodier, M., Ghislaine, C., Mirouze, J., Monnier, L. Human (recombinant DNA) and porcine NPH insulin are unequally effective in diabetic patients: A comparative study using continuous blood glucose monitoring. Acta Diabetol. Lat. 1984; 21: 211–217.

Rivier, J. Somatostatin: total solid phase synthesis. J. Am. Chem. Soc. 1974; 98: 2986–2992.

Rizza, R. A., Cryer, P. E., Gerich, J. E. Role of glucagon, catecholamines and growth hormone in human glucose counterregulation. J. Clin. Invest. 1979; 64: 62–71.

Rizza, R. A., Gerich, J. E., Haymond, M. W. Control of blood sugar in insulin-dependent diabetes: Comparison of an artificial endocrine pancreas, continuous subcutaneous insulin infusion and intensified conventional insulin therapy. N. Engl. J. Med. 1980; 303: 1313–1318.

Roland, J. M. Need stable diabetics mix their insulins? Diabetic Med. 1984; l: 51–53.

Rolleston, H. D. The endocrine organs in health and disease. London: Oxford University Press, 1936.

Rollo, J. An account of two cases of the diabetes mellitus, with remarks as they arose during the progress of the cure. London: C. Dilly, 1797.

Romans, R. G., Scott, D. A., Fisher, A. M. Preparation of crystalline insulin. Ind. Eng. Chem. 1940; 32: 908–910.

Root, A. M., Chance, R. E., Galloway, J. A. Immunogenicity of insulin. Diabetes 1972; 21 (Suppl. 2): 657–660.

Rosak, C., Althoff, P.-H., Enzmann, P., Schöffling, K. Comparative studies on intermediary metabolism and hormonal counterregulation following human insulin (recombinant DNA) and purified pork insulin in man. Diabetes Care 1982; 5 (Suppl. 2): 82–89.

Rosenbloom, A. L. Advances in commercial insulin preparations. Am. J. Dis. Child. 1974; 128: 631–633.

Ross, M. J. Production of medically important polypeptides using recombinant DNA technology. In: Gueriguian. J. L. (ed.), Insulins, growth hormone and recombinant DNA technology. New York: Raven Press 1981: 33–48.

Ross, J. W., Baker, R. S., Hooker, C. S., Johnson, I. S., Schmidtke, J. R., Smith, W. C. Procedure for detection of potential E. coli peptides (ECPs) in biosynthetic human insulin (BHI), antibodies to ECPs in patients treated with BHI and measurement of bacterial endotoxins in BHI. In: Gueriguian, J. L., Bransome, E. D., Outschoorn, A. S. (eds), Hormone drugs. Proceedings of the FDA–USP Workshop on Drug and Reference Standards for Insulins, Somatotropins and Thyroid-axis Hormones, Bethesda, Maryland. Rockville: USP Convention Inc., 1982: 127–138.

Roy, B., Chou, M. C. Y., Field, J. B. Time-action characteristics of Regular and NPH insulin in insulin treated diabetics. J. Clin. Endocrinol. Metab. 1980; 50: 475–479.

Rudman, D., Moffitt, S. D., Fernhoff, P. M., et al. Epinephrine deficiency in hypocorticotropic hypopituitary children. J. Clin. Endocrinol. Metab. 1981; 53: 722–729.

Ryle, A. P., Sanger, F., Smith, L. F., Kitai, R. The disulphide bonds of insulin. Biochem. J. 1955; 60: 541–546.

Sacca, L., Sherwin, R., Felig, P. Influence of somatostatin on glucagon and epinephrine-stimulated hepatic glucose output in the dog. J. Clin. Invest. 1980; 65: 682–689.

Saibene, V., Melandri, M., Brembilla, L., Spotti, D., Pozza, G. Comparison between multi-injection and continuous subcutaneous insulin therapy in insulin-dependent diabetic inpatients. Acta Diabetol. Lat. 1981; 18: 45–50.

Sailer, D., Ludwig, Th., Kolb, S. Comparison of the activity profiles of two fixed combinations of Regular/NPH human insulin (recombinant DNA) of different compositions with a fixed Regular/NPH porcine insulin combination (PPI) in insulin-dependent diabetic individuals. Diabetes Care 1982; 5: (Suppl. 2): 57–59.

Samuel, T. Differentiation between antibodies to protamines and somatic nuclear antigens by means of a comparative fluorescence study on swollen nuclei of spermatozoa and somatic cells. Clin. Exp. Immunol. 1977; 32: 290–298.

Santiago, J. V., Clemens, A. H., Clarke, W. L., Kipnis, D. M. Closed-loop and open-loop devices for blood glucose control in normal and diabetic subjects. Diabetes 1979; 28: 71–81.

Santiago, J. V., Clarke, W. L., Shah, D. S., Cryer, P. E. Epinephrine, norepinephrine, glucagon and growth hormone release in association with physiological decrements in the plasma glucose concentration in normal and diabetic man. J. Clin. Endocrinol. Metab. 1980; 51: 877–883.

Sathe, R. V. Diabetes in India – retrospect and prospect. J. Assoc. Phys. India 1969; 17: 387–398.

Schade, D. S., Eaton, R. P., Friedman, N., Spencer, W. The intravenous, intraperitoneal and subcutaneous routes of insulin delivery in diabetic man. Diabetes 1979; 28: 1069–1072.

Schade, D. S., Santiago, J. V., Skyler, J. S., Rizza, R. A. Intensive insulin therapy. Princeton: Excerpta Medica, 1983.

Schally, A., Dupont, A., Arimura, A., et al. Isolation and structure of somatostatin from porcine hypothalami. Biochemistry 1976; 15: 509–514.

Schatz, H., Pfeiffer, E. F. Release of immunoreactive and radioactively prelabelled endogenous (pro)-insulin from isolated islets of rat pancreas in the presence of exogenous insulin. J. Endocrinol. 1977; 74: 243–249.

Schiffrin, A., Belmonte, M. M. Comparison between continuous sub-cutaneous insulin infusion and multiple injections of insulin: a one year prospective study. Diabetes 1982; 31: 255–264.

Schlichtkrull, J. Insulin crystals I. Acta Chem. Scand. 1956; 10: 1455–1458.

Schlichtkrull, J. Insulin crystals IV. The preparation of nuclei seeds and monodisperse insulin crystal suspensions. Acta Chem. Scand. 1957; 11: 299–302.

Schlichtkrull, J. Insulin crystals. Chemical and biological studies on insulin crystals and insulin zinc suspensions. Thesis. Copenhagen: Ejnar Munksgaard, 1958.

Schlichtkrull, J. New insulin crystal suspensions with various timings of action and containing no added zinc. In: Oberdisse, K., Jahne, K. (eds), III Kongress der International Diabetes Federation, Düsseldorf, 21–25 July 1958. Stuttgart: Georg Thieme Verlag, 1959: 773–777.

Schlichtkrull, J., Funder, J., Munck, O. Clinical evaluation of a new insulin preparation. Demole, M. (ed.), 4e Congrès de la Fédération Internationale du Diabète Genève: Éditions Médecine et Hygiène 1961; 1: 303–305.

Schlichtkrull, J., Munck, O., Jersild, M. Insulin Rapitard and Insulin Actrapid. Acta Med. Scand. 1965; 177: 103–113.

Schlichtkrull, J., Brange, J., Ege, H., et al. Proinsulin and related proteins. Presented at the 5th Annual meeting of the European Association for the Study of Diabetes, Montpellier, 1969 (Abstract). Diabetologia 1970; 6: 80–81.

Schlichtkrull, J., Brange, J., Christiansen, A. H., Hallund, O., Heding, L. G., Jørgensen, K. H. Clinical aspects of insulin – antigenicity. Diabetes 1972; 21 (Suppl. 2): 649–656.

Schlichtkrull, J., Brange, J., Christiansen, Aa. H., et al. Monocomponent insulin and its clinical implications. Horm. Metab. Res. 1974; 5 (Suppl. l): 134–143.

Schlichtkrull, J., Pingel, M., Heding, L. G., Brange, J., Jørgensen, K. H. Insulin preparations with prolonged effect. In: Hasselblatt, A., Bruchhausen, F. V. (eds), Handbook of Experimental Pharmacology, New Series, Vol. XXXII/2. Berlin, Heidelberg, New York: Springer-Verlag, 1975: 729–777.

Schlichtkrull, J. The absorption of insulin. Acta Paediatr. Scand. 1977; Suppl. 270: 97–102.

Schlichtkrull, J. Insulin in perspective. IDF Bull. 1979; 24: 7–10.

Schlüter, K. J., Petersen, K-G., Borsche, A., Hobitz, H., Kerp, L. Effects of fully synthetic human insulin in comparison to porcine insulin in normal subjects. Horm. Metab. Res. 1981; 13: 657–659.

Schlüter, K. J., Petersen, K-G., Sontheimer, J., Enzmann, F., Kerp. L. Different counterregulatory responses to human insulin (recombinant DNA) and purified pork insulin. Diabetes Care 1982; 5 (Suppl. 2): 78–81.

Schlüter, K. J., Enzmann, F., Kerp. L. Different potencies of biosynthetic human and purified porcine insulin. Horm. Metab. Res. 1983a; 15: 271–274.

Schlüter, K. J., Kerp, L. Hormonelle Gegenregulation nach Humaninsulin und Schweineinsulin. Münch. Med Wochenschr. 1983b; 125 (Suppl. 1): 116–120.

Schmidt, D. D., Arens, A. Proinsulin vom Rind. Isolierung, Eigenschaften und seine Aktivierung durch Trypsin. Hoppe-Seyler's Z. Physiol. Chem. 1968; 349: 1157–1168.

Schmitt, E. W., Gattner, H. G. Verbesserte Darstellung von Des-alanyl B30 Insulin. Hoppe-Seyler's Z. Physiol. Chem. 1978; 359: 799–802.

Schultze, W. Die Bedeutung der Langerhanschen Inseln im Pankreas. Arch. Mikr. Anat. 1900; 56: 491–509.

Scott, E. L. The effect of pancreas extract on pancreatized dogs. MS Thesis No. T-10553, University of Chicago, 1911.

Scott, E. L. On the influence of intravenous injections of extract of pancreas on experimental pancreatic diabetes. Am. J. Physiol. 1912; 29: 306.

Scott, D. A. Crystalline insulin. Biochem. J. 1934; 28: 1592–1602.

Scott, D. A., Fisher, A. M. The effect of zinc salts on the action of insulin. J. Pharmacol. Exp. Ther. 1935; 55: 206–221.

Scott, D. A., Fisher, A. M. Studies on insulin with protamine. J. Pharmacol. Exp. Ther. 1936; 58: 78–92.

Selam, J. L., Slingeneyer, A., Hedon, B., Mares, P., Beraud, J. J., Mirouze, J. Long-term ambulatory peritoneal insulin infusion of brittle diabetes with portal pumps: comparison with intravenous and subcutaneous routes. Diabetes Care 1983; 6: 105–111.

Sestoft, L., Vølund, Aa., Gammeltoft, S., Birch, K., Hildebrandt, P. The biological properties of human insulin: subcutaneous absorption, receptor binding and clinical effect in diabetics assessed by a new statistical method. Acta Med. Scand. 1982; 212: 21–28.

Shamoon, H., Hendler, R., Sherwin, R. S. Altered responsiveness to cortisol, epinephrine and glucagon in insulin-infused juvenile onset diabetics: a mechanism for diabetic instability. Diabetes 1980; 29: 284–291.

Shapcott, D., O'Brien, D. A method for the isolation of insulin from single human pancreas. Diabetes 1970; 19: 831–836.

Sharpey-Schäfer, E. A. The endocrine organs. London 1916: 128.

Sheldon, J., Gurling, K. J., Hill, D. M., et al. Insulin: U–40, U–80 or U–100. (Letter). Br. Med. J. 1976; ii: 1319.

Sherwin, R. S., Kraemer, K. J., Tobin, J. D., et al. A model of the kinetics of insulin in man. J. Clin. Invest. 1974; 53: 1481–1492.

Sherwin, R., Hendler, R., DeFronzo, R., et al. Glucose homeostasis during prolonged suppression of insulin and glucagon by somatostatin. Proc. Natl. Acad. Sci. USA 1977a; 74: 348–352.

Sherwin, R., Tamborlane, W., Hendler, R., et al. Influence of glucagon replacement on the hyperglycaemic and hyperketonemic response to prolonged somatostatin infusion in normal man. J. Clin. Endocrinol. Metab. 1977b; 45: 1104–1107.

Sieber, P., Kamber, B., Hartmann, A., Jöhl, A., Riniker, B., Rittel, W. Totalsynthese von Humaninsulin unter gezielter Bildung der Disulfidbindungen. Helv. Chim. Acta 1974; 57: 2617–2621.

Siler, T., Vandenberg, G., Yen, S. Inhibition of growth hormone release in humans by somatostatin. J. Clin. Endocrinol. Metab. 1973; 37: 632–634.

Siperstein, M. D., Foster, D. W., Knowles, H. C. Jr., Levin, R., Madison, L. L., Roth, J. Control of blood glucose and diabetic vascular disease. (Editorial). N. Engl. J. Med. 1977; 296: 1060–1063.

Siperstein, M. D. Diabetic microangiopathy and the control of blood glucose. N. Engl. J. Med. 1983; 309: 1577–1579.

Skyler, J. S. Complications of diabetes mellitus: relationship to metabolic dysfunction. Diabetes Care 1979; 2: 499–509.

Skyler, J. S., Skyler, D. L., Seigler, D. E., O'Sullivan, M. J. Algorithms for adjustment of insulin dosage by patients who monitor blood glucose. Diabetes Care 1981; 4: 311–318.

Skyler, J. S., Miller, N. E., O'Sullivan, M. J., et al. Use of insulin in insulin-dependent diabetes mellitus. In: Skyler, J. S. (ed.), Insulin Update, 1982. Princeton: Excerpta Medica, 1982: 125–156.

Slama, G., Hautecouverture, M., Assan, R., Tchobroutsky, G. One to five days of continuous intravenous insulin infusion on seven diabetic patients. Diabetes 1974; 23: 732–738.

Slama, G., Buu, K. N. P., Tchobroutsky, G., et al. Plasma insulin and C-peptide levels during continuous subcutaneous insulin infusion. Diabetes Care 1979; 2: 251–255.

Smith, L. F. Isolation of insulin from pancreatic extracts using carboxymethyl and diethylaminoethyl celluloses. Biochim. Biophys. Acta 1964; 82: 231–236.

Sodoyez, J. C., Sodoyez-Goffaux, F. Effects of insulin antibodies on bioavailability of insulin: preliminary studies using ^{123}I-insulin in patients with insulin dependent diabetes. Diabetologia 1984; 27: 143–145.

Sönksen, P. H., Tompkins, C. V., Srivastava, M. C., Nabarro, J. D. N. A comparative study on the metabolism of human insulin and porcine proinsulin in man. Clin. Sci. Mol. Med. 1973; 45: 633–654.

Sönksen, P. H., Judd, S. L., Lowy, C. Home monitoring of blood glucose. Lancet 1980; i: 729–732.

Sonnenberg, G. E., Kemmer, F. W., Cüppers, H.-J., Berger, M. Subcutaneous use of regular human insulin (Novo): pharmacokinetics and continuous insulin infusion therapy. Diabetes Care 1983; 6 (Suppl. l): 35–39.

Spellacy, W. N., Goetz, F. C. Insulin antibodies in pregnancy. Lancet 1963; ii: 222–224.

Ssobolew, L. W. Die Bedeutung der Langerhanschen Inseln. Virchows. Arch. Pathol. Anat. 1902; 168: 91–128.

Starzynska, R., Seniow, S., Kodejszko, F., Kowalski, H., Starzynski, S., Depowska, B. Studies on the transport of insulin antibodies across the placenta to the fetus and their effect on the fetal pancreatic islet system. Acta Diabetologica Latina 1969; 6: 573–584.

Staten, M., Worcester, B., Szekeres, A., et al. Comparison of porcine and semi-synthetic human insulins using euglycaemic clamp-derived glucose-insulin dose-response curves in insulin-dependent diabetes. Metabolism 1984; 33: 132–135.

Steiner, D. F. Evidence for a precursor in the biosynthesis of insulin. Trans. N.Y. Acad. Sci. Series II 1967; 30: 60–68.

Steiner, D. F., Oyer, P. E. The biosynthesis of insulin and a probable precursor of insulin by a human islet cell adenoma. Proc. Natl. Acad. Sci. (Wash.) 1967; 57: 473–480.

Steiner, D. F., Hallund, O., Rubenstein, A., Cho, S., Bayliss, C. Isolation and properties of proinsulin, intermediate forms and other minor components from crystalline bovine insulin. Diabetes 1968; 17: 725–736.

Stimmler, L. Disappearance rate of insulin. (Letter). Lancet 1966; ii: 1078.

Stimmler, L., Mashiter, K., Snodgrass, G. J. A. I., Boucher, B., Abram, S. Insulin disappearance after intravenous injection and its effects on blood glucose in diabetic and non-diabetic children and adults. Clin. Sci. 1972; 42: 337–344.

Stout, R. W. Diabetes and atherosclerosis – the role of insulin. Diabetologia 1979; 16: 141–150.

Sundermann, S., Hauff, C., Cüppers, H. J., Broermann, C., Schutte, M., Berger, M. Absorption Kinetik und biologische Aktivität von semi-synthetischem Human-Insulin (Novo). Akt. Endokrin. Stoffw. 1981; 2: 116.

Surányi, L., Szalai, F. Influence of lecithin on insulin action. Klin. Wochenschr. 1930; 9: 2159.

Süsstrunk, H., Morell, B., Ziegler, W. H., Froesch, E. R. Insulin absorption from the abdomen and the thigh in healthy subjects during rest and exercise: blood glucose, plasma insulin, growth hormone, adrenaline and noradrenaline levels. Diabetologia 1982; 22: 171–174.

Swift, P. G. F., Kennedy, J. D., Gerlis, L. S. Change to U–100 insulin does not appear to affect insulin absorption. Br. Med. J. 1983; 286: 1015.

Szepesi, G., Gazdag, M. Improved high-performance liquid chromatographic method for the analysis of insulins and related compounds. J. Chromatogr. 1981; 218: 597–602.

Tamborlane, W., Sherwin, R., Hendler, R., et al. Metabolic effects of somatostatin in maturity-onset diabetes. N. Engl. J. Med. 1977; 297: 181–183.

Tamborlane, W. V., Sherwin, R. S., Genel, M., Felig, P. Reduction to normal of plasma glucose in juvenile diabetes by subcutaneous administration of insulin with a portable insulin pump. N. Engl. J. Med. 1979; 300: 573–578.

Tamborlane, W. V., Sherwin, R. S., Genel, M., Felig, P. Outpatient treatment of juvenile-onset diabetes with a preprogrammed portable subcutaneous insulin infusion system. Am. J. Med. 1980; 68: 190–196.

Tattersall, R. B. Home blood glucose monitoring. Diabetologia 1979; 16: 71–74.

Tattersall, R. B., Gale, E. Patient self-monitoring of blood glucose and refinement of conventional insulin treatment. Am. J. Med. 1981; 70: 177–182.

Tchobroutsky, G. Relation of diabetic control to development of microvascular complications. Diabetologia 1978; 15: 143–152.

Terabe, S., Konaka, R., Inouye, K. Separation of some polypeptide hormones by high-performance liquid chromatography. J. Chromatogr. 1979; 172: 163–177.

Teuscher, A. Treatment of insulin lipoatrophy with monocomponent insulin. Diabetologia 1974; 10: 211–214.

Teuscher, A. The place of the 'monocomponent' insulins in the therapy of diabetes mellitus (Translation). Schweiz. Med. Wochenschr. 1975; 105: 485–494.

Teuscher, A. Die biologische Wirkung von vollsynthetischem humanem Insulin bei Patienten mit Diabetes Mellitus. Schweiz Med. Wochenschr. 1979; 109: 743–747.

Thompson, E. O. P., O'Donnell, I. J. The chromatography of insulin on DEAE-cellulose in buffers containing 8 M urea. Austr. J. Biol. Sci. 1960; 13: 393–400.

Traisman, H. S., Newcomb, A. L. Management of juvenile diabetes mellitus. Saint Louis: C. V. Mosby Company, 1965.

Tranberg, K. G., Dencker, H. Modelling of plasma disappearance of unlabelled insulin in man. Am. J. Physiol. 1978; 235(b): E577–E585.

Trommer, C. A. Unterscheidung von Gummi, Dextrin, Traubenzucker und Rohrzucker. Ann. Chem. (Heidelberg) 1841; 39: 360–362.

Tuft, L. Insulin hypersensitiveness. Immunologic considerations and case reports. Am. J. Med. Sci. 1928; 176: 707–720.

Turner, R. C., Ward, E. A., Phillips, M. A., et al. Continuous subcutaneous insulin infusion or subcutaneous insulin injection (Letter). Lancet 1979; ii: 481.

Turner, R. C., Holman, R. R. Treatment of noninsulin-dependent diabetes with insulin. In: Skyler, J. S. (ed.), Insulin Update, 1982. Princeton: Excerpta Medica, 1982: 233–246.

Turner, R. C., Phillips, M., Jones, R., Dornan, T. L., Holman, R. R. Ultralente-based insulin regimens in insulin-dependent diabetics. In: Skyler, J. S. (ed.), Insulin Update, 1982. Princeton: Excerpta Medica, 1982: 157–174.

Turner, R. C., Phillips, M. A., Ward, E. A. Ultralente-based insulin regimens – clinical applications, advantages and disadvantages. Acta Med. Scand. 1983; Suppl. 671: 75–86.

Umber, F., Störring, F. K., Föllmer, W. Erfolge mit einem neuartigen Depotinsulin ohne Protaminzusatz (Surfen-Insulin). Klin. Wochenschr. 1938; 17: 443–446.

Unger, R., Ipp, E., Schusdziarra, V., et al. Hypothesis: Physiologic role of pancreatic somatostatin and the contribution of D-cell disorders to diabetes mellitus. Life Sci. 1977; 20: 2081–2086.

Unger, R. H. Meticulous control of diabetes: benefits, risks and precautions. Diabetes 1982; 31: 479–483.

United States Pharmacopeia: Insulin assay, 1980: 900–901.

Vale, W., Brazeau, P., Rivier, C., et al. Somatostatin: Recent Prog. Horm. Res. 1975; 34: 365–397.

Vander Hoogen, F. H. J., Hulst, S. G. Th., Zweens, J. Time-action profile of zinc human insulin (recombinant DNA) in young volunteers as compared with zinc porcine insulin (Monotard). Diabetes Care 1982; 5 (Suppl. 2): 71–72.

Viberti, G. C., Pickup, J. C., Keen, H., et al. Biosynthetic human insulin: Effect in healthy men on plasma glucose and non-esterified fatty acids in comparison with highly purified pork insulin. Diabetes Care 1981; 4 (Suppl. 2): 175–179.

Villa-Komaroff, L., Efstratiadis, A., Broome, S., et al. A bacterial clone synthesizing proinsulin. Proc. Natl. Acad. Sci. USA 1978; 75: 3727–3731.

Villalpando, S., Drash, A. Circulating glucagon antibodies in children who have insulin dependent diabetes mellitus. Diabetes 1979; 28: 294–299.

Vølund, Aa. Multivariate bioassay. Biometrics 1980; 36: 225–236.

Vølund, Aa., Pingel, M., Sørensen, E. Differential potency of pork and beef insulins in the USP rabbit bioassay system. In: Gueriguian, J. L., Bransome, E. D., Outschoorn, A. S. (eds.), Hormone drugs. Proceedings of the FDA-USP Workshop in Drug and Reference Standards for Insulins, Somatotropins and Thyroid-axis Hormones, Bethesda, Maryland. Rockville: USP Convention Inc., 1982: 208–215.

Wahren, J., Felig, P. Influence of somatostatin on carbohydrate disposal and absorption in diabetes mellitus. Lancet 1976; ii: 1213–1216.

Wahren, J., Efendič, S., Luft, R., et al. Influence of somatostatin on splanchnic glucose metabolism in post-absorptive and 60-hour fasted humans. J. Clin. Invest. 1977; 59: 299–307.

Waldhäusl, W., Bratusch-Marrain, P., Dudczak, R., et al. The diabetogenic action of somatostatin in healthy subjects and in maturity-onset diabetics. J. Clin. Endocrinol. Metab. 1977; 44: 876–883.

Walford, S., Gale, E. A. M., Allison, S. P., Tattersall, R. B. Self-monitoring of blood glucose: improvement of diabetic control. Lancet 1978; i: 732–735.

Walford, S., Allison, S. P., Kelly, U., Deverill, I., Reeves, W. G. Do antibodies influence insulin dose and diabetic control? (Abstract). Diabetologia 1980; 19: 565.

Walford, S., Allison, S. P., Reeves, W. G. The effect of insulin antibodies on insulin dose and diabetic control. Diabetologia 1982; 22: 106–110.

Ward, G. M., Simpson, R. W., Ward, E. A., Turner, R. C. Comparison of two twice-daily insulin regimens: Ultralente/Soluble and Soluble/Isophane. Diabetologia 1981; 21: 383–386.

Watkins, J. D., Williams, T. F., Martin, D. A., et al. A study of diabetic patients at home. Am. J. Public Health 1967; 57: 452–459.

Watkins, P. J. ABC of diabetes: Insulin treatment. Br. Med. J. 1982; 284: 1929–1932.

Weeke, J., Hansen, Aa. P., Lundbæk, K. The inhibition by somatostatin on the thyrotropin response to thyrotropin-releasing hormone in normal subjects. Scand. J. Clin. Lab. Invest. 1974; 33: 101–103.

Wehner, H., Huber, H., Kronenberg, K. H. The glomerular basement membrane of the rabbit kidney on long term treatment with heterologous insulin preparations of different purity. Diabetologia 1973; 9: 255–263.

Weinges, K., Ehrhardt, M., Enzmann, F. Comparison of biosynthetic human insulin and pork insulin in the Gerritzen Test. Diabetes Care 1981; 4 (Suppl. 2): 180–182.

Weinges, K., Ehrhardt, M., Nell, G., Enzmann, F. Pharmacodynamics of human insulin (recombinant DNA) – Regular, NPH and mixtures – obtained by the Gerritzen method in healthy volunteers. Diabetes Care 1982; 5 (Suppl. 2): 67–70.

Weir, G. C., Knowlton, S. D., Atkins, R. F., et al. Glucagon secretion from the perfused pancreas of streptozotocin-treated rats. Diabetes 1976; 25: 275–282.

Welinder, B. S., Andresen, F. H. Characterisation of insulin and insulin-like substances by high-performance liquid chromatography. In: Gueriguian, J. L., Bransome, E. D., Outschoorn, A. S. (eds), Hormone Drugs. Proceedings of the FDA-USP Workshop on Drug and Reference Standards for Insulins, Somatotropins and Thyroid-axis Hormones, Bethesda, Maryland. Rockville: USP Convention Inc., 1982: 163–177.

Wermer, P., Monguio, J. Antagonism of insulin and pituitrin. Clinical cases. Klin. Wochenschr. 1933; 12: 748.

Werther, G. A., Jenkins, P. A., Turner, R. C., Baum, J. D. Twenty-four hour metabolic profiles in diabetic children receiving insulin injections once or twice daily. Br. Med. J. 1980; 281: 414–418.

Wetzel, R. Application of recombinant DNA technology. Am. Sci. 1980; 68: 664–675.

Whitehouse, F. W., Lowrie, W. L., Redfern, E., Bryan, J. B. The Lente insulin triad. With emphasis on the use of "Lente" combinations. Ann. Intern. Med. 1961; 55: 894–902.

WHO Technical Report Series 565, Geneva 1975, p. 17.

WHO Expert Committee on Diabetes Mellitus: Second report. Technical Report Series No. 646. World Health Organisation, Geneva, 1980.

WHO Expert Committee on Biological Standardisation. Technical Report Series No 673:29, World Health Organisation, Geneva, 1982.

Williams, G., Pickup, J. C., Bowcock, S., Cooke, E., Keen, H. Subcutaneous aprotinin causes local hyperaemia. Diabetologia 1983; 24: 91–94.

Williams, G., Pickup, J. C., Collins, A. C. G., Keen, H. Prostaglandin E_1 accelerates subcutaneous insulin absorption in insulin-dependent diabetic patients. Diabetic Med. 1984; 1: 109–113.

Williams, J. R. A clinical study of the effects of insulin in severe diabetics. J. Metab. Res. 1922; 2: 729–751.

Willis, T. Pharmaceutice Rationalis sive diatriba de medicamentorum operationibus in humano corpore. London: Scott, 1674. Cap 3. Section 4.

Witters, L. A., Ohman, J. L., Weir, G. C., Raymond, L. W., Lowell, F. C. Insulin antibodies in the pathogenesis of insulin allergy and resistance. Am. J. Med. 1977; 63: 703–709.

World Health Organisation: Biomedical research: a revised code of ethics. WHO Chronicle 1976; 30: 360–362.

Wrenshall, G. A., Hetenyi, G., Feasby, W. R. The story of insulin. London: Bodley Head, 1962.

Wright, A. D., Walsh, C. H., Fitzgerald, M. G., Malins, J. M. Very pure porcine insulin in clinical practice. Br. Med. J. 1979; i: 25–27.

Yalow, R. S., Berson, S. A. Immunological specificity of human insulin: Application of immunoassay to insulin. J. Clin. Invest. 1961; 40: 2190–2198.

Yip, C. C., Logothetopoulus, J. A specific anti-proinsulin serum and the presence of proinsulin in calf serum. Proc. Natl. Acad. Sci. 1969; 62: 415–419.

Yue, D. K., Turtle, J. R. Antigenicity of 'monocomponent' pork insulin in diabetic subjects. Diabetes 1975; 24: 625–632.

Yue, D. K., Baxter, R. C., Turtle, J. R. C-peptide secretion and insulin antibodies as determinants of stability in diabetes mellitus. Metabolism 1978; 27: 35–44.

Zuelzer, G. L. Über Versuche einer specifischen Fermenttherapie des Diabetes. Z. Exp. Path. Ther. 1908; 5: 307–318.

Index